Advances in Trauma

Editor

LENA M. NAPOLITANO

CRITICAL CARE CLINICS

www.criticalcare.theclinics.com

Consulting Editor
JOHN A. KELLUM

January 2017 • Volume 33 • Number 1

ELSEVIER

1600 John F. Kennedy Boulevard • Suite 1800 • Philadelphia, Pennsylvania, 19103-2899

http://www.theclinics.com

CRITICAL CARE CLINICS Volume 33, Number 1
January 2017 ISSN 0749-0704, ISBN-13: 978-0-323-48257-8

Editor: Katie Pfaff
Developmental Editor: Casey Potter

Critical Care Clinics (ISSN: 0749-0704) is published quarterly by Elsevier Inc., 360 Park Avenue South, New York, NY 10010-1710. Months of issue are January, April, July, and October. Business and Editorial Offices: 1600 John F. Kennedy Blvd., Suite 1800, Philadelphia, PA 19103-2899. Customer Service Office: 6277 Sea Harbor Drive, Orlando, FL 32887-4800. Periodicals postage paid at New York, NY and additional mailing offices. Subscription prices are $221.00 per year for US individuals, $584.00 per year for US institution, $100.00 per year for US students and residents, $263.00 per year for Canadian individuals, $732.00 per year for Canadian institutions, $309.00 per year for international individuals, $732.00 per year for international institutions and $150.00 per year for Canadian and foreign students/ residents. To receive student/resident rate, orders must be accompanied by name of affiliated institution, date of term, and the signature of program/residency coordinator on institution letterhead. Orders will be billed at individual rate until proof of status is received. Foreign air speed delivery is included in all *Clinics* subscription prices. All prices are subject to change without notice. POSTMASTER: Send address changes to *Critical Care Clinics*, Elsevier Periodicals Customer Service, 11830 Westline Industrial Drive, St. Louis, MO 63146. **Customer Service: 1-800-654-2452 (US). From outside of the US, call 1-314-447-8871. Fax: 1-314-447-8029. E-mail: journalscustomerservice-usa@ elsevier.com (for print support) or journalsonlinesupport-usa@elsevier.com (for online support).**

Reprints. For copies of 100 or more of articles in this publication, please contact the Commercial Reprints Department, Elsevier Inc., 360 Park Avenue South, New York, NY 10010-1710. Tel.: 212-633-3874; Fax: 212-633-3820; E-mail: reprints@elsevier.com.

Critical Care Clinics is also published in Spanish by Editorial Inter-Medica, Junin 917, 1er A, 1113, Buenos Aires, Argentina.

Critical Care Clinics is covered in *MEDLINE/PubMed (Index Medicus), EMBASE/Excerpta Medica, Current Concepts/ Clinical Medicine, ISI/BIOMED,* and *Chemical Abstracts.*

Contributors

CONSULTING EDITOR

JOHN A. KELLUM, MD, MCCM
Professor of Critical Care Medicine, Medicine, Bioengineering and Clinical & Translational Science, Director, Center for Critical Care Nephrology; Vice Chair for Research, Department of Critical Care Medicine, University of Pittsburgh School of Medicine, Pittsburgh, Pennsylvania

EDITOR

LENA M. NAPOLITANO, MD, FACS, FCCP, MCCM
Professor of Surgery; Division Chief, Acute Care Surgery [Trauma, Burn, Critical Care, Emergency Surgery]; Associate Chair, Department of Surgery; Director, Trauma and Surgical Critical Care, University of Michigan Health System, Ann Arbor, Michigan

AUTHORS

GRANT V. BOCHICCHIO, MD, MPH
Department of Surgery, Washington University School of Medicine, St Louis, Missouri

PAUL M. CANTLE, MD, MBT, FRCSC
Department of Surgery, University of Texas Mcgovern Medical School, Houston, Texas

RONALD CHANG, MD
Center for Translational Injury Research, University of Texas Health Science Center, Houston, Texas

S. ARIANE CHRISTIE, MD
Research Fellow, General Surgery, Department of Surgery, San Francisco General Hospital, University of California, San Francisco, School of Medicine, San Francisco, California

MARK CIPOLLE, MD, PhD, FACS, FCCM
Director of Outcomes Research, Surgical Service Line, Department of Surgery, Christiana Care Health System, Professor of Surgery, Sidney Kimmel School of Medicine, Thomas Jefferson University, Wilmington, Delaware

MITCHELL J. COHEN, MD
Professor, Department of Surgery, San Francisco General Hospital, University of California, San Francisco, School of Medicine, San Francisco, California

BRYAN A. COTTON, MD, MPH, FACS, FRCPS(Glasg)
Department of Surgery, University of Texas Mcgovern Medical School, Houston, Texas

CRISTINA B. FEATHER, MD, MHS
Fellow, Surgical Critical Care, R Adams Cowley Shock Trauma Center, University of Maryland Medical Center, Baltimore, Maryland

EDUARDO GONZALEZ, MD
Department of Surgery, University of Colorado, Denver, Colorado

MARK R. HEMMILA, MD
MTQIP Program Director, Department of Surgery, University of Michigan Medical School, North Campus Research Complex, Ann Arbor, Michigan

JOHN B. HOLCOMB, MD
Department of Surgery, University of Texas Health Science Center, Houston, Texas

JILL L. JAKUBUS, PA-C, MHSA
MTQIP Program Manager, Department of Surgery, University of Michigan Medical School, North Campus Research Complex, Ann Arbor, Michigan

ERNEST E. MOORE, MD
Professor, Department of Surgery, Denver Health Medical Center, University of Colorado Denver; Editorial office, Journal of Trauma and Acute Care Surgery, Denver, Colorado

FREDERICK A. MOORE, MD
Professor of Surgery, University of Florida, Gainesville, Florida

HUNTER B. MOORE, MD
Department of Surgery, University of Colorado, Denver, Colorado

JONATHAN J. MORRISON, MBChB, PhD, FRCS
Department of Vascular Surgery, Queen Elizabeth University Hospital, Govan Road, Glasgow, United Kingdom

LENA M. NAPOLITANO, MD, FACS, FCCP, MCCM
Professor of Surgery; Division Chief, Acute Care Surgery [Trauma, Burn, Critical Care, Emergency Surgery]; Associate Chair, Department of Surgery; Director, Trauma and Surgical Critical Care, University of Michigan Health System, Ann Arbor, Michigan

RAMINDER NIRULA, MD, MPH
Department of Surgery, University of Utah, Salt Lake City, Utah

RICARDO J. RAMIREZ, MD
Department of Surgery, Washington University School of Medicine, St Louis, Missouri

ANGELA SAUAIA, MD, PhD
Professor of Public Health and Surgery, University of Colorado Denver, Denver, Colorado

LARA SENEKJIAN, MD, MSCI
Department of Surgery, University of Utah, Salt Lake City, Utah

PHILIP C. SPINELLA, MD
Department of Pediatrics, Washington University School of Medicine, St Louis, Missouri

DEBORAH M. STEIN, MD, MPH
Professor of Surgery, Medical Director, Chief, Neurotrauma Critical Care, Chief, Section of Trauma Critical Care, R Adams Cowley Shock Trauma Center, University of Maryland Medical Center, Baltimore, Maryland

JASON WEINBERGER, DO
Trauma/Surgical Critical Care Fellow, Department of Surgical Critical Care, R Adams Cowley Shock Trauma Center, University of Maryland Medical Center, Baltimore, Maryland

Contents

There have been many recent advances in the management of traumatic brain injury (TBI). Research regarding established and novel therapies is ongoing. Future research must not only focus on development of new strategies but determine the long-term benefits or disadvantages of current strategies. In addition, the impact of these advances on varying severities of brain injury must not be ignored. It is hoped that future research strategies in TBI will prioritize large-scale trials using common data elements to develop large registries and databases, and leverage international collaborations.

The resuscitation of traumatic hemorrhagic shock has undergone a paradigm shift in the last 20 years with the advent of damage control resuscitation (DCR). Major principles of DCR include minimization of crystalloid, permissive hypotension, transfusion of a balanced ratio of blood products, and goal-directed correction of coagulopathy. In particular, plasma has replaced crystalloid as the primary means for volume expansion for traumatic hemorrhagic shock. Predicting which patient will require DCR by prompt and accurate activation of a massive transfusion protocol, however, remains a challenge.

Noncompressible torso hemorrhage (NCTH) constitutes a leading cause of potentially preventable trauma mortality. NCTH is defined by high-grade injury present in one or more of the following anatomic domains: pulmonary, solid abdominal organ, major vascular or pelvic trauma, plus hemodynamic instability or the need for immediate hemorrhage control. Rapid operative management, as part of a damage control resuscitation strategy, remains the mainstay of treatment. However, endovascular techniques are evolving and may become more mainstream with the advent of hybrid rooms that can deliver concurrent open and radiologic/endovascular management of traumatic hemorrhage.

Exsanguinating torso hemorrhage is a leading killer of trauma patients. The most appropriate means of hemorrhage control must be used. Trauma surgeons should have expertise with all approaches for prompt hemorrhage control [laparotomy, thoracotomy, resuscitative endovascular balloon occlusion of the aorta (REBOA), and resuscitative thoracotomy]. REBOA is an exciting adjunct for hemorrhage control as it can be deployed quickly and placed percutaneously. Balloon inflation can vary dependent on patient physiology. REBOA is effective in hemorrhagic shock as a bridge to definitive hemostasis. Endovascular training is important for trauma surgeons caring for patients at high risk of death from traumatic hemorrhage.

Hemorrhage is the leading cause of preventable death in trauma. Damage control resuscitation relies on permissive hypotension, minimizing crystalloid use, and early implementation of massive transfusion protocols with established blood component ratios. These protocols improve the survival of the severely injured patient. Trauma physicians must quickly and accurately predict when a massive transfusion protocol should be activated. Several validated transfusion scores have been developed for this purpose. Many of these scores are useful for resuscitation research. One option, the ABC score, is an accurate, validated, and clinically useful score that is simple to calculate and rapidly obtained.

Following results from the CRASH-2 trial, tranexamic acid (TXA) gained considerable interest for the treatment of hemorrhage in trauma patients. Although TXA is effective at reducing mortality in patients presenting within 3 hours of injury, optimal dosing, timing of administration, mechanism, and pharmacokinetics require further elucidation. The concept of fibrinolysis shutdown in hemorrhagic trauma patients has prompted discussion of real-time viscoelastic testing and its potential role for appropriate patient selection. The results of ongoing clinical trials will help establish high-quality evidence for optimal incorporation of TXA in mature trauma networks in the United States and abroad.

Coagulopathy is common after injury and develops independently from iatrogenic, hypothermic, and dilutional causes. Despite considerable research on the topic over the past decade, trauma-induced coagulopathy (TIC) continues to portend poor outcomes, including decreased survival. We review the current evidence regarding the diagnosis and mechanisms underlying trauma induced coagulopathy and summarize the debates regarding optimal management strategy including product resuscitation, potential pharmacologic adjuncts, and targeted approaches to hemostasis. Throughout, we will identify areas of continued investigation and controversy in the understanding and management of TIC.

> Viscoelastic assays, such as thrombelastography (TEG) and rotational thrombelastometry (ROTEM), have emerged as point-of-care tools that can guide the hemostatic resuscitation of bleeding injured patients. This article describes the role of TEG in contemporary trauma care by explaining this assay's methodology, clinical applications, and result interpretation through description of supporting studies to provide the reader with an evidence-based user's guide. Although TEG and ROTEM are assays based on the same viscoelastic principle, this article is focused on data supporting the use of TEG in trauma, because it is available in trauma centers in North America; ROTEM is mostly available in Europe.

> The incidence of patients with trauma on novel oral anticoagulants (NOACs) for the treatment of thromboembolic disorders is increasing. In severe bleeding or hemorrhage into critical spaces, urgent reversal of this underlying pharmacologic coagulopathy becomes paramount. Optimal reversal strategy for commonly used NOACs is still evolving. Basic tenets of evaluation of patients with trauma and resuscitation remain the same. Clinical outcomes data in bleeding human patients with trauma are lacking, but are needed to establish efficacy and safety in these treatments. This article summarizes the available evidence and provides the optimal reversal strategy for bleeding patients with trauma on NOACs.

> Rib fractures are a frequently identified injury in the trauma population. Not only are multiple rib fractures painful, but they are associated with an increased risk of adverse outcomes. Pneumonia in particular can be devastating, especially to an elderly patient, but other complications such as prolonged ventilation and increased intensive care and hospital durations of stay have a negative impact on the patient. Computed tomography scan is the best modality to diagnosis rib fractures but the treatment of fractures is still evolving. Currently patient care involves a multidisciplinary approach that includes pain control, aggressive pulmonary therapy, and possibly surgical fixation.

> The development of organ dysfunction (OD) is related to the intensity and balance between trauma-induced simultaneous, opposite inflammatory responses. Early proinflammation via innate immune system activation may cause early OD, whereas antiinflammation, via inhibition of the adaptive immune system and apoptosis, may induce immunoparalysis, impaired healing, infections, and late OD. Patients discharged with low-level OD may develop the persistent inflammation-immunosuppression catabolism syndrome. Although the incidence of multiple organ failure

CRITICAL CARE CLINICS

Preface

Advances in Trauma-2016

Goal Zero Preventable Deaths After Injury

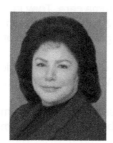

Lena M. Napolitano, MD, FACS, FCCP, MCCM
Editor

Trauma remains the leading cause of death for individuals aged 1 to 46 years, the third leading cause of death overall, and accounts for 30% of all life-years lost, with over 190,000 lives lost annually.[1] Trauma accounts for 41 million emergency department visits and over 2 million hospital admissions annually. The economic burden of trauma is more than $671 billion annually.[2] Despite an organized system of trauma care in the United States, from 2000 to 2010, the number of trauma deaths increased by 22.8% for those 25 years and older with a concurrent increase in the US population of 9.7%. The largest increase in trauma deaths was in 50- to 60-year-old individuals.[3]

So how can we provide optimal care to our trauma victims to ensure survival and optimal quality of life?

Standardization of evidence-based clinical care in trauma is of vital importance with a goal to improve trauma outcomes. Studies have documented low compliance rates (10%-40%) with standardized protocols in trauma. It has been confirmed that major deviations from guideline-based clinical care are associated with significantly higher mortality after injury and increased organ failure.[4,5] Although we have standardized trauma care in the initial hour after injury with use of Advanced Trauma Life Support, there is little standardization subsequently.[6]

A new report from the National Academies of Sciences, Engineering, and Medicine (NASEM) proposes a national trauma care system integrating military and civilian trauma systems to achieve zero preventable deaths after injury.[7] Recommendations encourage a culture of continuous learning and improvement, examination of unwarranted variation in practice, which has led to suboptimal patient outcomes, coordinated performance improvement and research to generate evidence-based best trauma care practices, structured quality improvement processes, and timely dissemination of trauma knowledge.[8] The American College of Surgeons Committee on

Crit Care Clin 33 (2017) xi–xiii
http://dx.doi.org/10.1016/j.ccc.2016.10.001
0749-0704/17/© 2016 Published by Elsevier Inc.

criticalcare.theclinics.com

Traumatic Brain Injury Advances

Deborah M. Stein, MD, MPH[a],*, Cristina B. Feather, MD, MHS[b],
Lena M. Napolitano, MD, FCCP, MCCM[c]

KEYWORDS

- Traumatic brain injury • Antiseizure prophylaxis • Hyperosmolar therapy
- Targeted temperature modulation • Intracranial pressure monitoring
- Decompressive craniectomy

KEY POINTS

- Antiseizure prophylaxis is beneficial only in the first 7 days after injury.
- Hyperosmolar therapy, with mannitol or hypertonic saline, can be used to control intracranial hypertension.
- Prevention of hyperthermia can prevent secondary brain injury. However, benefits of hypothermia are unclear.
- Intracranial pressure monitoring can aid in therapy.
- Decompressive craniectomy has not shown long-term benefits.

INTRODUCTION

Traumatic brain injury (TBI) continues to be a significant cause of mortality, morbidity, and economic burden globally.[1] Research on TBI over the last century has shown that a hallmark of treatment of TBI is prevention of secondary insults. Studies have shown that even brief episodes of hypoperfusion and hypoxemia can cause secondary injury and lead to worse short-term and long-term outcomes.[1–3] In order to improve medical care and patient outcomes, it is important to be knowledgeable of current literature regarding treatment of patients with TBI.

Disclosure: The authors have nothing to disclose.
[a] Neurotrauma Critical Care, Section of Trauma Critical Care, R Adams Cowley Shock Trauma Center, University of Maryland Medical Center, 22 South Greene Street, Baltimore, MD 21201, USA; [b] Surgical Critical Care, R Adams Cowley Shock Trauma Center, University of Maryland Medical Center, 22 South Greene Street, Baltimore, MD 21201, USA; [c] Division of Acute Care Surgery [Trauma, Burns, Surgical Critical Care, Emergency Surgery], Department of Surgery, Trauma and Surgical Critical Care, University of Michigan Health System, Room 1C340-UH, 1500 East Medical Center Drive, Ann Arbor, MI 48109-5033, USA
* Corresponding author.
E-mail address: dstein@umm.edu

PHARMACOLOGIC THERAPY
Posttraumatic Seizures Prophylaxis

Seizures in the acutely injured brain can increase intracranial pressure (ICP) and alter oxygen delivery to the brain.[1,4,5] In an attempt to prevent secondary brain injury, many investigators have studied the benefit of prophylaxis for posttraumatic seizures. A randomized, double-blind, placebo-controlled trial, published by Temkin and colleagues[6] in 1990, studied the role of phenytoin in prevention of early and late posttraumatic seizures. The trial included 404 patients, randomized to phenytoin or placebo treatment arms, for a treatment time of 12 months and a follow-up time of 24 months. The results showed a statistically significant difference in the rate of early posttraumatic seizures in the phenytoin group (3.6%) compared with the placebo group (14.2%).[6] There was no significant difference in the rate of posttraumatic seizures between the two groups from day 8 to end of follow-up. Overall, treatment with phenytoin was shown to be effective in decreasing the rate of posttraumatic seizures in the first 7 days of injury, but had no significant role in prevention of posttraumatic seizures after the first week of injury.[6] Notably, inclusion criteria allowed for a wide range of severity of TBI. Therefore, the difference in the benefit of treatment with phenytoin compared with placebo stratified by severity of TBI remains unclear.

As discussed by Temkin and colleagues,[6] treatment with phenytoin has some disadvantages; including several side effects and the need to monitor serum drug levels.[7] In the past decade, studies that compare the effectiveness of phenytoin with levetiracetam in prevention of early posttraumatic seizure prophylaxis have been conducted in an effort to provide an alternative pharmacologic therapy.[5,8] Zafar and colleagues[8] conducted a meta-analysis to compare the efficacies of phenytoin and levetiracetam in posttraumatic seizure prophylaxis. Eight studies comparing the 2 drugs were included in the meta-analysis: 2 randomized controlled trials (RCTs) and 6 observational studies. The meta-analysis showed no significant difference in the odds of seizures when comparing treatment with phenytoin and levetiracetam.[8]

Since publication of the Zafar and colleagues[8] study, a large multicenter prospective study comparing the efficacy of treatment with phenytoin with that of levetiracetam was completed by Inaba and colleagues.[9] This study, which included 813 patients, found no significant difference in rates of early posttraumatic seizures among patients treated with phenytoin compared with patients treated with levetiracetam.

The current Brain Trauma Foundation Guidelines recommend treatment with anticonvulsants within 7 days of injury.[1,10] Because this recommendation is based on the level II evidence outlined earlier, larger RCTs comparing efficacy of phenytoin with that of levetiracetam are needed to further delineate these recommendations. In addition, the importance of the severity of TBI and the use of anticonvulsants remains unclear, an important aspect to consider, because the long-term disadvantages related to seizure prophylaxis are poorly understood.[7]

Hyperosmolar Therapy

Hyperosmolar therapy is used to decrease high ICP in an effort to maintain cerebral blood flow and prevent secondary brain injury. The 2 most common pharmacologic interventions are mannitol and hypertonic saline. Mannitol increases cerebral blood flow by plasma expansion, decreasing the blood viscosity via deformed erythrocytes, and promotes osmotic diuresis.[1,11] Hypertonic saline promotes mobilization of water across the blood-brain barrier, and improved blood flow via plasma volume expansion.[1] Debate regarding the efficacy of these treatment modalities for increased ICP continues.

Kamel and colleagues[12] conducted a meta-analysis of RCTs comparing mannitol and hypertonic saline in the treatment of increased ICP. Five studies were included, with a total of 112 patients with a diagnosis of TBI, stroke, intracerebral hemorrhage, subarachnoid hemorrhage, or tumor resection. Treatment of increased ICPs with hypertonic saline was more favorable than treatment with mannitol, with a pooled relative risk of successful treatment with hypertonic saline compared with mannitol of 1.16 (95% confidence interval [CI], 1.00–1.33).[12] Importantly, the studies included had small sample sizes and a wide variety of intracranial disorders, limiting the application of the findings.

Mangat and colleagues[13] published a prospective observational study comparing the total ICP burden and cumulative ICP reduction among patients with severe TBI receiving monotherapy. Using propensity score matching, 35 patients treated with mannitol were matched with 35 patients treated with hypertonic saline. Cumulative and daily ICP burdens were calculated as percentages of days or hours with an acute ICP increase during ICP monitoring. Both the cumulative and daily ICP burdens were significantly lower in the patients receiving hypertonic saline compared with those treated with mannitol.[13] Although the patients were matched on factors most predictive of mortality specific to severe TBI, they were not matched on factors predicative of overall trauma mortality. In addition, the small sample size, absence of reporting of adverse effects of treatment, and lack of randomization prevents strong conclusions being made from this study.

Cottenceau and colleagues[14] conducted a RCT comparing equiosmolar doses of mannitol and hypertonic saline in the treatment of increased ICP. Forty-seven patients sustaining severe TBI were included in the study and randomized to mannitol or hypertonic saline treatment in the setting of acute increase of ICP. The difference in average time of increased ICP between the two treatment groups was not statistically significant.[14] The magnitude of ICP decrease from baseline was significantly higher in the subjects treated with hypertonic saline compared with those treated with mannitol.[14] Note that the largest changes in ICP were in patients with diffuse brain injury treated with hypertonic saline.[14] Although no definitive advantage of hypertonic saline versus mannitol in treatment of increased ICP was shown in this study, there was some evidence that injury pattern and severity are important.

A more recent meta-analysis, by Burgess and colleagues,[4] included 7 RCTs and 191 patients. As in the previous meta-analysis, treatment with hypertonic saline was more successful in treatment of increased ICP compared with treatment with mannitol.[4] There was no difference in 6-month mortality, and limited adverse events were reported.

In conclusion, intracranial hypertension can be harmful to the acutely injured brain, leading to decreased perfusion and secondary brain injury. It is important to maintain cerebral perfusion pressure and limit acute increases of ICP. At present, no large randomized controlled trial comparing treatment with mannitol and hypertonic saline in the setting of increased ICP in severe TBI has been completed. In addition, the significance of severity of injury or injury pattern in the treatment of acutely increased ICP is yet to be determined.

OTHER PHARMACOLOGIC THERAPY
Progesterone

Progesterone treatment was associated with robust positive effects in animal TBI models[15] and in 2 phase 2 RCTs.[16,17] However, 2 large phase 3 RCTs (the Study of a Neuroprotective Agent, Progesterone, in Severe Traumatic Brain Injury [SYNAPSE] and the Progesterone for the Treatment of Traumatic Brain Injury [PROTECT III] trial) did not confirm any clinical benefit of progesterone in TBI treatment.[18,19]

Erythropoietin

Erythropoietin (EPO) showed high therapeutic potential as a neuroprotective agent in animal studies, but failed in recently completed clinical trials. However, in an RCT of 200 patients with severe TBI (EPO, n = 102; placebo, n = 98) enrolled within 6 hours of injury, EPO failed to improve favorable outcomes by 20% at 6 months.[20] The EPO-TBI study randomized 606 patients with moderate or severe TBI to EPO or placebo and reported that EPO did not reduce the number of patients with severe neurologic dysfunction (Extended Glasgow Outcome Scale [GOS-E] level 1–4) or increase the incidence of deep venous thrombosis of the lower extremities and had no effect on 6-month mortality (11% EPO vs 16% placebo; RR [risk ratio], 0.68; 95% CI, 0.44–1.03; $P = .07$).[21]

A meta-analysis of 5 RCTs with 915 patients showed that EPO significantly reduced mortality (RR, 0.69; 95% CI, 0.49–0.96; $P = .03$) and shortened hospitalization time ($P<.0001$) for patients with TBI. However, no differences in favorable neurologic outcome and deep vein thrombosis were identified. The investigators suggested that EPO is beneficial for patients with TBI in terms of reducing mortality and shortening hospitalization time without increasing the risk of deep vein thrombosis. However, its effect on improving favorable neurologic outcomes did not reach statistical significance. Therefore, more well-designed RCTs are necessary to ascertain the optimum dosage and time window of EPO treatment of patients with TBI.[22]

Amantadine

Amantadine hydrochloride acts as an N-methyl-D-aspartate antagonist and indirect dopamine agonist. Small RCTs have suggested that amantadine was effective in improving functional outcomes after TBI. A placebo-controlled RCT[23] of amantadine for severe TBI randomized 184 patients who were in a vegetative or minimally conscious state 4 to 16 weeks after TBI and who were receiving inpatient rehabilitation to receive amantadine or placebo for 4 weeks. Amantadine accelerated the pace of functional recovery during active treatment as measured by the Disability Rating Scale.

At present, there is no single pharmacologic therapy that unequivocally improves clinical functional outcomes after TBI, but several agents have potential benefit and should be investigated further.[24,25] Potential pharmacologic therapy for TBI matched with pathophysiologic events is shown in **Fig. 1**. Given the recent failures in clinical translation of therapies in TBI, new approaches (such as a rigorous multicenter preclinical drug and circulating biomarker screening consortium, Operation Brain Trauma Therapy [OBTT]) may be helpful in the development of successful pharmacologic strategies for TBI.[26]

NONPHARMACOLOGIC THERAPY
Targeted Temperature Modulation

Hyperthermia can cause secondary brain injury in the setting of TBI by increasing vascular permeability, and promoting edema and inflammation.[27] In the clinical setting, mild hyperthermia has been associated with poorer outcomes and longer intensive care unit stays.[28,29] As a result of these findings, interest in targeted temperature modulation (TTM) to prevent hyperthermia in TBI has grown.[30,31]

The European Study of Therapeutic Hypothermia (32°C–35°C) for ICP Reduction after TBI (Eurotherm3235 Trial) was designed to further define the association of hypothermia and functional outcome in patients with TBI.[32,33] Patients with a sustained ICP of greater than 20 mm Hg despite other therapeutic maneuvers (n = 387) were randomized to hypothermia (32°C–35°C) plus standard care or standard care alone. Guidelines for induction of hypothermia and rewarming were determined a priori.[33] Hypothermia was titrated to ICP, and patients were considered rewarmed after 48 hours of

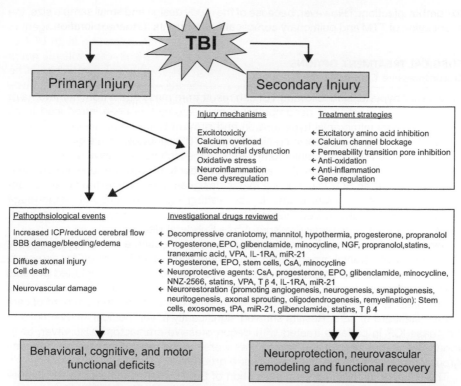

Fig. 1. TBI pathophysiology and recovery phases and potential pharmacologic treatment strategies. BBB, blood-brain barrier; CsA, cyclosporine A; IL-1RA, interleutin-1 receptor antagonist; miR-21, microRNA-21; NNZ-2566, synthetic analogue of the endogenous N-terminus tripeptide glycine-proline-glutamate; NGF, nerve growth factor; Tβ4, thymosin beta 4; tPA, tissue plasminogen activator; VPA, valproic acid. (*From* Xiong Y, Zhang Y, Mahmood A, et al. Investigational agents for treatment of traumatic brain injury. Expert Opin Investig Drugs 2015;24(6):743–60.)

treatment or until ICP was controlled. The trial was terminated early, because signs of harm within the treatment arm were appreciated.[33] Although there were statistically significantly fewer failures of therapy to control acutely increased ICP in the hypothermia group, the treatment group had a lower GOS-E at 6 months compared with the control arm.[33] Two randomized trials in the pediatric population showed similar results of worse outcomes in the hypothermia treatment groups.[30] Of note, the patients treated with the standard-of-care protocol in the Eurotherm3235 Trial received normothermic TTM, confounding the results. In addition, although hypothermia did not improve functional outcome, there was an observed decrease in ICP in the treatment arm.[33,34]

A second RCT is underway (Prophylactic Hypothermia Trial to Lessen Traumatic Brain Injury [POLAR]). Instead of comparing hypothermia with standard of care, prophylactic hypothermia is compared with normothermic TTM.[35] This study may be able to provide improved insights into the benefit of TTM in the clinical setting.

Of note, 1 small retrospective study evaluated the effect of TTM compared with standard of care on clinical complications. O'Phelan and colleagues[36] reported a statistically significant increase in the rate of pulmonary complications in patients treated with TTM compared with standard of care. This difference was explained by the inhibition of fever to combat infection.[36] However, because of the study design and small sample size, the association of TTM and pulmonary complications warrants further exploration.

SURGICAL TREATMENT OPTIONS
Decompressive Craniectomy

Intracranial hypertension following TBI can result from mass effect from hematoma or contusion. The practice of decompressive craniectomy has been introduced in an effort to control intracranial hypertension and prevent further brain injury.[37,38] The 3 clinical trials for decompressive craniectomy for TBI are reviewed in **Fig. 2**.

Primary decompressive craniectomy refers to the technique of leaving the resected bone flap out after evacuation of a hematoma in order to prevent intracranial hypertension.[39] Presently an RCT is underway that is designed to determine the benefit of primary decompressive craniectomy in the setting of acute subdural hemorrhage (RESCUE-ASDH [Randomized Evaluation of Surgery with Craniectomy for Uncontrollable Elevation of Intracranial Pressure-Acute Subdural Hematoma]).

Secondary decompressive craniectomy involves resecting a bone flap specifically to decrease intracranial hypertension when there is no other indication for neurosurgical intervention. The DECRA (Decompressive Craniectomy) trial included patients who had refractory increased ICPs between 15 minutes and 1 hour of onset.[40] A total of 155 patients were randomized to decompressive craniectomy and standard of care versus standard of care. Results showed significantly fewer medical interventions to decrease ICP in patients treated with decompressive craniectomy. However, at 6-month follow-up, functional outcome was worse in the decompressive craniectomy group compared with the standard-of-care group.[40]

The RESCUEicp (Randomized Evaluation of Surgery with Craniectomy for Uncontrollable Elevation of Intracranial Pressure) trial (n=408) compared secondary

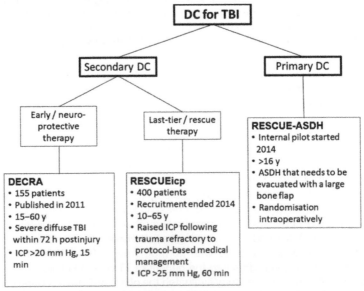

Fig. 2. Randomized trials of decompressive craniectomy (DC) for TBI. (*From* Kolias AG, Adams H, Timofeev I, et al. Decompressive craniectomy following traumatic brain injury: developing the evidence base. Br J Neurosurg 2016;30(2):246–50.)

decompressive craniectomy to optimal medical management.[41,42] In contrast to the DECRA trial, decompressive craniectomy was only performed if ICP remained elevated (ICP > 25 mm Hg for 1-12 hours) despite Stage I [optimal medical management (head elevation, ventilation, sedation, analgesia, neuromuscular blockade)] and Stage 2 (ventriculostomy, inotropes, mannitol, hypertonic saline, loop diuretics, hypothermia) treatment. At 6-months, decompressive craniectomy resulted in lower mortality (26.9% vs. 48.9%) than medical management, but higher rates of vegetative state (8.5% vs. 2.1%), lower severe disability (21.9% vs. 14.4%) and upper severe disability (15.4% vs. 8.0%). Future studies are required to determine which patients will benefit with mortality reduction but minimize risk for vegetative state and poor functional outcomes.[43]

INTRACRANIAL PRESSURE MONITORING

Current guidelines recommend ICP monitoring in patients with severe TBI and a confirmatory radiographic evidence of intracranial disorder, or patients with a normal computed tomography (CT) scan, but more than 40 years of age, with evidence of posturing, or systolic blood pressure less than 90 mm Hg.[1] Guidelines advocate the early treatment of ICP because increased severity and longer duration of increased ICP are associated with poor outcome. Management of increased ICP includes standardized strategies that use a so-called staircase approach with an escalating treatment intensity.[44] The American College of Surgeons TBI Guidelines recommend a 3-tier approach for management of increased ICP (**Boxes 1–3**).[45]

The value of ICP monitoring in medical decision making and patient outcomes was evaluated in the BEST:TRIP (Benchmark Evidence of South American Trials: Treatment of Intracranial Pressure) trial.[46,47] Chesnut and colleagues[46] hypothesized that routine ICP monitoring in severe TBI would decrease mortality and improve neurologic outcome. Patients with severe TBI presenting to 6 trauma centers in South America were included and randomized to ICP monitoring with goal ICP less than 20 mm Hg, or a serial imaging–clinical examination protocol.[47] A total of 324 patients were included, with 92% follow-up rate. There was no mortality or clinical outcome benefit observed when comparing patients in the ICP-monitoring group with patients in the serial imaging–clinical examination protocol group.[46] Pitfalls of this study include limited prehospital care resources, leading

---

Box 1
Three-tiered management of ICP in TBI: tier 1

Tier 1

- Head of bed elevated at 30° (reverse Trendelenburg) to improve cerebral venous outflow.

- Sedation and analgesia using recommended short-acting agents (eg, propofol, fentanyl, midazolam) in intubated patients.

- Ventricular drainage performed intermittently. Continuous drainage is not recommended unless an additional ICP monitor is placed, because, when the drain is open, it does not accurately reflect the ICP.

- Repeat CT imaging and neurologic examination should be considered to rule out the development of a surgical mass lesion and guide treatment.

If ICP remains greater than or equal 20 to 25 mm Hg, proceed to tier 2.
From American College of Surgeons Trauma Quality Improvement Program. Best practices in the management of traumatic brain injury. Available at: https://www.facs.org/~/media/files/quality%20programs/trauma/tqip/traumatic%20brain%20injury%20guidelines.ashx. Accessed May 1, 2016.

Box 2
Three-tiered management of ICP in TBI: tier 2

Tier 2

- In patients with a parenchymal ICP monitor an EVD should be considered to allow for intermittent cerebrospinal fluid drainage.

- Hyperosmolar therapy should be given intermittently as needed for ICP increase and not on a routine schedule.
  - Mannitol should be administered in intermittent boluses (0.25–1 g/kg body weight). Care should be taken in hypovolemic patients when osmotic diuresis is instituted with mannitol. The serum sodium level and osmolality must be assessed frequently (every 6 hours) and additional doses should be held if serum osmolality exceeds 320 mOsm/L. Mannitol may also be held if there is evidence of hypovolemia.
  - Hypertonic saline may be administered in intermittent boluses of 3% sodium chloride solution (250 mL over 30 minutes) or other concentrations (eg, 30 mL of 23.4%). Serum sodium level and osmolality must be assessed frequently (every 6 hours) and additional doses should be held if serum sodium exceeds 160 mEq/L.

- Cerebral autoregulation should be assessed (see text). If the patient is not autoregulating, the CPP goal should be decreased to reduce ICP (to no less than 50 mm Hg). Additional neuromonitoring (eg, Pbto$_2$, Sjvo$_2$, CBF) may help determine optimal CPP.

- Paco$_2$ goal of 30 to 35 mm Hg should be maintained, as long as brain hypoxia is not encountered. Additional neuromonitoring (eg, Pbto$_2$, Sjvo$_2$, CBF) may help determine optimal Paco$_2$.

- Repeat CT imaging and neurologic examination should be considered to rule out development of a surgical mass lesion and guide treatment.

- Neuromuscular paralysis achieved with a bolus test dose of a neuromuscular blocking agent should be considered if the above measures fail to adequately decrease ICP and restore CPP. If there is a positive response, continuous infusion of a neuromuscular blocking agent should be used (tier 3).

If ICP remains greater than or equal to 20 to 25 mm Hg proceed to tier 3.
Abbreviations: CBF, cerebral blood flow; CPP, cerebral perfusion pressure; EVD, external ventricular drain; Pbto$_2$, perfusion and brain tissue oxygenation; Sjvo$_2$, jugular venous oxygen saturation.
From American College of Surgeons Trauma Quality Improvement Program. Best practices in the management of traumatic brain injury. Available at: https://www.facs.org/~/media/files/quality%20programs/trauma/tqip/traumatic%20brain%20injury%20guidelines.ashx. Accessed May 1, 2016.

---

to a survival bias. In addition, there was a high mortality after 14 days of injury in both groups, attributable to limited postdischarge resources. In addition, the non-ICP group had a higher incidence of treatment with barbiturates and hypertonic saline, indicating an advantage of ICP monitors to better target other therapeutic measures.[46]

Yuan and colleagues[48] completed a meta-analysis evaluating the association of ICP monitoring and mortality in patients with severe TBI. Fourteen studies were included: 13 observational studies and 1 RCT (Chesnut and colleagues,[46] 2012). There was no measured association between ICP monitoring and mortality benefit in pooled analysis and subgroup analysis.[48] Importantly, there was a large degree of heterogeneity among the included studies with regard to outcome measurements and protocols to control intracranial hypertension.

Noninvasive intracranial monitoring is an emerging technique. Transcranial Doppler ultrasonography (TCD) has been described to estimate ICP. This technique relies on arterial waveform variability, and has a wide range of reported accuracy compared

---

Box 3
Three-tiered management of ICP in TBI: tier 3

Tier 3 (includes potential salvage therapies)

- Decompressive hemicraniectomy or bilateral craniectomy should only be performed if treatments in tiers 1 and 2 are not sufficient or are limited by development of side effects of medical treatment.

- Neuromuscular paralysis via continuous infusion of a neuromuscular blocking agent can be used if there is a positive response to a bolus dose. The infusion should be titrated to maintain at least 2 twitches (out of a train of 4) using a peripheral nerve stimulator. Adequate sedation must be used.

- Barbiturate or propofol (anesthesia dosage) coma may be induced for patients who have failed to respond to aggressive measures to control malignant intracranial hypertension, but it should only be instituted if a test dose of barbiturate or propofol results in a decrease in ICP, thereby identifying the patient as a responder. Hypotension is a frequent side effect of high-dose therapy with these agents. Meticulous volume resuscitation should be ensured and infusion of vasopressor/inotropes may be required. Prolonged use or high dose of propofol can lead to propofol infusion syndrome. Continuous electroencephalogram may be used to ensure targeting of the infusion to burst suppression.

- Hypothermia (<36°C) is not currently recommended as an initial TBI treatment. Hypothermia should be reserved for rescue or salvage therapy after reasonable attempts at ICP control after the previous tier 3 treatments have failed.

From American College of Surgeons Trauma Quality Improvement Program. Best practices in the management of traumatic brain injury. Available at: https://www.facs.org/~/media/files/quality%20programs/trauma/tqip/traumatic%20brain%20injury%20guidelines.ashx. Accessed May 1, 2016.

---

with invasive methods ICP monitoring.[49] The reliability of TCD continues to be refined. However, currently it is not standard of care for ICP monitoring.

It is well understood that intracranial hypertension can produce severe effects to the already injured brain. However, there continues to be a lack of evidence to guide management on how best to monitor intracranial hypertension, and with what threshold intervention should be initiated.[50] Furthermore, hospital-level compliance with evidence-based guidelines for ICP monitoring and craniotomy had minimal association with risk-adjusted outcomes in patients with severe TBI.[51]

UPDATED BRAIN TRAUMA FOUNDATION GUIDELINES SEVERE TBI

The updated Guidelines (Fourth Edition)[52] have modified some recommendations based on new evidence, and include the following:

- ***ICP monitoring:*** Management of severe TBI patients using information from ICP monitoring is recommended to reduce in-hospital and 2-week post-injury mortality.
- ***ICP thresholds:*** Treating ICP > 22 mm Hg is recommended because values above this level are associated with increased mortality,.
- ***Cerebral perfusion pressure (CCP) monitoring:*** Management of severe TBI patients using guidelines-based recommendations for CPP monitoring is recommended to decreased 2-week mortality.
- ***CPP thresholds:*** The recommended target CPP value for survival and favorable outcomes is between 60 and 70 mm Hg. Whether 60 or 70 mm Hg is the minimum optimal CPP threshold is unclear and may depend upon the autoregulatory status of the patient.

Table 1
Complications of therapeutic interventions for TBI

Interventions	Complications
Seizure Prophylaxis	
Phenytoin	Adverse drug reactions Must follow serum drug levels
Levetiracetam	Cost Adverse drug reactions
Hyperosmolar Therapy	
Mannitol	Intravascular volume depletion Rebound increased ICP
Hypertonic saline	Hypernatremia Volume expansion
Temperature Modulation	
Hypothermia	Rebound increased ICP during rewarming Altered metabolism
Normothermia	Need for pharmacologic and physiologic intervention Pulmonary complications
ICP Monitoring	
Invasive	Bleeding Infection
Noninvasive	Reliability
Decompressive craniectomy	Poor long-term functional outcome

TREATMENT COMPLICATIONS

Treatment complications are listed in **Table 1**.

EVALUATION OF OUTCOME AND LONG-TERM RECOMMENDATIONS

Most current studies include patients with severe TBIs, and measure long-term functional outcomes at 6 months using The GOS-E. However, the association of severity of injury and current treatment modalities is not well described. In addition, follow-up is limited and complications of therapy are poorly reported.

SUMMARY

There have been many recent advances in the management of TBI. Research regarding established therapies, such as antiseizure prophylaxis, and novel therapies, such as TTM, is ongoing. Future research must not only focus on development of new strategies but determine the long-term benefits or disadvantages of current strategies. In addition, the impact of these advances on varying severities of brain injury must not be ignored. It is hoped that future research strategies in TBI will prioritize large-scale trials using common data elements to develop large registries and databases led by the Federal Interagency Traumatic Brain Injury Research (FITBIR) informatics system as a partnership between the National Institutes of Health (NIH) and Department of Defense (DOD), and leverage international collaborations such as the International Initiative for Traumatic Brain Injury Research (InTBIR).

REFERENCES

1. Brain Trauma Foundation, American Association of Neurological Surgeons, Congress of Neurological Surgeons. Guidelines for the management of severe traumatic brain injury. J Neurotrauma 2007;24(Suppl 1):S1–106.

2. Stein DM, Hu PF, Brenner M, et al. Brief episodes of intracranial hypertension and cerebral hypoperfusion are associated with poor functional outcome after severe traumatic brain injury. J Trauma 2011;71(2):364–73 [discussion: 373–4].

3. Badri S, Chen J, Barber J, et al. Mortality and long-term functional outcome associated with intracranial pressure after traumatic brain injury. Intensive Care Med 2012;38(11):1800–9.

4. Burgess S, Abu-Laban RB, Slavik RS, et al. A systematic review of randomized controlled trials comparing hypertonic sodium solutions and mannitol for traumatic brain injury: implications for emergency department management. Ann Pharmacother 2016;50(4):291–300.

5. Szaflarski JP, Sangha KS, Lindsell CJ, et al. Prospective, randomized, single-blinded comparative trial of intravenous levetiracetam versus phenytoin for seizure prophylaxis. Neurocrit Care 2010;12(2):165–72.

6. Temkin NR, Dikmen SS, Wilensky AJ, et al. A randomized, double-blind study of phenytoin for the prevention of post-traumatic seizures. N Engl J Med 1990; 323(8):497–502.

7. Bhullar IS, Johnson D, Paul JP, et al. More harm than good: antiseizure prophylaxis after traumatic brain injury does not decrease seizure rates but may inhibit functional recovery. J Trauma Acute Care Surg 2014;76(1):54–60 [discussion: 60–1].

8. Zafar SN, Khan AA, Ghauri AA, et al. Phenytoin versus Leviteracetam for seizure prophylaxis after brain injury - a meta analysis. BMC Neurol 2012;12:30.

9. Inaba K, Menaker J, Branco BC, et al. A prospective multicenter comparison of levetiracetam versus phenytoin for early posttraumatic seizure prophylaxis. J Trauma Acute Care Surg 2013;74(3):766–71 [discussion: 771–3].

10. Kruer RM, Harris LH, Goodwin H, et al. Changing trends in the use of seizure prophylaxis after traumatic brain injury: a shift from phenytoin to levetiracetam. J Crit Care 2013;28(5):883.e9-13.

11. Wakai A, McCabe A, Roberts I, et al. Mannitol for acute traumatic brain injury. Cochrane Database Syst Rev 2013;(8):CD001049.

12. Kamel H, Navi BB, Nakagawa K, et al. Hypertonic saline versus mannitol for the treatment of elevated intracranial pressure: a meta-analysis of randomized clinical trials. Crit Care Med 2011;39(3):554–9.

13. Mangat HS, Chiu YL, Gerber LM, et al. Hypertonic saline reduces cumulative and daily intracranial pressure burdens after severe traumatic brain injury. J Neurosurg 2015;122(1):202–10.

14. Cottenceau V, Masson F, Mahamid E, et al. Comparison of effects of equiosmolar doses of mannitol and hypertonic saline on cerebral blood flow and metabolism in traumatic brain injury. J Neurotrauma 2011;28(10):2003–12.

15. Deutsch ER, Espinoza TR, Atif F, et al. Progesterone's role in neuroprotection, a review of the evidence. Brain Res 2013;1530:82–105.

16. Wright DW, Kellermann AL, Hertzberg VS, et al. ProTECT: a randomized clinical trial of progesterone for acute traumatic brain injury. Ann Emerg Med 2007;49: 391–402.

Optimal Fluid Therapy for Traumatic Hemorrhagic Shock

Ronald Chang, MD[a],*, John B. Holcomb, MD[b]

KEYWORDS

- Massive transfusion protocol • Hemorrhagic shock • Damage control resuscitation

KEY POINTS

- Hemorrhage is the leading cause of preventable trauma deaths and occurs rapidly (median 2–3 hours after presentation).
- Early activation of a predefined massive transfusion protocol improves outcomes for the patient with exsanguinating hemorrhage, although accurate identification remains a challenge.
- Large infusions of crystalloid are dangerous for patients with traumatic hemorrhagic shock, and even relatively small volumes of crystalloid may be harmful.
- Plasma should be used as the primary means of volume expansion for resuscitation of trauma patients with hemorrhagic shock.
- Although the exact mechanisms underlying the benefits of plasma are unclear, it is likely more than simple replacement of volume and clotting factors.

INTRODUCTION

Hemorrhage is a top cause of death after injury and is the leading cause of potentially preventable trauma deaths.[1–3] In contrast to other causes of trauma death, such as traumatic brain injury (TBI), multiple organ dysfunction syndrome (MODS), and sepsis, exsanguination occurs rapidly with a median time to death of 2 to 3 hours after presentation.[4,5] Advances in the treatment of hemorrhagic shock have historically been made during times of armed conflict: major milestones include the first blood banks during World War I, the development of dried plasma during World War II, recognition of a close association between shock and coagulopathy during the Vietnam War,[6] and the advent of damage control resuscitation (DCR) during the recent wars in

R. Chang is supported by a T32 fellowship (grant no. 5T32GM008792) from NIGMS. The authors have no relevant financial conflicts of interest.
[a] Center for Translational Injury Research, University of Texas Health Science Center, 6410 Fannin Street, Suite 1100, Houston, TX 77030, USA; [b] Department of Surgery, University of Texas Health Science Center, 6410 Fannin Street, Suite 1100, Houston, TX 77030, USA
* Corresponding author. 6410 Fannin Street, Suite 1100, Houston, TX 77030.
E-mail address: ronald.chang@uth.tmc.edu

Afghanistan and Iraq. DCR was a paradigm shift in the management of traumatic hemorrhagic shock and is a major focus of this article.

As the management of trauma evolves over time, experts are discovering more and more that resuscitation of the severely injured patient (the normalization of deranged physiology and correction of the shock state) has as much impact on patient outcome as surgical treatment of the injured tissues. Development of an optimal resuscitation strategy with attention to the type, quantity, and timing of fluid therapy is of paramount importance to any clinician caring for trauma patients presenting with hemorrhagic shock.

PATIENT EVALUATION OVERVIEW

A small minority (1%–3%) of patients presenting to a major urban trauma center will require substantial blood product transfusion following injury, typically referred to as massive transfusion (MT). Traditionally, MT had been arbitrarily defined as transfusion of at least 10 units of packed red blood cells (PRBCs) within 24 hours. Early identification of the trauma patient who will require MT is difficult but nonetheless essential because early activation of a predefined MT protocol (MTP) is associated with decreased blood product waste,[7] as well as reduced incidence of organ failure and other complications.[8]

Several scoring systems have been proposed to predict need for MT but early iterations, such as the Trauma Associated Severe Hemorrhage (TASH) score[9] and the McLaughlin score,[10] relied on laboratory values that are not available until some time after presentation. In 2010, Cotton and colleagues[11] published a multicenter validation study of the Assessment of Blood Consumption (ABC) score, which gives 1 point for each of the following: penetrating mechanism, systolic blood pressure (SBP) less than 90 mm Hg, heart rate greater than 120 beats per minute, and positive Focused Abdominal Sonography in Trauma (FAST) examination (**Boxes 1** and **2**).

A score of 2 or more is predictive of MT with a sensitivity of 75% to 90%, specificity of 67% to 88%, and overall accuracy of 84% to 87% for all trauma patients. Importantly, the ABC score requires no laboratory data, can be determined within minutes of patient arrival, and can be easily recalculated over time. The American College of Surgeons (ACS) Trauma Quality Improvement Program (TQIP) Massive Transfusion in Trauma Guidelines now recommends use of the ABC score of 2 or more for MTP activation.

Pommerening and colleagues[12] examined the reliability of physician gestalt in predicting need for MT by performing a secondary analysis on subjects from the Prospective, Observational, Multicenter, Major Trauma Transfusion (PROMMTT) study. Of note, entry into this study required transfusion of at least 1 PRBC unit within the first 6 hours, and subjects who died within 30 minutes of presentation were excluded.

Box 1
Assessment of blood consumption score. Score of 2 or more points predicted need for massive transfusion within 24 hours with sensitivity 75% to 90%, specificity 67% to 86%, and overall accuracy 84% to 86%

- Penetrating mechanism (no = 0; yes = 1)
- Emergency department SBP less than 90 mm Hg (no = 0; yes = 1)
- Emergency department heart rate greater than 120 bpm (no = 0; yes = 1)
- Positive Focused Abdominal Sonography in Trauma (FAST) examination (no = 0; yes = 1)

Box 2
Initiate massive transfusion protocol (MTP) if one or more of the following criteria are met

- ABC score of 2 or more
- Persistent hemodynamic instability
- Active bleeding requiring operation or angioembolization
- Blood transfusion in the trauma bay

Adapted from ACS TQIP. Massive Transfusion in Trauma Guidelines. American College of Surgeons. Available at: https://www.facs.org/%7E/media/files/quality%20programs/trauma/tqip/massive%20transfusion%20in%20trauma%20guildelines.ashx. Accessed April 13, 2016.

Therefore, included subjects were at overall intermediate risk for requiring MT, whereas subjects at the 2 extremes were excluded. In this subject group, investigators found that physician gestalt and several scoring systems, including ABC, performed relatively poorly, achieving modest sensitivities and specificities of 65% to 70%. Independent predictors of a false-negative physician gestalt were bleeding in the pelvis and relatively normal blood gas parameters.

Viscoelastic assays of coagulation (thromboelastography [TEG] and rotational thromboelastometry [ROTEM]) can be used to diagnose and monitor trauma-induced coagulopathy. Because clinically meaningful results can be available within minutes of trauma patient arrival, TEG and ROTEM have been proposed as predictors of need for MT. Prospective observational studies by Cotton and colleagues[13] and Davenport and colleagues[14] found that admission TEG and ROTEM parameters available within 5 minutes of assay initiation more accurately predicted MT compared with the slower conventional coagulation assays (CCAs).

One difficulty in conducting MT research is that the traditional definition on which much of the literature is based ($\geq$10 PRBC units within 24 hours) is woefully inadequate: it does not capture the intensity of resuscitative efforts and is prone to survivor bias.[15] In particular, rapidly hemorrhaging patients are excluded when they exsanguinate before reaching the threshold, whereas less critically ill patients are included when they accrue units steadily over 24 hours. In response, newer definitions of MT that delineate use of blood products within a narrower timeframe have gained acceptance. For example, the concept of the critical administration threshold (CAT), defined as the transfusion of at least 3 PRBC units within any 1-hour time window within the first 24 hours,[16] has been prospectively validated in trauma subjects and found to be a more sensitive predictor of mortality than the traditional MT definition.[17] An advantage of CAT is that it can be obtained prospectively. Studies have shown that patients who reach CAT soon after presentation or who reach CAT multiple times have increased mortality,[16,17] and CAT may serve as an indicator to proceed with abbreviated instead of definitive laparotomy.[18]

PHARMACOLOGIC TREATMENT OPTIONS

The term damage control originated in the United States Navy to describe the protocol used to save a ship that has suffered catastrophic structural damage from sinking, placing a heavy emphasis on the limitation and containment of fires and flooding.[19] This term was adopted by trauma surgeons to describe the use of abbreviated surgeries to rapidly temporize life-threatening injuries (namely, hemorrhage) with delay of definitive repair until after adequate resuscitation. Damage control surgery is

The goal of permissive hypotension is to maintain only the minimal blood pressure necessary to perfuse the vital organs. The rationale, which Cannon recognized a century ago, is that elevations in blood pressure before surgical hemostasis is achieved may compromise a tenuous clot and exacerbate blood loss. Much of the evidence for this practice comes from animal studies. In a swine model of uncontrolled hemorrhage, Sondeen and colleagues[49] demonstrated that there was a reproducible mean arterial blood pressure of 64 plus or minus 2 mm Hg at which the clot was popped and rebleeding occurred. A meta-analysis identified 9 animal studies that investigated hypotensive resuscitation after hemorrhage, all of which reported decreased mortality with a pooled relative risk of 0.37 (95% CI 0.33–0.71) in animals undergoing hypotensive fluid resuscitation compared with those undergoing normotensive resuscitation.[50]

Comparatively, there are fewer such studies in human subjects. Bickell and colleagues[51] published the first such study in 1994. They randomized 289 subjects after penetrating torso injury to standard fluid resuscitation, which was begun prehospital, or delayed fluid resuscitation, which was begun in the operating room. The investigators reported significantly improved survival in the delayed resuscitation group (70% vs 62%). However, subsequent studies have reported mixed results. In 2002, Dutton and colleagues[52] randomized 110 subjects with hemorrhagic shock in the emergency department to initial fluid resuscitation with high (100 mm Hg) and low (70 mm Hg) SBP goals and reported no mortality difference between groups. A multicenter pilot trial by ROC randomized 192 prehospital hypotensive trauma subjects to high (110 mm Hg) and low (70 mm Hg) SBP goals and reported improved 24-hour survival in the low SBP group after blunt trauma (97% vs 82%) but no difference after penetrating trauma (81% vs 81%).[53] Significantly, all of the randomized trials cited excluded patients with significant head injury.

The ideal target blood pressure for the initial resuscitation of hemorrhagic shock before definitive hemorrhage control remains unclear. There are currently no concrete recommendations from any of the leading trauma organizations. An open question is how low and for how long the blood pressure can be kept before the harm outweighs the benefit. Another consideration is the head-injured patient, for whom even a single episode of hypotension may substantially increase TBI-related morbidity and mortality.[54] Finally, previous studies used crystalloid to achieve blood pressure goals and there are currently little data regarding hypotensive resuscitation with blood products such as plasma. However, the available data suggest permissive hypotension is probably safe for short periods of time (in the absence of TBI) until definitive hemorrhage control can be achieved.

Optimal Transfusion of Blood Products

In the mid-seventeenth century, Richard Lower performed the first successful animal-to-animal blood transfusion when he demonstrated that a dog hemorrhaged nearly to the point of death could be completely restored by the transfusion of another dog's blood.[55] In the early nineteenth century, English obstetrician James Blundell performed the first successful human-to-human blood transfusion to save the life of a woman with postpartum hemorrhage.[56] However, several barriers, including infections secondary to lack of sterile technique, no understanding of the different blood types, and catheter thrombosis due to deficient knowledge of anticoagulants, made blood transfusion prohibitively dangerous and difficult. It was not until the early twentieth century when these barriers were overcome that blood transfusions could become routine. For the next 50 years, transfusion of whole blood was the norm. By the 1970s, however, component therapy had replaced whole blood transfusions to maximize the efficient utilization of donated blood and to limit the spread of blood-borne pathogens.

Plasma

Early definitive hemorrhage control and MT with DCR are the preferred treatment of the trauma patient in severe hemorrhagic shock. The actual composition of an MTP has changed drastically over the last 20 years. Before the advent of DCR, a trauma patient undergoing MT would have received stepwise resuscitation with crystalloid, artificial colloids, and PRBCs. Not until 1 to 2 blood volumes have already been replaced would plasma and platelets be given.[57] This all changed after the shift to DCR, which began in earnest with the landmark study by Borgman and colleagues[58] in 2007, a retrospective study of 246 massively transfused military trauma subjects treated at a US combat support hospital in Iraq. The investigators separated subjects into 3 groups by ratio of plasma to PRBC: low (median ratio 1:8), medium (median ratio 1:2.5), and high (median ratio 1:1.4). The all-cause mortality for the 3 groups were 65%, 34%, and 19%, respectively, whereas the mortality due to hemorrhage were 93%, 78%, and 37%, respectively. Every 1 unit increase in the ratio of plasma to PRBC was associated with an OR of 8.6 (95% CI 2.1–35.2) improved likelihood of survival. The same year, Johansson and colleagues[59] demonstrated that early transfusion of high ratios of plasma and platelets in subjects who underwent repair of a ruptured abdominal aortic aneurysm had significantly improved 30 day survival (66% vs 44%) compared with historical controls.

Further observational data describing the benefit of early high plasma ratios followed for civilian trauma patients.[60–63] In particular, the PROMMTT study was a multicenter prospective observational trial that analyzed 905 bleeding trauma subjects who received at least 1 PRBC unit within 6 hours, at least 3 PRBCs units within 24 hours, and survived for at least 30 minutes after arrival.[4] PROMMTT demonstrated that early utilization of higher ratios of plasma and platelets to PRBCs was associated with decreased in-hospital mortality. Specifically, every unit increase in the plasma to PRBC and platelet to PRBC ratios within the first 6 hours (when hemorrhage was the primary cause of death) was associated with an adjusted hazard ratio of 0.31 (95% CI 0.16–0.58) and 0.55 (95% CI 0.31–0.98) of in-hospital mortality, respectively. After the first 24 hours when other causes of death increased in incidence, ratios of plasma and platelets to PRBCs were no longer significantly associated with mortality.

The first randomized control trial investigating the optimal ratio of blood products was the Pragmatic, Randomized Optimal Platelet and Plasma Ratios (PROPPR) study, a multicenter study that randomized 680 severely injured, bleeding trauma subjects to resuscitation with a 1:1:1 or 1:1:2 ratio of plasma, platelets, and PRBC.[5] The investigators found no differences in 24-hour or 30-day mortality. However, subjects in the higher plasma and platelets ratio (1:1:1) group had significantly increased achievement of hemostasis (86% vs 78%) and decreased death due to bleeding (9% vs 15%) compared with the low ratio (1:1:2) group. Other studies have demonstrated improved subject outcomes after implementation of DCR principles. Shrestha and colleagues[64] have shown increased likelihood of successful nonoperative management and survival in civilian subjects with high-grade liver injuries after blunt trauma. In the military setting, soldiers injured in combat are also surviving with more severe injuries after implementation of DCR.[65] Based on these studies, the ACS TQIP Massive Transfusion in Trauma Guidelines recommend DCR in patients who meet MTP triggers (Box 4).[66]

The underlying mechanism behind these benefits, however, is unclear. Restoration of intravascular volume and correction of coagulopathy are clearly important aspects.

Box 4
If massive transfusion protocol (MTP) trigger criteria are met, initiate damage control resuscitation (DCR)

- Begin universal blood product infusion rather than crystalloid or colloid solutions.
- Transfuse universal red blood cells (RBCs) and plasma in a ratio between 1:1 and 1:2 (plasma/RBC).
- Transfuse 1 single donor apheresis or random donor platelet pool for each 6 units of RBC.
- Blood products should be automatically sent by the transfusion service in established ratios.
- Subsequent coolers should be delivered at 15-minute intervals until the MTP has been terminated.
- The goal is to keep at least 1 MTP cooler ahead for the duration of the MTP activation.

Adapted from ACS TQIP. Massive Transfusion in Trauma Guidelines. American College of Surgeons. Available at: https://www.facs.org/%7E/media/files/quality%20programs/trauma/tqip/massive%20transfusion%20in%20trauma%20guildelines.ashx. Accessed April 13, 2016.

In animal models of hemorrhagic shock, plasma-based resuscitation mitigated hyperfibrinolysis[67] and platelet dysfunction[68] compared with crystalloid resuscitation. However, proteins involved with coagulation represent only a small fraction of the human plasma proteome. Besides restoration of intravascular volume and clotting factors, another benefit is likely repair of endothelial injury. Severe trauma,[69] as well as several other inflammatory conditions, including diabetes,[70] sepsis,[71] and ischemia-reperfusion,[72] are known to result in injury to the endothelium with loss of microvascular integrity, resulting in extravasation of intravascular fluid into the interstitial space. Liberal resuscitation with crystalloids and artificial colloids increases hydrostatic pressure without repairing the endothelial injury, resulting in edema and the edema-related complications that were common in the pre-DCR era (**Fig. 1**). In contrast, in vitro[73–75] and animal models[76,77] of hemorrhagic shock demonstrate that plasma restores microvascular integrity, in part by repair of the endothelial glycocalyx layer (EGL). In a large animal model of concomitant hemorrhagic shock and TBI, resuscitation with fresh frozen plasma (FFP) resulted in less secondary brain injury compared with resuscitation with crystalloid or artificial colloid, likely secondary to restoration of cerebral endothelium.[78] In trauma patients, there are strong correlations between increasing circulating levels of glycocalyx components (a marker for EGL injury) and trauma severity, coagulopathy, and mortality,[69,79,80] although it remains unclear if these relationships are causative or merely associative.

Clinicians have long recognized that time is against the bleeding trauma patient and that faster initiation of lifesaving interventions improves outcomes. In light of this, key logistical hurdles must be overcome to expedite the delivery of plasma. Blood banks stock FFP, which has a shelf of life of up to 1 year at −18°C but requires 20 to 30 minutes of thaw time before use, limiting immediate availability. Options to make plasma readily available for emergency use include stocking thawed plasma and liquid plasma. After FFP is thawed, the most labile clotting factors (V and VIII) maintain 65% of their activity at the end of its 5 day shelf life.[81] Liquid plasma, on the other hand, is never frozen and includes a preservative to maintain stability of most clotting factors for up to 26 days. Toward the end of its shelf life, most clotting factors maintain 88% activity and in vitro studies demonstrate that never-frozen liquid plasma has a better coagulation profile than thawed plasma.[82]

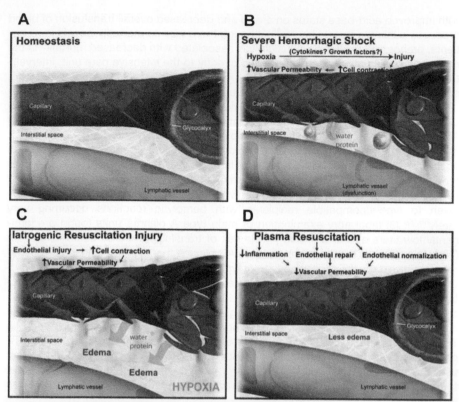

Fig. 1. Proposed effect of hemorrhagic shock and crystalloid versus plasma resuscitation on the microvasculature. (*A*) Homeostasis before injury. (*B*) Hemorrhagic shock results in shedding of endothelial glycocalyx layer (EGL) components, resulting in endothelial injury, microvascular permeability, and leakage of fluid into the interstitial space. (*C*) Crystalloids increase hydrostatic pressure in the presence of persistent endothelial injury, resulting in edema. (*D*) Plasma restores intravascular volume while restoring the EGL and repairing endothelial injury, limiting edema. (*From* Pati S, Matijevic N, Doursout MF. Protective effects of fresh frozen plasma on vascular endothelial permeability, coagulation, and resuscitation after hemorrhagic shock are time dependent and diminish between days 0 and 5 after thaw. J Trauma 2010;69(Suppl 1):S61; with permission.)

Another logistical hurdle affecting speed of delivery is storage location. For example, a before-and-after study demonstrated that moving 4 units of universal-donor thawed plasma from the blood bank to the emergency department was independently associated with decreased time to first plasma transfusion, decreased usage of PRBCs (coefficient −2.9, 95% CI −5.7 to −0.2) and plasma (coefficient −2.7, 95% CI −5.4 to −0.1) within the first 24 hours, and decreased mortality (OR 0.43, 95% CI 0.19–0.96).[83] The multicenter PROPPR study demonstrated the feasibility of high-level trauma centers to rapidly deliver universal donor plasma to hemorrhaging trauma patients quickly and consistently with minimal wastage.[84]

In the last several years, many investigators have proposed transitioning hospital interventions for trauma patients to the prehospital phase of care, including plasma. A retrospective study that analyzed 1677 severely injured trauma patients who were transported by helicopter found that in-flight plasma transfusion was associated with improved acid-base status on arrival and decreased overall transfusion of blood products within the first 24 hours.[85] Although there was no mortality benefit in all patients, prehospital plasma transfusion was associated with decreased mortality in the most critically ill patients (those admitted directly to the intensive care unit, interventional radiology, operating room, or morgue). Randomized trials to study the impact of prehospital plasma in ground[86] and aeromedical transport[87] are on-going.

A final logistic consideration is that individuals with the universal plasma donor AB blood type make up only 4% of the population of the United States.[88] The scarcity of AB plasma has been further exacerbated by the widespread adoption of DCR principles. To circumvent this shortage, the use of type A plasma has been proposed as an alternative. The rationale is that (1) 85% of individuals in the United States have either type A or type O blood,[88] making type A plasma compatible with the almost all potential recipients; (2) the plasma transfused with type O apheresis platelets is routinely given to type-incompatible recipients with hemolytic reactions occurring very rarely[89,90]; (3) laboratory examination of male type A plasma units found predominantly low titers of anti-B[91]; and (4) the risk of transfusion-related acute lung injury (TRALI) is currently much higher with type AB plasma than type A.[92] Based on limited retrospective data, the emergency use of type A plasma seems safe.[93–95] As this practice becomes widespread,[96] more accurate data about the safety profile of this practice will soon become available.

Previous studies had raised concerns regarding the safety of increased plasma use, citing potentially increased risk of developing inflammatory complications such as TRALI, ARDS, and MODS.[97–99] Analysis of the prospectively acquired PROMMTT dataset did not demonstrate an independent association between blood product use and moderate-to-severe hypoxemia.[37] Indeed, the PROPPR randomized trial found no difference in inflammatory or transfusion-related complications between the high-ratio and low-ratio groups.[5]

Platelets
The inclusion of platelets with a balanced MTP approach is intuitive to more accurately mimic the whole blood that was lost. Retrospective studies[60,100,101] report increased survival in massively transfused patients who received high ratios of platelets to PRBCs. PROMMTT provided prospective observational data demonstrating that every unit increase in the platelet to PRBC ratio decreased the hazard ratio of mortality within the first 6 hours by 0.55 (95% CI 0.31–0.98).[4] As was the case with plasma, this relationship parallels the risk of death from hemorrhage and became weaker with time, such that the platelet to PRBC ratio after 24 hours was no longer significantly associated with mortality. In the PROPPR randomized trial,[5] subjects in the high plasma and platelets ratio group had lower death due to hemorrhage, although the independent effects of plasma and platelets cannot be disentangled in this study. The most recent guidelines from the ACS Committee on Trauma recommend transfusing 1 unit of platelets (what was previously known as a 6-pack of platelets) for every 6 PRBC units.[102]

Fresh whole blood
Fresh whole blood (FWB) can be stored at room temperature for up to 8 hours and at 6°C of less for 24 to 48 hours, depending on institutional guidelines.[103] Although economic and other considerations have all but eliminated the civilian use of FWB, several factors make FWB an attractive option for the resuscitation of hemorrhagic shock. First, the diluting effect secondary to the anticoagulants and additives in each blood product component reduces the hematocrit, factor activity, and platelet count of a

1:1:1 ratio of component therapy compared with a unit of FWB (**Table 1**).[104] An in vitro study compared the parameters of FWB and reconstituted whole blood (1:1:1 ratio component therapy) and reported findings similar to the theoretic calculations.[105] Second, the use of FWB would preclude the loss of quality of blood product components due to storage time.[106–108] Indeed, use of blood products with increased storage duration is associated with increased mortality and morbidity.[109–111] Third, use of FWB would reduce the number of donors to which the recipient is exposed and may reduce the risk of blood-borne pathogens. Finally, transfusion of 1 whole blood unit is logistically simpler than transfusion of multiple components and may reduce harm from administrative errors.

The limited availability of refrigeration and potential shortages of blood product components means that FWB will always have a niche in the austere environment. Military experience with the transfusion of FWB is extensive, dating as far back as World War I, and includes the transfusion of over 9000 whole blood units during the recent military conflicts in Afghanistan and Iraq.[112] Two retrospective analyses of combat casualties treated at a combat support hospital[113] and by forward surgical teams[114] reported improved survival in patients who received FWB compared with component therapy (PRBC and FFP only, no platelets due to a shortage). Lingering questions regarding the use of FWB include warm versus cold storage, shelf life, and the ability to rapidly screen FWB units for infectious agents and type compatability,[103] although some have advocated the use of low anti-A/B titer type O whole blood as an alternative to type specificity.[115]

Establishing the ability to rapidly and safely transfuse FWB for trauma patients requires changes to donor blood processing at regional blood banks. Donor whole blood could be theoretically held for its shelf life (24–48 hours) and subsequently processed into components if not transfused as FWB. The authors recently performed a pilot study that demonstrated the feasibility of modified whole blood therapy in a civilian trauma setting[116]; however, the whole blood units used in the study were leukoreduced and platelet-poor, meaning patients still required transfusions of apheresis platelets.

Goal-directed correction of coagulopathy

Perturbations of different aspects of TEG and ROTEM tracings point to deficiencies in different components of coagulation, and this allows using blood products or other adjuncts to correct these deficiencies in a targeted manner. The use of TEG and ROTEM in liver transplantation[117] and cardiac surgery[118] has been shown to reduce blood product use with similar or improved patient outcomes. In the case of the relatively stable trauma patient, in whom surgical hemorrhage control is achieved and MTP is deactivated, the use of TEG and ROTEM to guide further blood product utilization is intuitive and an important component of DCR.[57] A recent single-institution

---

Table 1
Calculated parameters of fresh whole blood versus reconstituted whole blood with 1 packed red blood cell unit (335 mL with hematocrit of 55%), 1 platelet unit (5.5×10^{10} platelets in 50 mL), and 1 fresh frozen plasma unit (80% coagulation factor activity)

	Fresh Whole Blood	1:1:1 Component Therapy
Hematocrit (%)	38–50	29
Platelets ($\times 10^9$/L)	150–400	88
Coagulation factor activity (%)	100	65

randomized controlled trial (n = 111) reported that use of a goal-directed, TEG-guided MTP compared with MTP guided by CCAs to resuscitate severely injured patients was associated with improved survival (11/56 deaths TEG vs 20/55 deaths CCA, P = .049).[66] Data regarding the use of blood products and other therapeutics in response to abnormalities of different TEG/ROTEM parameters, are presented elsewhere in this issue.

However, the role of coagulation assays to guide transfusion of blood products during MTP in lieu of fixed ratios is unclear and controversial.[119,120] Although it was not designed to answer this question, analysis of data from the PROPPR randomized trial demonstrated subjects randomized to the low (1:1:2) plasma and platelet ratio group were transfused additional units of plasma and platelets in a laboratory-driven, goal-directed fashion after MTP was deactivated, such that the cumulative ratio of blood products used approached 1:1:1 by 24 hours,[5] suggesting that the optimal ratio may be close to 1:1:1 regardless of how it is arrived at. Direct comparisons between fixed ratio versus goal-directed MTP are lacking in the literature,[121,122] although other investigators argue that the 2 strategies are not mutually exclusive.[123]

TREATMENT RESISTANCE AND COMPLICATIONS
Cryoprecipitate and Fibrinogen Concentrate

Cryoprecipitate, collected as the precipitate of plasma after a freeze-thaw cycle, is enriched in factors VIII and XIII, von Willebrand factor, fibronectin, and fibrinogen. These factors are theoretically replaced at physiologic levels by plasma during the course of MT, and the discussion regarding the use of cryoprecipitate focuses on the need for additional boluses of these components, particularly fibrinogen. Although previous data suggested a critical fibrinogen threshold of 100 mg/dL (1.0 g/L), more recent studies found significant bleeding at this level,[124,125] indicating the need for a higher cutoff. Currently, the ACS Committee on Trauma recommends transfusing cryoprecipitate to maintain fibrinogen at 180 mg/dL or greater,[102] whereas European guidelines describe a minimum cutoff of 150 to 200 mg/dL.[126]

An analysis of blood samples from 52 massively transfused patients found that fibrinogen was commonly the first factor to reach critically low levels.[127] A review of 1332 massively transfused combat casualties found that use of cryoprecipitate within the first 24 hours was independently associated with improved survival.[128] These data suggest a potential benefit with early delivery of fibrinogen, either by fibrinogen concentrate (off-label use in the United States) or cryoprecipitate. A randomized controlled trial to evaluate the use of prehospital fibrinogen concentrate (Fibrinogen in Trauma-induced coagulopathy [FlinTIC])[129] is ongoing.

Continued Hemorrhage

Continued hemorrhage despite adequate surgical control and DCR is secondary to worsening trauma-induced coagulopathy. Although DCR is designed to treat coagulopathy directly, adjunctive measures may also be used. We defer discussion of treatment of coagulopathy, in this issue.

Transfusion-Related Acute Lung Injury

The most notable complication resulting from blood product transfusion is TRALI, characterized by inflammatory-mediated pulmonary edema resulting in hypoxia within hours of transfusion.[130] Although any blood product may precipitate TRALI, the risk was historically highest with plasma.[92] Recognizing that a significant source of TRALI cases were precipitated by plasma donated by multiparous women who likely

III. Tissue oxygenation, type of fluid and temperature management

R13
Tissue oxygenation
***
A target systolic blood pressure of 80–90 mm Hg should be employed until major bleeding has been stopped in the initial phase following trauma without brain injury. A mean arterial pressure ≥80 mm Hg should be maintained in patients with severe TBI.

R14
Restricted volume replacement
***
A restricted volume replacement strategy should be used to achieve target blood pressure until bleeding can be controlled.

R15
Vasopressors and inotropic agents
***
In addition to fluids, vasopressors should be administered to maintain target blood pressure in the presence of life-threatening hypotension. An inotropic agent should be infused in the presence of myocardial dysfunction.

R16
Type of fluid
***
Use of isotonic crystalloid solutions should be initiated in the hypotensive bleeding trauma patient. Hypotonic solutions such as Ringer's lactate should be avoided in patients with severe head trauma. Excessive use of 0.9% NaCl solution might be avoided and use of colloids might be restricted.

R17
Erythrocytes
***
Treatment should aim to achieve a target Hb of 7–9 g/dL.

R18
Temperature management
***
Early application of measures to reduce heat losses and warm the hypothermic patient should be employed to achieve and maintain normothermia.

IV. Rapid control of bleeding

R19
Damage control surgery
***
Damage control surgery should be employed in the severely injured patient presenting with deep haemorrhagic shock, signs of ongoing bleeding and coagulopathy. Severe coagulopathy, hypothermia, acidosis, inaccessible major anatomic injury, a need for time-consuming procedures or concomitant major injury outside the abdomen should also trigger a damage control approach. Primary definitive surgical management should be employed in the haemodynamically stable patient in the absence of any of these factors.

R20
Pelvic ring closure and stabilisation
***
Patients with pelvic ring disruption in haemorrhagic shock should undergo immediate pelvic ring closure and stabilisation.

R21
Packing, embolisation & surgery
***
Patients with ongoing haemodynamic instability despite adequate pelvic ring stabilisation should undergo early preperitoneal packing, angiographic embolisation and/or surgical bleeding control.

R22
Local haemostatic measures
***
Topical haemostatic agents should be employed in combination with other surgical measures or with packing for venous or moderate arterial bleeding associated with parenchymal injuries.

V. Initial management of bleeding and coagulopathy

R23
Coagulation support
***
Monitoring and measures to support coagulation should be initiated immediately upon hospital admission.

R24
Initial resuscitation
***
Initial management of patients with expected massive haemorrhage should include either plasma (FFP or pathogen-inactivated plasma) in a plasma-RBC ratio of at least 1:2 as needed or fibrinogen concentrate and RBC according to Hb level.

R25
Antifibrinolytic agents
***
TXA should be administered as early as possible to the trauma patient who is bleeding or at risk of significant haemorrhage at a loading dose of 1 g infused over 10 min, followed by an i.v. infusion of 1 g over 8 h. TXA should be administered to the bleeding trauma patient within 3 h after injury. Protocols for the management of bleeding patients might consider administration of the first dose of TXA en route to the hospital.

Fig. 2. Summary of treatment modalities for the bleeding trauma patient. (*Adapted from* Rossaint R, Bouillon B, Cerny V, et al. The European guideline on management of major bleeding and coagulopathy following trauma: fourth edition. Crit Care 2016;20:100.)

24. Shoemaker WC, Appel P, Bland R. Use of physiologic monitoring to predict outcome and to assist in clinical decisions in critically ill postoperative patients. Am J Surg 1983;146(1):43–50.

25. Shoemaker WC, Appel PL, Kram HB, et al. Prospective trial of supranormal values of survivors as therapeutic goals in high-risk surgical patients. Chest 1988;94(6):1176–86.

26. Shah SK, Uray KS, Stewart RH, et al. Resuscitation-induced intestinal edema and related dysfunction: state of the science. J Surg Res 2011;166(1):120–30.

27. Balogh Z, McKinley BA, Cocanour CS, et al. Supranormal trauma resuscitation causes more cases of abdominal compartment syndrome. Arch Surg 2003; 138(6):637–42.

28. Cotton BA, Guy JS, Morris JA Jr, et al. The cellular, metabolic, and systemic consequences of aggressive fluid resuscitation strategies. Shock 2006;26(2): 115–21.

29. Lang F, Busch GL, Ritter M, et al. Functional significance of cell volume regulatory mechanisms. Physiol Rev 1998;78(1):247–306.

30. Häussinger D, Schliess F, Warskulat U, et al. Liver cell hydration. Cell Biol Toxicol 1997;13(4–5):275–87.

31. Tseng GN. Cell swelling increases membrane conductance of canine cardiac cells: evidence for a volume-sensitive Cl channel. Am J Physiol 1992;262(4 Pt 1):C1056–68.

32. Velmahos GC, Demetriades D, Shoemaker WC, et al. Endpoints of resuscitation of critically injured patients: normal or supranormal? A prospective randomized trial. Ann Surg 2000;232(3):409–18.

33. Lobo DN, Bostock KA, Neal KR, et al. Effect of salt and water balance on recovery of gastrointestinal function after elective colonic resection: a randomised controlled trial. Lancet 2002;359(9320):1812–8.

34. Brandstrup B, Tønnesen H, Beier-Holgersen R, et al. Effects of intravenous fluid restriction on postoperative complications: comparison of two perioperative fluid regimens: a randomized assessor-blinded multicenter trial. Ann Surg 2003; 238(5):641–8.

35. Biffl WL, Moore EE, Burch JM, et al. Secondary abdominal compartment syndrome is a highly lethal event. Am J Surg 2001;182(6):645–8.

36. Kasotakis G, Sideris A, Yang Y, et al. Aggressive early crystalloid resuscitation adversely affects outcomes in adult blunt trauma patients: an analysis of the Glue Grant database. J Trauma Acute Care Surg 2013;74(5):1215–22.

37. Robinson BR, Cotton BA, Pritts TA, et al. Application of the Berlin definition in PROMMTT patients: the impact of resuscitation on the incidence of hypoxemia. J Trauma Acute Care Surg 2013;75(1 Suppl 1):S61–7.

38. Ley EJ, Clond MA, Srour MK, et al. Emergency department crystalloid resuscitation of 1.5 L or more is associated with increased mortality in elderly and non-elderly trauma patients. J Trauma 2011;70(2):398–400.

39. Brown JB, Cohen MJ, Minei JP, et al. Goal-directed resuscitation in the prehospital setting: a propensity-adjusted analysis. J Trauma Acute Care Surg 2013; 74(5):1207–12.

40. Velasco IT, Pontieri V, Rocha e Silva M Jr, et al. Hyperosmotic NaCl and severe hemorrhagic shock. Am J Physiol 1980;239(5):H664–73.

41. Mazzoni MC, Borgstrom P, Arfors KE, et al. Dynamic fluid redistribution in hyperosmotic resuscitation of hypovolemic hemorrhage. Am J Physiol 1988;255(3 Pt 2):H629–37.

42. Junger WG, Rhind SG, Rizoli SB, et al. Resuscitation of traumatic hemorrhagic shock patients with hypertonic saline-without dextran-inhibits neutrophil and endothelial cell activation. Shock 2012;38(4):341–50.
43. Pascual JL, Ferri LE, Seely AJ, et al. Hypertonic saline resuscitation of hemorrhagic shock diminishes neutrophil rolling and adherence to endothelium and reduces in vivo vascular leakage. Ann Surg 2002;236(5):634–42.
44. Rizoli SB, Rhind SG, Shek PN, et al. The immunomodulatory effects of hypertonic saline resuscitation in patients sustaining traumatic hemorrhagic shock: a randomized, controlled, double-blinded trial. Ann Surg 2006;243(1):47–57.
45. Bulger EM, Cuschieri J, Warner K, et al. Hypertonic resuscitation modulates the inflammatory response in patients with traumatic hemorrhagic shock. Ann Surg 2007;245(4):635–41.
46. Bulger EM, May S, Kerby JD, et al. Out-of-hospital hypertonic resuscitation after traumatic hypovolemic shock: a randomized, placebo controlled trial. Ann Surg 2011;253(3):431–41.
47. Delano MJ, Rizoli SB, Rhind SG, et al. Prehospital resuscitation of traumatic hemorrhagic shock with hypertonic solutions worsens hypocoagulation and hyperfibrinolysis. Shock 2015;44(1):25–31.
48. Cannon WB, Fraser J, Cowell EB. The preventive treatment of wound shock. JAMA 1918;70(9):618–21.
49. Sondeen JL, Coppes VG, Holcomb JB. Blood pressure at which rebleeding occurs after resuscitation in swine with aortic injury. J Trauma 2003;54(5 Suppl):S110–7.
50. Mapstone J, Roberts I, Evans P. Fluid resuscitation strategies: a systematic review of animal trials. J Trauma 2003;55(3):571–89.
51. Bickell WH, Wall MJ, Pepe PE, et al. Immediate versus delayed fluid resuscitation for hypotensive patients with penetrating torso injuries. N Engl J Med 1994;331(17):1105–9.
52. Dutton RP, Mackenzie CF, Scalea TM. Hypotensive resuscitation during active hemorrhage: impact on in-hospital mortality. J Trauma 2002;52(6):1141–6.
53. Schreiber MA, Meier EN, Tisherman SA, et al. A controlled resuscitation strategy is feasible and safe in hypotensive trauma patients: results of a prospective randomized pilot trial. J Trauma Acute Care Surg 2015;78(4):687–95.
54. Chesnut RM, Marshall LF, Klauber MR, et al. The role of secondary brain injury in determining outcome from severe head injury. J Trauma 1993;34(2):216–22.
55. Learoyd P. The history of blood transfusion prior to the 20th century–part 1. Transfus Med 2012;22(5):308–14.
56. Learoyd P. The history of blood transfusion prior to the 20th century–part 2. Transfus Med 2012;22(6):372–6.
57. Johansson PI, Stensballe J, Oliveri R, et al. How I treat patients with massive hemorrhage. Blood 2014;124(20):3052–8.
58. Borgman MA, Spinella PC, Perkins JG, et al. The ratio of blood products transfused affects mortality in patients receiving massive transfusions at a combat support hospital. J Trauma 2007;63(4):805–13.
59. Johansson PI, Stensballe J, Rosenberg I, et al. Proactive administration of platelets and plasma for patients with a ruptured abdominal aortic aneurysm: evaluating a change in transfusion practice. Transfusion 2007;47(4):593–8.
60. Holcomb JB, Wade CE, Michalek JE, et al. Increased plasma and platelet to red blood cell ratios improves outcome in 466 massively transfused civilian trauma patients. Ann Surg 2008;248(3):447–58.

61. Teixeira PG, Inaba K, Shulman I, et al. Impact of plasma transfusion in massively transfused trauma patients. J Trauma 2009;66(3):693–7.
62. Mitra B, Mori A, Cameron PA, et al. Fresh frozen plasma (FFP) use during massive blood transfusion in trauma resuscitation. Injury 2010;41(1):35–9.
63. Peiniger S, Nienaber U, Lefering R, et al. Balanced massive transfusion ratios in multiple injury patients with traumatic brain injury. Crit Care 2011;15(1):R68.
64. Shrestha B, Holcomb JB, Camp EA, et al. Damage-control resuscitation increases successful nonoperative management rates and survival after severe blunt liver injury. J Trauma Acute Care Surg 2015;78(2):336–41.
65. Langan NR, Eckert M, Martin MJ. Changing patterns of in-hospital deaths following implementation of damage control resuscitation practices in US forward military treatment facilities. JAMA Surg 2014;149(9):904–12.
66. Gonzalez E, Moore EE, Moore HB, et al. Goal-directed hemostatic resuscitation of trauma-induced coagulopathy: a pragmatic randomized clinical trial comparing a viscoelastic assay to conventional coagulation assays. Ann Surg 2016;263(6):1051–9.
67. Moore HB, Moore EE, Morton AP, et al. Shock-induced systemic hyperfibrinolysis is attenuated by plasma-first resuscitation. J Trauma Acute Care Surg 2015; 79(6):897–903.
68. Sillesen M, Johansson PI, Rasmussen LS, et al. Fresh frozen plasma resuscitation attenuates platelet dysfunction compared with normal saline in a large animal model of multisystem trauma. J Trauma Acute Care Surg 2014;76(4): 998–1007.
69. Rahbar E, Cardenas JC, Baimukanova G, et al. Endothelial glycocalyx shedding and vascular permeability in severely injured trauma patients. J Transl Med 2015;13:117.
70. Nieuwdorp M, Mooij HL, Kroon J, et al. Endothelial glycocalyx damage coincides with microalbuminuria in type 1 diabetes. Diabetes 2006;55(4):1127–32.
71. Liang Y, Li X, Zhang X, et al. Elevated levels of plasma TNF-α are associated with microvascular endothelial dysfunction in patients with sepsis through activating the NF-κB and p38 mitogen-activated protein kinase in endothelial cells. Shock 2014;41(4):275–81.
72. Rehm M, Bruegger D, Christ F, et al. Shedding of the endothelial glycocalyx in patients undergoing major vascular surgery with global and regional ischemia. Circulation 2007;116(17):1896–906.
73. Haywood-Watson RJ, Holcomb JB, Gonzalez EA, et al. Modulation of syndecan-1 shedding after hemorrhagic shock and resuscitation. PLoS One 2011;6(8): e23530.
74. Wataha K, Menge T, Deng X, et al. Spray-dried plasma and fresh frozen plasma modulate permeability and inflammation in vitro in vascular endothelial cells. Transfusion 2013;53(Suppl 1):80S–90S.
75. Peng Z, Pati S, Potter D, et al. Fresh frozen plasma lessens pulmonary endothelial inflammation and hyperpermeability after hemorrhagic shock and is associated with loss of syndecan 1. Shock 2013;40(3):195–202.
76. Kozar RA, Peng Z, Zhang R, et al. Plasma restoration of endothelial glycocalyx in a rodent model of hemorrhagic shock. Anesth Analg 2011;112(6):1289–95.
77. Potter DR, Baimukanova G, Keating SM, et al. Fresh frozen plasma and spray-dried plasma mitigate pulmonary vascular permeability and inflammation in hemorrhagic shock. J Trauma Acute Care Surg 2015;78(6 Suppl 1):S7–17.

78. Jin G, DeMoya MA, Duggan M, et al. Traumatic brain injury and hemorrhagic shock: evaluation of different resuscitation strategies in a large animal model of combined insults. Shock 2012;38(1):49–56.

79. Johansson PI, Stensballe J, Rasmussen LS, et al. A high admission syndecan-1 level, a marker of endothelial glycocalyx degradation, is associated with inflammation, protein C depletion, fibrinolysis, and increased mortality in trauma patients. Ann Surg 2011;254(2):194–200.

80. Ostrowski SR, Johansson PI. Endothelial glycocalyx degradation induces endogenous heparinization in patients with severe injury and early traumatic coagulopathy. J Trauma Acute Care Surg 2012;73(1):60–6.

81. Downes KA, Wilson E, Yomtovian R, et al. Serial measurement of clotting factors in thawed plasma stored for 5 days. Transfusion 2001;41(4):570.

82. Matijevic N, Wang YW, Cotton BA, et al. Better hemostatic profiles of never-frozen liquid plasma compared with thawed fresh frozen plasma. J Trauma Acute Care Surg 2013;74(1):84–90.

83. Radwan ZA, Bai Y, Matijevic N, et al. An emergency department thawed plasma protocol for severely injured patients. JAMA Surg 2013;148(2):170–5.

84. Novak DJ, Bai Y, Cooke RK, et al. Making thawed universal donor plasma available rapidly for massively bleeding trauma patients: experience from the Pragmatic, Randomized Optimal Platelets and Plasma Ratios (PROPPR) trial. Transfusion 2015;55(6):1331–9.

85. Holcomb JB, Donathan DP, Cotton BA, et al. Prehospital transfusion of plasma and red blood cells in trauma patients. Prehosp Emerg Care 2015;19(1):1–9.

86. Moore EE, Chin TL, Chapman MC, et al. Plasma first in the field for postinjury hemorrhagic shock. Shock 2014;41(Suppl 1):35–8.

87. Brown JB, Guyette FX, Neal MD, et al. Taking the blood bank to the field: the design and rationale of the Prehospital Air Medical Plasma (PAMPer) trial. Prehosp Emerg Care 2015;19(3):343–50.

88. American Red Cross. Blood Types. 2010. Available at: http://givebloodgivelife.org/education/bloodtypes.php. Accessed April 14, 2016.

89. Mair B, Benson K. Evaluation of changes in hemoglobin levels associated with ABO-incompatible plasma in apheresis platelets. Transfusion 1998;38:51–5.

90. Karafin MS, Blagg L, Tobian AAR, et al. ABO antibody titers are not predictive of hemolytic reactions due to plasma-incompatible platelet transfusions. Transfusion 2012;48:2087–93.

91. Stubbs JR, Zielinski MD, Berns KS, et al. How we provide thawed plasma for trauma patients. Transfusion 2015;55(8):1830–7.

92. Eder AF, Dy BA, Perez JM, et al. The residual risk of transfusion-related acute lung injury at the American Red Cross (2008-2011): limitations of a predominantly male-donor plasma mitigation strategy. Transfusion 2013;53(7):1442–9.

93. Zielinski MD, Johnson PM, Jenkins D, et al. Emergency use of prethawed Group A plasma in trauma patients. J Trauma Acute Care Surg 2013;74(1):69–74.

94. Zielinski MD, Schrager JJ, Johnson P, et al. Multicenter comparison of emergency release group A versus AB plasma in blunt-injured trauma patients. Clin Transl Sci 2015;8(1):43–7.

95. Chhibber V, Green M, Vauthrin M, et al. Is group A thawed plasma suitable as the first option for emergency release transfusion? (CME). Transfusion 2014;54:1751–5.

96. Dunbar NM, Yazer MH, Biomedical Excellence for Safer Transfusion (BEST) Collaborative. A possible new paradigm? A survey-based assessment of the

use of thawed group A plasma for trauma resuscitation in the United States. Transfusion 2016;56(1):125–9.

97. Watson GA, Sperry JL, Rosengart MR, et al. Fresh frozen plasma is independently associated with a higher risk of multiple organ failure and acute respiratory distress syndrome. J Trauma 2009;67(2):221–7.

98. Johnson JL, Moore EE, Kashuk JL, et al. Effect of blood products transfusion on the development of postinjury multiple organ failure. Arch Surg 2010;145(10): 973–7.

99. Inaba K, Branco BC, Rhee P, et al. Impact of plasma transfusion in trauma patients who do not require massive transfusion. J Am Coll Surg 2010;210(6): 957–65.

100. Gunter OL Jr, Au BK, Isbell JM, et al. Optimizing outcomes in damage control resuscitation: identifying blood product ratios associated with improved survival. J Trauma 2008;65(3):527–34.

101. Holcomb JB, Zarzabal LA, Michalek JE, et al. Increased platelet:RBC ratios are associated with improved survival after massive transfusion. J Trauma 2011; 71(2 Suppl 3):S318–28.

102. Committee on Trauma of the American College of Surgeons. ACS TQIP massive transfusion in trauma guidelines. Chicago: American College of Surgeons; 2015. Available at: https://www.facs.org/~/media/files/quality%20programs/trauma/ tqip/massive%20transfusion%20in%20trauma%20guildelines.ashx. Accessed April 13, 2016.

103. Spinella PC, Reddy HL, Jaffe JS, et al. Fresh whole blood use for hemorrhagic shock: preserving benefit while avoiding complications. Anesth Analg 2012; 115(4):751–8.

104. Kauvar DS, Holcomb JB, Norris GC, et al. Fresh whole blood transfusion: a controversial military practice. J Trauma 2006;61(1):181–4.

105. Ponschab M, Schöchl H, Gabriel C, et al. Haemostatic profile of reconstituted blood in a proposed 1:1:1 ratio of packed red blood cells, platelet concentrate and four different plasma preparations. Anaesthesia 2015;70(5):528–36.

106. Kiraly LN, Underwood S, Differding JA, et al. Transfusion of aged packed red blood cells results in decreased tissue oxygenation in critically injured trauma patients. J Trauma 2009;67(1):29–32.

107. Arslan E, Sierko E, Waters JH, et al. Microcirculatory hemodynamics after acute blood loss followed by fresh and banked blood transfusion. Am J Surg 2005; 190(3):456–62.

108. Lozano ML, Rivera J, Gonzalez-Conejero R, et al. Loss of high-affinity thrombin receptors during platelet concentrate storage impairs the reactivity of platelets to thrombin. Transfusion 1997;37(4):368–75.

109. Inaba K, Lustenberger T, Rhee P, et al. The impact of platelet transfusion in massively transfused trauma patients. J Am Coll Surg 2010;211(5):573–9.

110. Spinella PC, Carroll CL, Staff I, et al. Duration of red blood cell storage is associated with increased incidence of deep vein thrombosis and in hospital mortality in patients with traumatic injuries. Crit Care 2009;13(5):R151.

111. Weinberg JA, McGwin G Jr, Vandromme MJ, et al. Duration of red cell storage influences mortality after trauma. J Trauma 2010;69(6):1427–31.

112. Chandler MH, Roberts M, Sawyer M, et al. The US military experience with fresh whole blood during the conflicts in Iraq and Afghanistan. Semin Cardiothorac Vasc Anesth 2012;16(3):153–9.

113. Spinella PC, Perkins JG, Grathwohl KW, et al. Warm fresh whole blood is independently associated with improved survival for patients with combat-related traumatic injuries. J Trauma 2009;66(4 Suppl):S69–76.
114. Nessen SC, Eastridge BJ, Cronk D, et al. Fresh whole blood use by forward surgical teams in Afghanistan is associated with improved survival compared to component therapy without platelets. Transfusion 2013;53(Suppl 1):107S–13S.
115. Strandenes G, Berséus O, Cap AP, et al. Low titer group O whole blood in emergency situations. Shock 2014;41(Suppl 1):70–5.
116. Cotton BA, Podbielski J, Camp E, et al. A randomized controlled pilot trial of modified whole blood versus component therapy in severely injured patients requiring large volume transfusions. Ann Surg 2013;258(4):527–32.
117. Wang SC, Shieh JF, Chang KY, et al. Thromboelastography-guided transfusion decreases intraoperative blood transfusion during orthotopic liver transplantation: randomized clinical trial. Transplant Proc 2010;42(7):2590–3.
118. Weber CF, Gorlinger K, Meininger D, et al. Point-of-care testing: a prospective, randomized clinical trial of efficacy in coagulopathic cardiac surgery patients. Anesthesiology 2012;117(3):531–47.
119. Kelly JM, Callum JL, Rizoli SB. 1:1:1-warranted or wasteful? even where appropriate, high ratio transfusion protocols are costly: early transition to individualized care benefits patients and transfusion services. Expert Rev Hematol 2013;6(6):631–3.
120. Kashuk JL, Moore EE, Sawyer M, et al. Postinjury coagulopathy management: goal directed resuscitation via POC thrombelastography. Ann Surg 2010;251(4):604–14.
121. Nascimento B, Callum J, Tien H, et al. Effect of a fixed-ratio (1:1:1) transfusion protocol versus laboratory-results-guided transfusion in patients with severe trauma: a randomized feasibility trial. CMAJ 2013;185(12):583–9.
122. Tapia NM, Chang A, Norman M, et al. TEG-guided resuscitation is superior to standardized MTP resuscitation in massively transfused penetrating trauma patients. J Trauma Acute Care Surg 2013;74(2):378–85.
123. Ho AM, Holcomb JB, Ng CS, et al. The traditional vs "1:1:1"approach debate on massive transfusion in trauma should not be treated as a dichotomy. Am J Emerg Med 2015;33(10):1501–4.
124. Charbit B, Mandelbrot L, Samain E, et al. The decrease of fibrinogen is an early predictor of the severity of postpartum hemorrhage. J Thromb Haemost 2007;5(2):266–73.
125. Karlsson M, Ternstrom L, Hyllner M, et al. Prophylactic fibrinogen infusion reduces bleeding after coronary artery bypass surgery. A prospective randomised pilot study. Thromb Haemost 2009;102(1):137–44.
126. Rossaint R, Bouillon B, Cerny V, et al. The European guideline on management of major bleeding and coagulopathy following trauma: fourth edition. Crit Care 2016;20(1):100.
127. Chambers LA, Chow SJ, Shaffer LE. Frequency and characteristics of coagulopathy in trauma patients treated with a low- or high-plasma-content massive transfusion protocol. Am J Clin Pathol 2011;136(3):364–70.
128. Morrison JJ, Ross JD, Dubose JJ, et al. Association of cryoprecipitate and tranexamic acid with improved survival following wartime injury: findings from the MATTERs II Study. JAMA Surg 2013;148(3):218–25.
129. Maegele M, Zinser M, Schlimp C, et al. Injectable hemostatic adjuncts in trauma: fibrinogen and the FlinTIC study. J Trauma Acute Care Surg 2015;78(6 Suppl 1):S76–82.

required, the cycle of exsanguination and ischemic organ dysfunction will have been halted.

This is referred to as *compressible* hemorrhage and is found in accessible sites, such as the extremities, where either a pressure dressing or tourniquet can be applied. Following from the military lessons of the past decade, mortality from compressible hemorrhage is theoretically preventable with rapid hemostasis and resuscitation.[6] However, where a hemorrhagic focus is inaccessible and therefore *noncompressible*, it is more difficult to break the cycle of bleeding and organ dysfunction.[7]

Hemorrhage from within the torso exemplifies the problem of *noncompressible* hemorrhage, where in general, formal surgical intervention is required for hemostasis. As hemorrhage is a time-dependent pathology, this can be difficult to achieve before significant and/or irreversible ischemic organ damage has occurred.

Noncompressible torso hemorrhage (NCTH) can be highly lethal and has seen significant changes in management in the past decade. This review aims to present the state of current practice and future research efforts.

DEFINITION OF NONCOMPRESSIBLE TORSO HEMORRHAGE

Despite recognition of the mortality burden associated with NCTH, there has been little done to define and codify this injury pattern so as to guide identification and management. Such efforts have been the cornerstone of other similarly important, but unrelated pathologies, such as sepsis and septic shock, in which clear definitions have proved critical to recognition and treatment.[8] A standardized NCTH definition enables research efforts to be harnessed and therapeutic approaches specifically targeted.[5]

Several facets need to be considered when defining NCTH: anatomic injury pattern, physiology, and the clinical need for intervention. All of these factors play an important role in decision making and should be reflected in any formal description.[9]

Anatomic injury pattern is an important basic consideration. Trauma patients are frequently polytraumatized, making the prioritization of critical treatments challenging. For example, a patient presenting with signs of hypovolemic shock and a trivial torso injury should prompt a meticulous search for alternate source of hemorrhage. Similarly, anatomic disruption must be coupled with a marker of hemorrhagic shock, providing evidence of failing homeostasis and the sequelae of reduced perfusion. This is critical, as the findings of "hemodynamic instability" significantly influence the need for aggressive hemostatic intervention.

However, whereas severe hemodynamic instability is easily recognized, many patients occupy a middle ground, in which they have sufficient reserve to compensate for a significant insult. Should this physiologic reserve be exhausted, such patients can decompensate in a rapid and life-threatening manner.[4] Clinician judgment is therefore very important and on occasion, hemostatic intervention may be deemed necessary despite relatively normal physiology. Furthermore, depending on data collection mechanisms, physiologic data can be poorly collected. Consequently, the addition of a procedural marker for the need for immediate hemorrhage control serves as another marker of NCTH.[9]

Morrison and Rasmussen[5] sought to use this scheme to define NCTH in trauma as the presence of hemorrhage due to vascular disruption from 1 or more of 4 anatomic categories (**Box 1, Table 1**). They included 4 anatomic domains of high-grade injury, associated with bleeding, with preexisting abbreviated injury scale (AIS) codes: complex pelvic fracture, major vascular, solid organ, and pulmonary injury. This was coupled to physiologic indicators of hemorrhagic shock (systolic blood pressure

---

Box 1
Adjuncts for treatment of noncompressible torso hemorrhage (NCTH)

Pelvic binder or sheet wrap for pelvic fracture stabilization

Pelvic preperitoneal packing

Resuscitative balloon occlusion of the aorta (REBOA)

Resuscitative thoracotomy

Abdominal aortic junctional tourniquet (AAJT)

Endovascular angioembolization of traumatic hemorrhage

Correction of coagulopathy and fibrinolysis, blood products, tranexamic acid

Intra-abdominal hemostatic foam (research only)

[SBP] <90 mm Hg) and/or the need for immediate hemorrhage control (eg, exploratory laparotomy for splenectomy).

This NCTH definition was largely driven by military experience, where the notion of *compressible* hemorrhage was well established.[7] Recognition of this had led to innovation in the fields of novel hemostatic compounds and tourniquet design, specifically targeting *compressible* hemorrhage, which has resulted in a significant reduction in mortality.[10]

The NCTH definition from Morrison and Rasmussen[5] has demonstrated its utility in the interrogation of registries, which is discussed in the subsequent "Epidemiology" section.[11–13] Importantly, this definition is not meant to be restrictive, but more a concept to aid clinicians and researchers, and thus can be interpreted/modified pragmatically. For example, the use of an SBP less than 90 mm Hg as a sole physiologic measure of shock is open to discussion; one could advocate for the inclusion of a lactate measurement, higher SBP, or other similar metabolic metric.[14–16] Likewise, hemorrhage control procedures are not specified in detail, as this field is continuing to evolve with the development of new techniques.

EPIDEMIOLOGY OF NONCOMPRESSIBLE TORSO HEMORRHAGE

It is challenging to determine the exact rate of traumatic NCTH from the literature, as many studies report from disparate clinical settings, injury types, and specialty perspectives. This section endeavors to represent a contemporary overview from pertinent clinical areas.

Prehospital Setting

This is a frequently neglected, but critical, phase of trauma care.[17] Prompt attendance at the scene by a medically trained person can on occasion provide a window for the

---

Table 1
Definition of noncompressible torso hemorrhage (NCTH): presence of hemorrhage due to vascular disruption from 1 or more of 4 anatomic categories

Criteria for Noncompressible Torso Hemorrhage		
Anatomic	AND Physiologic	Procedural
1. Pulmonary		Need for immediate
2. Solid organ injury	Systolic blood pressure <90 mm Hg	hemorrhage control
3. Major vascular trauma	Lactate >4 mmol/L	
4. Pelvic fracture		

delivery of critical hemostatic intervention. Due to the challenges of an austere, and occasionally hostile scene, data collection is frequently sparse. However, preventable death analyses have been performed, which helps to inform this picture.

The most comprehensive analysis has been performed by Davis and colleagues,[18] who assessed 512 prehospital deaths that occurred in 2011 and used a peer-review panel to assign a cause of death. Neurotrauma constituted the great cause of death (36%), followed by hemorrhage (34%), asphyxia (15%), and combined hemorrhage/neurotrauma (15%). Death was thought to be potentially preventable in 29.0% of cases and hemorrhage was a component in 64.5% of cases.

In-Hospital Setting

The data from this setting is much more detailed. Preventable death analyses from trauma centers in both the United States and Canada confirm that NCTH is the leading cause of potentially preventable death.[19,20] Teixeira and colleagues[19] analyzed an 8-year period from California and identified a potentially preventable mortality rate of 2.5%, where bleeding was the largest source of mortality (39.2%). Similar findings were reported by Tien and colleagues[20] from Canada, where 16% of hemorrhage deaths were found to be potentially preventable due to delays in identifying the bleeding focus. Hemorrhage from blunt pelvic injury was the leading cause of exsanguination in these preventable deaths.

Kisat and colleagues[11] reported the only civilian study that used the definition of NCTH proposed by Morrison and Rasmussen.[5] These investigators used the NTDB (National Trauma Databank) to define the incidence of NCTH and the mortality associated with each anatomic domain. Of patients presenting with torso injury, 8.2% were identified as having evidence of NCTH. The mortality was 44.6% within this group, illustrating the high mortality burden of NCTH. The most lethal injury was major torso vessel injury (odds ratio [OR] 1.54, 95% confidence interval [CI] 1.33–1.78), followed by pulmonary injury (OR 1.32, 95% CI 1.18–1.48). Lower mortality was found in patients with pelvic injury (OR 0.80, 95% CI 0.65–0.98).

Military Setting

Conflict from the past decade has acted as a catalyst to reappraise the role of hemorrhage in preventable death. One of the first studies to provide insight into NCTH as a specific clinical problem was by Holcomb and colleagues,[21] who analyzed 82 fatalities early in the Iraq and Afghan Wars. NCTH was the cause of death in 50% of patients judged to have sustained potentially survivable injuries.

Several similar studies have been reported; however, the most comprehensive was reported by Eastridge and colleagues[6] who assessed 10 years of US military deaths (2001–2011) and identified 1 in 4 as potentially survivable. Of these, 61.3% died due to torso hemorrhage and 87% of deaths occurred before hospital admission.

This prompted a more detailed characterization of military NCTH by Stannard and colleagues[13] and Morrison and colleagues[12] who analyzed both US and UK mortality.[12,13] Stannard and colleagues[13] used the US Department of Defense Trauma Registry and identified an incidence of torso injury of 12.7%, of which 17.1% had evidence of ongoing hemorrhage. Major arterial and pulmonary injuries were identified as the most mortal injury complexes. Morrison and colleagues[12] used the UK Joint Theater Trauma Registry, which included an analysis of patients who died before hospital admission. The overall case fatality rate was 85.5%, with only 25.0% of patients actually surviving to hospital discharge.

SETTING, RESOURCE, AND INSTITUTIONAL CONSIDERATIONS

As trauma care increases in complexity, considerations concerning the setting in which patients are resuscitated and the resources required to deliver certain interventions can pose challenges. Articles such as the current review frequently focus on cutting edge techniques that are evolving, but the reality can be different in many institutions.

The fundamental principle is to match the clinical needs of the patient, with the clinical capability of the treating facility.[22] Within trauma care, there is a clear volume-outcome relationship with regard to minimum case number, thus consideration must be given to concentrating complex cases within a specified regional center.[23–25] This is generally the model adopted by most inclusive trauma systems; however, there is significant variation across North America and the rest of the world.

Centers that aim to treat patients with NCTH must be able to provide end-to-end care, which at minimum includes an emergency department, operating rooms, radiology (diagnostic and interventional) and an intensive care unit (ICU) supported by laboratory and transfusion facilities. These facilities can be in different areas of the hospital, which can necessitate multiple patient transfers. Clinicians managing NCTH need to factor in the logistical difficulties of delivering a resuscitation in a region of the hospital that is less well resourced. A typical example is the use of interventional radiology (IR), which has become an indispensable hemostatic tool, but may not be well suited to supporting clinicians looking after critical patients.

An option, so as to mitigate the risk of such an approach, is to consider moving resources to the patient. This has been described in the civilian literature as the "operating room resuscitation," in which critical casualties were taken directly to the operating room and the resuscitation, surgical, and critical care phases commenced within that room. This was pioneered by Rhodes and colleagues[26] in the late 1980s, who felt that bluntly injured, hypotensive patients had the most to gain by this approach.

This strategy fell out of favor due to problems with resources, combined with limited appreciable mortality improvement, but has recently been reexamined by the military. Reports from combat support hospitals based in Southern Afghanistan described a philosophy in which a critical patient could be fast-tracked straight to the operating room to undergo an aggressive team-based resuscitation, which included parallel surgery.[27] Generally, these were patients presenting with multiple amputations and torso trauma, in whom hemorrhage control and the restoration of volume was critical to sustaining life.

This philosophy has been extended and modified in the civilian setting with the development of the Resuscitation with Angiography, Percutaneous Therapy Operative Repair (RAPTOR)[28] suite or Trauma Hybrid Operating Room (THOR),[29] where concurrent operative and endovascular intervention can be performed. However, the number of appropriate patients is small: a recent analysis of a level 1 trauma center identified that only 64 (7%) of 911 hypotensive patients required such an approach.[30] Although clearly such a facility has great potential, the philosophy has drawbacks, specifically in relation to "overtriage" of patients: should your selected patient not require complex and time-critical intervention, then you have the potential to block an important resource.

INVESTIGATIONS IN NONCOMPRESSIBLE TORSO HEMORRHAGE

Information is critical to decision making in trauma, especially in blunt injury; however, this cannot be acquired at the expense of timely intervention in a deteriorating patient: the yield must justify the risk. Patients with NCTH are by definition hemodynamically unstable, and the traditional approach has been to minimize diagnostic investigations (rapid chest and pelvic radiography, FAST examination, basic blood tests, and blood typing) and to quickly determine hemorrhage source so as to expedite appropriate surgical exploration for hemorrhage control, as hemorrhage is a time-dependent pathology.

In general, a minimalist approach remains true today, especially in the setting of penetrating trauma; however, depending on the institutional capability and configuration, rapidly acquired axial imaging can help with decision making and prognostication. Computed tomography (CT) is a technique that has evolved significantly in terms of quality and speed of acquisition. A further change has been the location of CT facilities; many scanners are now housed within an emergency department, with a minority of portable scanners available in resuscitation bays.

The greatest benefit of CT is in blunt trauma, in which imaging enables a more complete characterization of injury pattern, which can include the identification of clinically occult injuries. Findings from such imaging can significantly alter management; for example, objective evidence of traumatic brain injury may prompt a surgeon to treat a bleeding spleen with removal, rather than to attempt salvage. Equally, the identification of subtle stigmata of duodenal injury such as retroperitoneal air, can prevent delayed recognition of a hollow organ injury and the ensuring sepsis.

Within the literature in the past 5 years, several studies from Germany and Japan have demonstrated a survival advantage when rapid whole-body CT scanning is used in unstable patients with blunt trauma. Huber-Wagner and colleagues[31] compared the outcome of 9233 patients undergoing CT with 7486 patients who did not. Whole-body CT was an independent predictor of improved survival (OR 0.73; 95% CI 0.60–0.90). Similar findings have been reported in Japan, where the benefit of CT appears to greatest in the most severely injured patients. In a logistic regression, CT was identified as an independent predictor of survival (OR 7.22; 95% CI 1.76–29.60).[32]

RESUSCITATION IN NONCOMPRESSIBLE TORSO HEMORRHAGE
Damage Control Resuscitation

An understanding of "damage control" philosophy is crucial for clinicians managing NCTH.[33] The original concept of damage control surgery (DCS) was based on the naval principle of repair-at-sea, in which function is sacrificed over salvage, until definitive repair is possible.[34] In the patient context, the traditionally view has been that patients in the operating room with deranged physiology are likely to deteriorate further if definitive repair of their injuries is attempted. This frequently manifests as the lethal triad of acidosis, hypothermia, and coagulopathy, which can initiate an irretrievable cycle that ultimately leads to death.

Therefore, in this setting, temporizing maneuvers are used, where viscera are packed, vascular shunts are inserted, bowel is left in discontinuity, and the cavity temporarily closed. This is followed by a period of resuscitation in the ICU where physiology is normalized, before returning to the operating room for definitive repair.[35]

This approach was first described in 1989 by Rotondo and colleagues,[34] in which the paralleled resuscitation involved large volumes of crystalloid and packed red blood cell (PRBC) transfusions. It has subsequently become clear that such resuscitation can in fact promote the lethal triad (See Mitchell J. Cohen and S. Ariane Christie's article, "Coagulopathy of Trauma," in this issue.) Evidence has since emerged from the military setting, that a balanced resuscitation strategy using equal PRBC, freshfrozen plasma, and platelet transfusions is associated with improved survival (See Ronald Chang and John B. Holcombs' article, "Optimal Fluid Therapy for Traumatic Hemorrhagic Shock," in this issue.) When this is combined with minimal crystalloid administration, active warming, permissive hypotension, and expeditious hemorrhage control, it is collectively referred to as damage control resuscitation (DCR).[36]

Several military and civilian groups have sought to investigate the impact of DCR on DCS. Morrison and colleagues[37] assessed the presence of acidosis, coagulopathy, and hypothermia before and after DCS in a cohort of severely injured combat casualties. Interestingly, aggressive DCR was found to improve all of these parameters intraoperatively, although this was a single-arm series without a control group.

Within the civilian literature, DCR, in conjunction with DCS, has been found to confer a survival advantage. Both Cotton and colleagues[38] and Duchesne and colleagues[39] compared the outcomes of a cohort of DCS patients before and after the adoption of a DCR protocol. Both studies found a reduction in crystalloid and blood product use, in addition to a mortality improvement.

Resuscitative Aortic Occlusion

The aim of resuscitation is to sustain vital function and, as the previous section describes, this is generally initiated with intravenous blood products and/or drugs. Once this process has commenced and the patient is considered "less unstable," the required hemostatic intervention is initiated; for example, exploratory laparotomy. Certainly, most patients with NCTH do benefit from the transfusion of products before intervention, as this improves oxygen delivery, treats coagulopathy, and permits some physiologic resilience while hemorrhage control is obtained. However, for patients presenting in extremis, a different approach is required, as transfusion alone is unlikely to improve hemodynamic stability.

In patients presenting with profound shock or circulatory arrest due to hemorrhage, resuscitative aortic occlusion can help with efforts to sustain or restore the spontaneous circulation.[40] Aortic occlusion increases systemic vascular, improving coronary and cerebral perfusion, while simultaneously providing inflow control to the vasculature below the level of occlusion.[41] This hemodynamic profile is highly beneficial to patients in hemorrhagic shock.

The most common level of occlusion is at the thoracic aorta, although lower levels of occlusion can be performed provided the hemorrhagic focus remains distal to the occlusion. The downside to this procedure relates to the associated ischemia-reperfusion injury once the occlusion is released. This has been well characterized in animal models, and the reperfusate includes a mixture of lactic acid, potassium, and proinflammatory cytokines.[42] The immediate cardiovascular consequences include negative inotropy (acidemia and hypocalcemia) and dysrhythmias (hyperkalemia), all of which contribute to a reduction in cardiac output.

Medium to long-term problems relate to direct ischemic organ damage (eg, renal failure following thoracic aortic occlusion) or indirect organ injury, such as acute respiratory distress syndrome due to the associated systemic inflammatory response syndrome.[42] These effects can be minimized by short occlusion times, prompt hemostasis, and the restoration of circulating volume. The burden of organ failure that is associated with this maneuver is considerable, and critical care physicians play a crucial role in supporting these patients (See "Postinjury Inflammation and Organ Dysfunction," article by Angela and colleagues in this issue.)[43]

Resuscitative aortic occlusion can be accomplished by several means; most commonly via open surgical approaches.[5] The left thoracotomy enables access to the thoracic aorta, which also permits the control of intrathoracic hemorrhage and the delivery of internal massage should they be required.[44] Usefully, this procedure can be performed with fairly minimal surgical equipment, making it suitable for use in the prehospital or emergency department setting.

NCTH. The left antero-lateral thoracotomy, between the fourth and fifth rib interspace, is perhaps the most straightforward incision to perform and can be accomplished in the supine position. This permits access to the left chest, allowing the surgeon to open the pericardium, compress the aorta, and access the left lung. However, despite the ease of incision, access to the pulmonary hilum, aortic arch, and arch vessels is poor.

Extension of the left anterolateral thoracotomy incision over the sternum into the right chest (clamshell thoracotomy) affords access to both hemi-thoraces and the mediastinal structures, but is an exceptionally morbid incision. In the postoperative phase of care, it is not uncommon for patients to experience significant pain and to incur pulmonary complications. In Europe, the clamshell has become the standard incision for RT, which is probably justified, as many practitioners are nonsurgeons seeking to decompress tamponade, but wherever possible, surgeons should seek to anticipate and reduce morbidity.

The posterolateral thoracotomy affords the best access to the pulmonary hilum, but necessitates a lateral position on the operating table, which in NCTH may be problematic. A median sternotomy incision allows for excellent cardiac and great vessel access, but requires specialty surgical instruments (eg, pneumatic or oscillating sternal saw, Gigli saw wire, or Lebsche sternum knife). The thorax is a cavity in which there are multiple access options, all of which must be carefully considered before making an incision. A poorly placed incision can increase the challenge of hemostasis considerably.

Abdominal Access

Unlike the chest, the number of options for abdominal access is limited. Most viscera can be accessed from a midline incision, and this remains the incision of choice for trauma laparotomy. Where more specific diagnostic information is available (eg, following CT scanning) specific incisions can be considered to target specific organs, but this is infrequently the case in the management of traumatic hemorrhage.

Endovascular Access

As this modality increases in clinical use, arterial access is becoming increasingly important. The most commonly accessed artery is the common femoral artery, which can be found at the midinguinal point. Several puncture techniques are described: blind puncture, ultrasound-guided, and the surgical cut-down.

A blind technique is not encouraged in NCTH, as the pulse may be weak and the risk of missing the artery is high. An ultrasound-guided puncture is best for experienced practitioners, as this ensures the common femoral artery is punctured rather than the superficial or deep branches. However, in the setting of profound hemodynamic instability, an open cut-down may be best.

This can be accomplished through a small, vertical groin incision (4–6 cm) at the midinguinal point. There is nothing but subcutaneous tissue between the skin and the artery and the dissection must be sufficient to enable discreet palpation of artery, sufficient to allow the safe puncture with a needle. Formal vascular control is not required at this stage, but will be required when the procedure is concluded.

Arterial access in the groin is an excellent tool to have in patients with NCTH. Not only does this provide for a platform for endovascular intervention, but also for continuous blood pressure monitoring and serial blood gas analysis with which to assess the response to therapy and resuscitation. Clearly the latter 2 can be performed by using a conventional arterial line in the radial position, but in NCTH and hemorrhagic shock, smaller arteries are more difficult to cannulate due to peripheral vasoconstriction.

ORGAN-SPECIFIC APPROACHES
Pulmonary Injury

Having gained access to the chest, thorough inspection should be undertaken to identify the bleeding focus. When considering pulmonary injuries, the location of the injury is important; peripherally located injuries are easier to manage than hilar injuries.

Where a peripheral segment has been traumatized and is bleeding, this can be excised in a nonanatomical fashion by using a linear stapler. This is usually the case in blunt trauma, whereas in penetrating trauma, the hemorrhage is usually emanating from a wound tract. This tract can be opened using a linear stapler passed through the injury, termed tractotomy, and opened to reveal the bleeding vessel. These can then be directly sutured to achieve hemostasis.

When the bleeding is more centrally placed, a hilar injury must be suspected, which can be a significant challenge to manage. An initial maneuver is to pinch the hilum between the thumb and forefinger. This will give the anesthesiologist time to catch up with the resuscitation, while permitting you time to plan the next step. In general, the next step is to mobilize the lung, by dividing the inferior pulmonary ligament. This can commence deep in the chest and consists of a pleural reflection from the lung medially, onto the mediastinum. Ideally, this mobilization is commenced with dissecting scissors and then swept cranially by a digit up to the hilum. The first structure to be encountered at the hilum while performing this is the inferior pulmonary vein, thus it is important to be careful. There are often other congenital and age-related adhesions that can be taken down with sharp dissection as required.

Having mobilized the lung, various methods of control can be performed. The lung twist is a fairly radical maneuver, in which the entire lung is rotated, twisting and tamponading the pulmonary vasculature. Another option is to wrap a Foley catheter around the hilum twice and apply some traction. Once hilar control is achieved, the injury must be further inspected and a decision made around treatment options. These include primary repair of a bleeding vessel, suture ligation, anatomic lobectomy, or in extreme circumstances, pneumonectomy.

Trauma pneumonectomy is a procedure of last resort and can be performed by using a stapling device. The physiologic consequences are extreme, with more than half of patients going into right heart and respiratory failure with severe hypoxemia. Extracorporeal membrane oxygenation (ECMO) should be considered early in these patients.[56]

Solid Organ Injury

The first maneuver following a laparotomy for hemorrhage control should be to undertake 4-quadrant packing. Care should be taken during this to determine the main focus of bleeding, and the nonhemorrhagic quadrants should be unpacked first. This should leave the surgeon with an anatomic zone of injury to consider, so that the necessary hemostatic maneuver is planned and prepared for.

In terms of solid organ injury, management of splenic injury in an exsanguinating patient is relatively simple: splenectomy. Splenic hemostasis also can be achieved endovascularly, but this is contingent on the deployment of rapid and time-conscious interventional skills. If such a maneuver was to be contemplated, it would be best undertaken in a RAPTOR/THOR room, where there is the option to rapidly convert from endovascular to an open approach. The evidence base for such an approach is currently weak.

Evidence of renal trauma is manifest as a retroperitoneal zone II hematoma (**Fig. 2**), which is located laterally in the retroperitoneum. In blunt trauma, this can be managed conservatively, unless there is evidence of ongoing bleeding, such as an

	Mechanism of Injury	
	BLUNT	**PENETRATING**
Zone I (centromedial)	Explore	Explore
Zone II (lateral)	Selective	Explore
Zone III (pelvic)	Selective	Explore

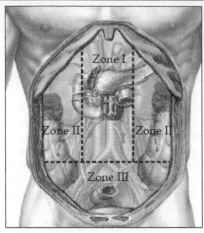

Fig. 2. Retroperitoneal zones of trauma.

expansile hematoma. In the setting of NCTH, this is likely to be the case, and exploration of the hematoma is likely to result in a nephrectomy. If there is time, it is prudent to check for a contralateral organ, as in the setting of a single kidney, greater attempts should be made at conservation. This includes the option of selective angioembolization, but the same messages as discussed in the previous paragraph apply.

In penetrating trauma and a zone II hematoma, there is a greater emphasis on exploration, as there may be violation of the collecting system. When faced with torrential bleeding, nephrectomy is the only real option, but repair may be considered if control is adequate. Drains also should be placed in the perinephric and retroperitoneum if repair is undertaken, in case of a urine leak.

Liver trauma is a complex subject; however, packing is the mainstay treatment. On occasion, control of liver inflow via a Pringle maneuver is helpful to confirm an arterial or portal venous origin to the bleeding. Direct ligation of bleeding vessels within the liver parenchyma can be facilitated by finger fracture hepatotomy. A particularly feared injury is the juxta-hepatic venous injury, in which a Pringle maneuver is of limited help. Several methods of hemorrhage control exist, including total hepatic vascular isolation, but these are rarely practiced.

Major Vascular Injury

The principle of vascular repair is simple; the practice is often far less straightforward. The principle consists of obtaining proximal and distal control of the injured vessel, with the option of either primary repair, shunt, interposition graft, bypass, or ligation. The latter is very much a procedure of last resort, but should never be forgotten; aside from the suprahepatic cava, all major vessels can be ligated if needs must.

In terms of important exposures, surgeons must be facile with the left and right medial visceral rotations, which enable access to the abdominal aorta and inferior vena cava, respectively. These rotations are used for mandatory exploration of a central zone hematoma. The difference with each of these maneuvers compared with a standard colonic mobilization is that the kidney is also included, to permit exposure of the respective great vessel.

On occasions, uninjured vessels need to be divided so as to facilitate access to an injured vessel. This is true of the arch vessels, where the left brachiocephalic vein can be divided, without the need for reconstruction. The iliac artery may also be divided to enable access to the iliac vein; however, the artery does need reconstruction at the end of the case.

Standard de Bakey vascular clamps can used to control arterial injuries, but in general venous injury is best controlled with swab-sticks. This requires active assistants (note the pleural) and ideally 2 high-capacity suctions. Critically, in any penetrating injury, make sure that both sides of the vessel are examined, which may entail enlarging the anterior defect to inspect the posterior wall.

Temporary vascular shunts are a very useful option in the unstable patient with multiple injuries, in whom definitive repair would take too long.[57,58] Vessels ranging from the aorta through to visceral arteries like the superior mesenteric artery can all be shunted if required. The optimal vascular conduit to use depends on what you have available. Ultimately, tubing from a blood-giving set or similar is sufficient and patients do not require any form of systemic anticoagulation. Arterial shunts can remain in place for up to 24 hours before definitive arterial repair is required.

When considering definitive vascular repair, the conduit of choice is in general autologous vein, especially when the field has been contaminated. The long saphenous vein is an ideal caliber for most vascular repairs; however, when a larger vessel, such as the aorta, requires repair, superficial femoral vein is another option. This can be harvested from the above-knee position, up to the confluence with the profunda vein without any significant consequence to the limb.

Endovascular intervention currently has a limited role in unstable patients with major torso vascular trauma. This may change as the experience from RAPTOR/THOR hybrid operating rooms and similar paradigms of care build the evidence base. The most useful adjunct currently is in balloon occlusion providing proximal control, similar to the principles discussed in relation to REBOA.

Pelvic Trauma

This constitutes a particularly challenging injury type, in which there are multiple therapeutic options available, depending on the mechanism, and clinical and radiological findings.[59,60] Hemorrhage can originate from fragile venous plexuses that overly the sacrum and accounts for most of the bleeding, along with disrupted boney ends. Arterial bleeding is found in a minority of patients, which can be manifest as a blush of contrast on CT or angiography, associated with ongoing hypotension and a large hematoma.

Boney stabilization should be addressed by the application of a pelvic binder, sited over the greater trochanters. In the past, there has been substantial focus on the application of an external-fixator or C-clamp, but these are now used less frequently.[60] Once boney stabilization has been achieved and DCR is under way, some venous bleeding will stop as a stable clot is formed. This will be evident if the patient responds favorably to transfusion.

However, if the patient continues to deteriorate or only transiently responds to DCR, then ongoing pelvic venous bleeding or an arterial source should be suspected. The presence of a contrast blush on CT is highly predictive of arterial bleeding and those

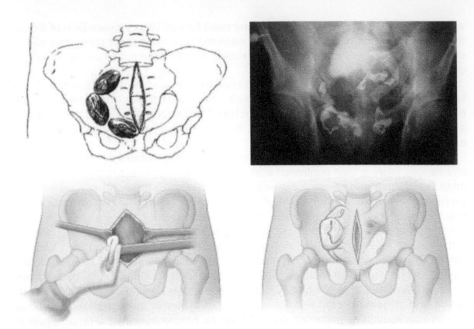

Fig. 3. Preperitoneal pelvic packing for pelvic trauma/hemorrhage. Preperitoneal packing (from ACSSurgery.com): "Preperitoneal pelvic packing (PPP) is performed through a 6 to 8 cm midline incision made from the pubic symphysis cephalad, with division of the midline fascia. The pelvic hematoma often dissects the preperitoneal and paravesical space down to the presacral region, facilitating PPP; alternatively, blunt digital dissection opens the preperitoneal space for packing. Three standard surgical laparotomy pads are placed on each side of the bladder, deep within the preperitoneal space, and the fascia is closed with O-PDS suture and the skin with staples." (*From* Cothren CC, Osborn PM, Moore EE, et al. Preperitoneal pelvic packing for hemodynamically unstable pelvic fractures: a paradigm shift. J Trauma 2007;62(4):834–9; [discussion: 839–42]; with permission, and ACSSurgery.com.)

patients should undergo endovascular intervention with pelvic angiography and/or embolization. Ideally, any embolization would be achieved selectively, rather than nonselective internal iliac artery embolization. Certainly, nonselective bilateral internal iliac artery embolization should be discouraged due to the potential consequences of buttock ischemia.

In patients in whom a pelvic arterial bleeding source is not suspected, or indeed if the institution does not have an endovascular capability, preperitoneal pelvic packing (**Fig. 3**) is a useful adjunct. This is achieved either via a Pfannenstiel or midline incision, down to the peritoneum, which remains unopened. The plane between the rectus muscle and peritoneum is developed, which will sweep back into the retroperitoneum. In the setting of a pelvic fracture, this dissection has usually been performed by the hematoma. Within this space, 2 to 3 laparotomy packs are placed on each side.

SUMMARY

NCTH is a leading cause of potentially preventable trauma mortality. It can be defined by high-grade injury present in one or more of the following anatomic domains: pulmonary, solid abdominal organ, major vascular, or pelvic trauma; plus hemodynamic instability or the need for immediate hemorrhage control. Rapid operative management, as part of a DCR strategy, remains the mainstay of treatment. However, endovascular techniques are evolving and may become more mainstream with the advent of hybrid rooms that can deliver concurrent open and radiologic/endovascular management.

REFERENCES

1. Kauvar DS, Lefering R, Wade CE. Impact of hemorrhage on trauma outcome: an overview of epidemiology, clinical presentations, and therapeutic considerations. J Trauma 2006;60(6 Suppl):S3–11.
2. Kauvar DS, Wade CE. The epidemiology and modern management of traumatic hemorrhage: US and international perspectives. Crit Care 2005;9(Suppl 5):S1–9.
3. Holcomb JB, del Junco DJ, Fox EE, et al. The prospective, observational, multi-center, major trauma transfusion (PROMMTT) study: comparative effectiveness of a time-varying treatment with competing risks. JAMA Surg 2013;148(2):127–36.
4. Gutierrez G, Reines H, Wulf-Gutierrez ME. Clinical review: hemorrhagic shock. Crit Care 2004;8(5):1–9.
5. Morrison JJ, Rasmussen TE. Noncompressible torso hemorrhage: a review with contemporary definitions and management strategies. Surg Clin North Am 2012;92(4):843–58.
6. Eastridge BJ, Mabry RL, Seguin P, et al. Death on the battlefield (2001-2011): im-plications for the future of combat casualty care. J Trauma Acute Care Surg 2012; 73(6 Suppl 5):S431–7.
7. Blackbourne LH, Czarnik J, Mabry R, et al. Decreasing killed in action and died of wounds rates in combat wounded. J Trauma 2010;69(Suppl 1):S1–4.
8. Singer M, Deutschman CS, Seymour CW, et al. The third international consensus definitions for sepsis and septic shock (sepsis-3). JAMA 2016;315(8):801–10.
9. Gruen RL, Brohi K, Schreiber M, et al. Haemorrhage control in severely injured patients. Lancet 2012;380(9847):1099–108.
10. Kotwal RS, Montgomery HR, Kotwal BM, et al. Eliminating preventable death on the battlefield. Arch Surg 2011;146(12):1350–8.
11. Kisat M, Morrison JJ, Hashmi ZG, et al. Epidemiology and outcomes of non-compressible torso hemorrhage. J Surg Res 2013;184(1):414–21.
12. Morrison JJ, Stannard A, Rasmussen TE, et al. Injury pattern and mortality of noncompressible torso hemorrhage in UK combat casualties. J Trauma Acute Care Surg 2013;75(2 Suppl 2):S263–8.
13. Stannard A, Morrison JJ, Scott DJ, et al. The epidemiology of noncompressible torso hemorrhage in the wars in Iraq and Afghanistan. J Trauma Acute Care Surg 2013;74(3):830–4.
14. Eastridge BJ, Salinas J, McManus JG, et al. Hypotension begins at 110 mm Hg: redefining "hypotension" with data. J Trauma 2007;63(2):291–7 [discussion: 297–9].
15. Hasler RM, Nuesch E, Juni P, et al. Systolic blood pressure below 110 mm Hg is associated with increased mortality in blunt major trauma patients: multicentre cohort study. Resuscitation 2011;82(9):1202–7.
16. Hasler RM, Nuesch E, Juni P, et al. Systolic blood pressure below 110 mmHg is associated with increased mortality in penetrating major trauma patients: multi-centre cohort study. Resuscitation 2012;83(4):476–81.
17. Chaudery M, Clark J, Wilson MH, et al. Traumatic intra-abdominal hemorrhage control: has current technology tipped the balance toward a role for prehospital intervention? J Trauma Acute Care Surg 2015;78(1):153–63.

18. Davis JS, Satahoo SS, Butler FK, et al. An analysis of prehospital deaths: who can we save? J Trauma Acute Care Surg 2014;77(2):213–8.
19. Teixeira PG, Inaba K, Hadjizacharia P, et al. Preventable or potentially preventable mortality at a mature trauma center. J Trauma 2007;63(6):1338–46 [discussion: 1346–7].
20. Tien HC, Spencer F, Tremblay LN, et al. Preventable deaths from hemorrhage at a level I Canadian trauma center. J Trauma 2007;62(1):142–6.
21. Holcomb JB, McMullin NR, Pearse L, et al. Causes of death in U.S. Special Operations Forces in the global war on terrorism: 2001-2004. Ann Surg 2007;245(6):986–91.
22. Davenport RA, Tai N, West A, et al. A major trauma centre is a specialty hospital not a hospital of specialties. Br J Surg 2010;97(1):109–17.
23. MacKenzie EJ, Rivara FP, Jurkovich GJ, et al. A national evaluation of the effect of trauma-center care on mortality. N Engl J Med 2006;354(4):366–78.
24. Garwe T, Cowan LD, Neas BR, et al. Directness of transport of major trauma patients to a level I trauma center: a propensity-adjusted survival analysis of the impact on short-term mortality. J Trauma 2011;70(5):1118–27.
25. Metcalfe D, Bouamra O, Parsons NR, et al. Effect of regional trauma centralization on volume, injury severity and outcomes of injured patients admitted to trauma centres. Br J Surg 2014;101(8):959–64.
26. Rhodes M, Brader A, Lucke J, et al. Direct transport to the operating room for resuscitation of trauma patients. J Trauma 1989;29(7):907–13 [discussion: 913–5].
27. Tai NR, Russell R. Right turn resuscitation: frequently asked questions. J R Army Med Corps 2011;157(3 Suppl 1):S310–4.
28. Ball CG, Kirkpatrick AW, D'Amours SK. The RAPTOR: resuscitation with angiography, percutaneous techniques and operative repair. Transforming the discipline of trauma surgery. Can J Surg 2011;54(5):E3–4.
29. Holcomb JB, Fox EE, Scalea TM, et al. Current opinion on catheter-based hemorrhage control in trauma patients. J Trauma Acute Care Surg 2014;76(3):888–93.
30. Fehr A, Beveridge J, D'Amours SD, et al. The potential benefit of a hybrid operating environment among severely injured patients with persistent hemorrhage: how often could we get it right? J Trauma Acute Care Surg 2016;80(3):457–60.
31. Huber-Wagner S, Biberthaler P, Haberle S, et al. Whole-body CT in haemodynamically unstable severely injured patients–a retrospective, multicentre study. PLoS One 2013;8(7):e68880.
32. Wada D, Nakamori Y, Yamakawa K, et al. Impact on survival of whole-body computed tomography before emergency bleeding control in patients with severe blunt trauma. Crit Care 2013;17(4):R178.
33. Jansen JO, Thomas R, Loudon MA, et al. Damage control resuscitation for patients with major trauma. BMJ 2009;338:b1778.
34. Rotondo MF, Schwab CW, McGonigal MD, et al. 'Damage control': an approach for improved survival in exsanguinating penetrating abdominal injury. J Trauma 1993;35(3):375–82 [discussion: 382–3].
35. Rotondo MF, Zonies DH. The damage control sequence and underlying logic. Surg Clin North Am 1997;77(4):761–77.
36. Duchesne JC, McSwain NE Jr, Cotton BA, et al. Damage control resuscitation: the new face of damage control. J Trauma 2010;69(4):976–90.
37. Morrison JJ, Ross JD, Poon H, et al. Intra-operative correction of acidosis, coagulopathy and hypothermia in combat casualties with severe haemorrhagic shock. Anaesthesia 2013;68(8):846–50.

38. Cotton BA, Reddy N, Hatch QM, et al. Damage control resuscitation is associated with a reduction in resuscitation volumes and improvement in survival in 390 damage control laparotomy patients. Ann Surg 2011;254(4):598–605.
39. Duchesne JC, Kimonis K, Marr AB, et al. Damage control resuscitation in combination with damage control laparotomy: a survival advantage. J Trauma 2010; 69(1):46–52.
40. Dunn EL, Moore EE, Moore JB. Hemodynamic effects of aortic occlusion during hemorrhagic shock. Ann Emerg Med 1982;11(5):238–41.
41. White JM, Cannon JW, Stannard A, et al. Endovascular balloon occlusion of the aorta is superior to resuscitative thoracotomy with aortic clamping in a porcine model of hemorrhagic shock. Surgery 2011;150(3):400–9.
42. Morrison JJ, Ross JD, Markov NP, et al. The inflammatory sequelae of aortic balloon occlusion in hemorrhagic shock. J Surg Res 2014;191(2):423–31.
43. Sagraves SG, Toschlog EA, Rotondo MF. Damage control surgery—the intensivist's role. J Intensive Care Med 2006;21(1):5–16.
44. Hunt PA, Greaves I, Owens WA. Emergency thoracotomy in thoracic trauma—a review. Injury 2006;37(1):1–19.
45. Stannard A, Eliason JL, Rasmussen TE. Resuscitative endovascular balloon occlusion of the aorta (REBOA) as an adjunct for hemorrhagic shock. J Trauma 2011;71(6):1869–72.
46. Biffl WL, Fox CJ, Moore EE. The role of REBOA in the control of exsanguinating torso hemorrhage. J Trauma Acute Care Surg 2015;78(5):1054–8.
47. Davies GE, Lockey DJ. Thirteen survivors of prehospital thoracotomy for penetrating trauma: a prehospital physician-performed resuscitation procedure that can yield good results. J Trauma 2011;70(5):E75–8.
48. Sadek S, Lockey DJ, Lendrum RA, et al. Resuscitative endovascular balloon occlusion of the aorta (REBOA) in the pre-hospital setting: an additional resuscitation option for uncontrolled catastrophic haemorrhage. Resuscitation 2016;107: 135–8.
49. Lyon M, Shiver SA, Greenfield EM, et al. Use of a novel abdominal aortic tourniquet to reduce or eliminate flow in the common femoral artery in human subjects. J Trauma Acute Care Surg 2012;73(2 Suppl 1):S103–5.
50. Taylor DM, Coleman M, Parker PJ. The evaluation of an abdominal aortic tourniquet for the control of pelvic and lower limb hemorrhage. Mil Med 2013;178(11): 1196–201.
51. Rago A, Duggan MJ, Marini J, et al. Self-expanding foam improves survival following a lethal, exsanguinating iliac artery injury. J Trauma Acute Care Surg 2014;77(1):73–7.
52. Rago AP, Larentzakis A, Marini J, et al. Efficacy of a prehospital self-expanding polyurethane foam for noncompressible hemorrhage under extreme operational conditions. J Trauma Acute Care Surg 2015;78(2):324–9.
53. Taviloglu K, Yanar H. Current trends in the management of blunt solid organ injuries. Eur J Trauma Emerg Surg 2009;35(2):90–4.
54. Demetriades D, Hadjizacharia P, Constantinou C, et al. Selective nonoperative management of penetrating abdominal solid organ injuries. Ann Surg 2006; 244(4):620–8.
55. Matsumoto J, Lohman BD, Morimoto K, et al. Damage control interventional radiology (DCIR) in prompt and rapid endovascular strategies in trauma occasions (PRESTO): a new paradigm. Diagn Interv Imaging 2015;96(7–8):687–91.
56. Arlt M, Philipp A, Voelkel S, et al. Extracorporeal membrane oxygenation in severe trauma patients with bleeding shock. Resuscitation 2010;81(7):804–9.

57. Gifford SM, Aidinian G, Clouse WD, et al. Effect of temporary shunting on extremity vascular injury: an outcome analysis from the Global War on Terror vascular injury initiative. J Vasc Surg 2009;50(3):549–55 [discussion: 555–6].
58. Taller J, Kamdar JP, Greene JA, et al. Temporary vascular shunts as initial treatment of proximal extremity vascular injuries during combat operations: the new standard of care at Echelon II facilities? J Trauma 2008;65(3):595–603.
59. Costantini TW, Coimbra R, Holcomb JB, et al. Current management of hemorrhage from severe pelvic fractures: results of an American Association for the Surgery of Trauma multi-institutional trial. J Trauma Acute Care Surg 2016;80(5): 717–25.
60. Cullinane DC, Schiller HJ, Zielinski MD, et al. Eastern Association for the Surgery of Trauma practice management guidelines for hemorrhage in pelvic fracture–update and systematic review. J Trauma 2011;71(6):1850–68.

Resuscitative Endovascular Balloon Occlusion of the Aorta: Indications, Outcomes, and Training

 CrossMark

Lena M. Napolitano, MD, FCCP, MCCM

KEYWORDS

- Resuscitative endovascular balloon occlusion of aorta • Hemorrhagic shock
- Aortic occlusion • Aortic balloon • Noncompressible torso hemorrhage
- Resuscitative thoracotomy

KEY POINTS

- Resuscitative endovascular balloon occlusion of aorta (REBOA) is an adjunct to trauma hemorrhage control; it provides early aortic occlusion to improve blood pressure and stabilize patients to undergo definitive hemorrhage control.
- The 2 main indications for REBOA use in trauma are hemorrhagic shock related to pelvic hemorrhage or abdominal/torso hemorrhage.
- REBOA is deployed in aortic zone III for pelvic hemorrhage and zone I for abdominal or truncal hemorrhage; zone II is a zone of no occlusion.
- After REBOA placement and balloon inflation, definitive hemostasis must be achieved either in the operating room, hybrid suite, or interventional radiology.
- Appropriate implementation of REBOA requires adequate endovascular inventory (a REBOA kit) and a clear concise REBOA protocol so that the REBOA procedure is standardized. Advanced education and training are required for all practitioners responsible for REBOA insertion.

INTRODUCTION

Aortic balloon occlusion has been successfully used for ruptured abdominal aortic aneurysm control with increased survival,[1] aortoenteric fistula aortic hemorrhage control,[2] postpartum or abdominal/pelvic surgery hemorrhage,[3] hemoperitoneum owing to splenic artery aneurysm,[4] gastrointestinal hemorrhage, and for control of vascular injuries. Aortic balloon occlusion for treatment of ruptured abdominal aortic aneurysm is now the standard of care.[5] However, the use of resuscitative endovascular balloon occlusion of the aorta (REBOA) in trauma is relatively new. REBOA is an adjunct to trauma hemorrhage control, providing early aortic occlusion to improve blood

Division of Acute Care Surgery [Trauma, Burns, Surgical Critical Care, Emergency Surgery], Department of Surgery, Trauma and Surgical Critical Care, University of Michigan Health System, Room 1C340-UH, 1500 East Medical Center Drive, Ann Arbor, MI 48109-5033, USA
E-mail address: lenan@umich.edu

Crit Care Clin 33 (2017) 55–70
http://dx.doi.org/10.1016/j.ccc.2016.08.011   criticalcare.theclinics.com

pressure and transiently stabilize patients to undergo definitive hemorrhage control. REBOA must be in the armamentarium of the trauma surgeon to assist in achieving prompt hemostasis.

HISTORY

Resuscitative balloon occlusion of the aorta for the treatment of traumatic hemorrhagic shock was first reported in 1954 by Lieutenant Colonel Carl W. Hughes, US Army (Walter Reed Army Medical Center) in 3 critically injured soldiers (**Fig. 1**). It was reported that, "It was arbitrarily decided that the catheter would be used only in moribund cases with evidence of intra-abdominal bleeding in which blood pressure could not be obtained after administration of 10 units of blood."[6] All patients died from major injuries and he recommended earlier use of aortic balloon occlusion may be beneficial.

In 1986, a preliminary report of the use of Percluder occluding aortic balloon in 23 patients included 15 trauma patients. Although all patients had an increase in arterial pressure with aortic occlusion, only 2 of the 15 trauma patients (13%) were long-term survivors.[7]

In 1989, Shaftan and colleagues[8] reported the use of intraaortic balloon occlusion in penetrating abdominal trauma in 21 patients with variable outcomes: group 1 (n = 5) cardiac rhythm, no systolic blood pressure (SBP), no survivors; group 2 (n = 6) SBP of less than 80 mm Hg, 3 survivors (50%); and group 3 (n = 10), hemodynamic deterioration to SBP of 80 mm Hg, 4 survivors (40%). These early REBOA patient series were fraught with problems related to delayed implementation of REBOA and prolonged aortic occlusion.

A recent systematic review of REBOA use in the management of hemorrhagic shock identified 41 studies with 857 total patients. Clinical settings included postpartum hemorrhage (n = 5), upper gastrointestinal bleeding (n = 3), pelvic surgery (n = 8), trauma (n = 15), and ruptured aortic aneurysm (n = 10). The overall mortality rate was 49.4%. REBOA did increase the SBP by 53 mm Hg in all patients.[9] However, it is not possible to determine whether REBOA had any positive impact on the ultimate outcome from these reports.

The first report of intraaortic balloon occlusion without fluoroscopy for the treatment of life-threatening hemorrhagic shock from pelvic fracture in 13 patients was published

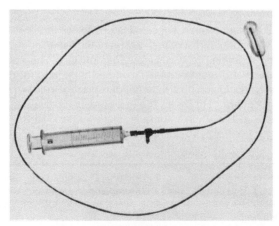

Fig. 1. Lt. Col. Carl W. Hughes' original balloon catheter for aortic occlusion. (*From* Hughes CW. Use of an intra-aortic balloon catheter tamponade for controlling intra-abdominal hemorrhage in man. Surgery 1954;36:65–8.)

in 2010, with successful placement of all aortic balloons and significant increase in SBP by 70 mm Hg.[10] Angiography confirmed arterial injury in 92% of patients requiring embolization and the survival rate was 46%. This report was the first to demonstrate that REBOA placement was life saving in that it permitted hemodynamic stabilization for safe transport to angiography. The survival rate was inversely related to duration of balloon inflation and the mean injury severity score.

Since 2010, there has been extensive experience with REBOA for the treatment of ruptured abdominal aortic aneurysm, significant improvements in technology, and increased endovascular education. The time is right to expand the use of REBOA into the trauma settings for the treatment of hemorrhagic shock, in particular owing to noncompressible torso hemorrhage and pelvic fracture hemorrhage.

RESUSCITATIVE ENDOVASCULAR BALLOON OCCLUSION OF THE AORTA PROCEDURE

REBOA can be a life-saving adjunct for the treatment of hemorrhagic shock and appropriate knowledge of the critical steps of the procedure is required. REBOA will be deployed in aortic zone III (from the lowest renal artery to the aortic bifurcation) for pelvic hemorrhage and aortic zone I (take-off of the left subclavian artery to the celiac trunk) for abdominal or truncal hemorrhage. Aortic zone II (from the celiac trunk to the lowest renal artery) is a zone of no occlusion (**Fig. 2**).

Appropriate implementation of REBOA requires adequate endovascular inventory (a REBOA kit) and a clear concise REBOA protocol (**Fig. 3**) so that the REBOA procedure is standardized. Advanced education and training are required for all practitioners who will be responsible for REBOA insertion.

Two catheters are used for REBOA in the United States—the CODA balloon catheter (Cook Medical, Bloomington, IN) and the ER-REBOA™ catheter (Prytime Medical Devices, Inc., Boerne, TX; **Fig. 4**). The CODA balloon catheter comes in 9 and 10 Fr sizes, and requires a stiff guidewire for placement and arterial sheaths of 12 or 14 Fr for insertion. Use of the large introducer sheaths mandates open arterial repair after sheath removal.

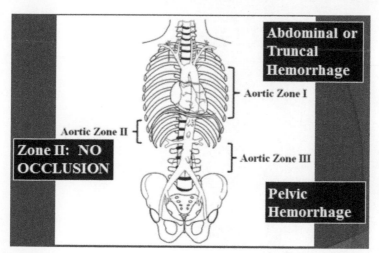

Fig. 2. Aortic zones for REBOA balloon inflation. If abdominal or truncal hemorrhage, the REBOA balloon is inflated in zone I; for pelvic hemorrhage, the REBOA balloon is inflated in zone III. REBOA, resuscitative endovascular balloon occlusion of the aorta. Zone 1: take-off of the left subclavian artery down to the celiac trunk; Zone 2: from the celiac trunk to the lowest renal artery; Zone 3: from the lowest renal artery to the aortic bifurcation.

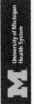

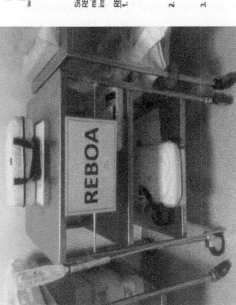

Resuscitative Endovascular Balloon Occlusion of the Aorta (REBOA) as Adjunct for Hemorrhagic Shock

Similar to resuscitative thoracotomy with aortic clamping for traumatic arrest due to hemorrhage, REBOA is used for temporary aortic occlusion. REBOA supports proximal aortic pressure and minimizes hemorrhage until hemorrhage control and hemostasis are obtained. REBOA can be used instead of resuscitative thoracotomy in hemorrhagic shock.

REBOA Steps:

1. Arterial access and Sheath Placement
   a. Ultrasound-guided femoral arterial access with Micropuncture kit (21 gauge needle, 4 or 5 French catheter and dilator, 0.018 inch guidewire)
   b. Or Femoral arterial cut-down, proximal/distal control for direct puncture
   c. Upsize to 12/14-French Introducer Sheath with Amplatz guidewire (0.035 in)
   d. Confirm Amplatz guidewire position in proximal aorta – digital radiography
2. Balloon selection and positioning
   a. Cook Medical CODA Balloon 10 Fr (32 mm diameter, 120cm length)
   b. Cook Medical CODA Balloon 9 Fr (can use with 12 Fr Introducer sheath)
   c. Compliant, low-atmosphere, high volume balloon, max diameter 40 mm
3. Balloon inflation
   a. Use the minimal pressure to gain wall apposition, to prevent aortic injury.
   b. 30-60cc syringe – fill with NS or ½ NS/Contrast for visualization and hand-inflate. Balloon maximum inflation volume is 40cc (9Fr, max 30cc volume).
   c. All attempts should be made to minimize the time of balloon inflation
4. Balloon deflation
   a. Intermittent deflation of REBOA can be used to optimize visceral perfusion, goal SBP > 90 mm Hg
5. Sheath removal – Primary arterial repair needed after 14Fr sheath removal

REBOA INTRA-AORTIC PLACEMENT

The placement of the balloon is determined by the location of the injury and ongoing hemorrhage:

Zone 1 Descending Thoracic Aorta (origin of left subclavian artery to celiac artery) is used for truncal hemorrhage control

Zone 2 Para-visceral Aorta (celiac artery to lowest renal artery): NO-OCCLUSION ZONE

Zone 3 Infra-renal Aorta (lowest renal artery to aortic bifurcation) for pelvic hemorrhage and junctional bleeding.

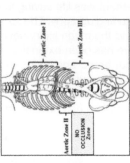

References:
1. Stannard A, Eliason JL, Rasmussen TE. Resuscitative endovascular balloon occlusion of the aorta (REBOA) as an adjunct for hemorrhagic shock. J Trauma. 2011 Dec;71(6):1869-72.
2. Brenner ML, Moore LJ, DuBose JJ, Tyson GH, McNutt MK, Albarado RP, Holcomb JB, Scalea TM, Rasmussen TE. A clinical series of resuscitative endovascular balloon occlusion of the aorta for hemorrhage control and resuscitation. J Trauma Acute Care Surg. 2013 Sep;75(3):506-511.
3. Markov NP, Percival TJ, Morrison JJ, Ross JD, Scott DJ, Spencer JR, Rasmussen TE. Physiology of a novel endovascular occlusion device: UK. Surgery (ESTARS™) Course. Curriculum Development, Content Validation and Program Assessment. American Association for the Surgery of Trauma; 2013. Abstract 90. 72nd Annual Meeting of the AAST and Clinical Congress of Acute Care Surgery. San Francisco, CA.
4. White JM, Cannon JW, Stannard A, Markov NP, Spencer JR, Rasmussen TE. Endovascular balloon occlusion of the aorta is superior to resuscitative thoracotomy with aortic clamping in a model of hemorrhagic shock. Surgery 2011;150(3):400-9.
5. Hughes CW. Use of intra-aortic balloon catheter tamponade for controlling intra-abdominal hemorrhage in man. Surgery 1954;36:65-68.

Fig. 3. REBOA kit and cart in Royal London Hospital emergency department. University of Michigan REBOA protocol. REBOA, resuscitative endovascular balloon occlusion of the aorta. (*Courtesy of University of Michigan Health System, Ann Arbor, MI.*)

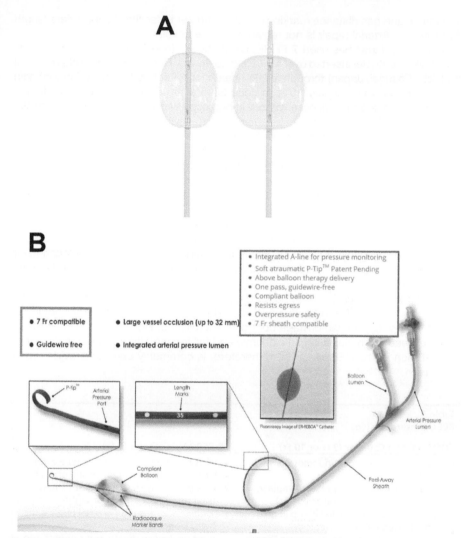

Fig. 4. REBOA catheters available for use in Trauma. (*A*) Cook CODA Balloon catheter, can occlude aortic diameters up to 40 mm. A 9 Fr CODA balloon catheter requires a 12 Fr arterial sheath. A 10 Fr Coda balloon requires a 14 Fr arterial sheath. Both require open primary arterial repair after sheath removal (www.cookmedical.com). (*B*) ER-REBOA™ Catheter (approved by the US Food and Drug Administration in October 2015), can occlude aortic diameters of up to 32 mm. It requires a 7 Fr arterial sheath. No guidewire is required for placement. It has length markings on the catheter, integrated arterial pressure lumen for arterial pressure monitoring, and does not require arterial repair after sheath removal (ER7232A; available: www.pryormedical.com). (*Courtesy of* Prytime Medical, Lakewood, CO; http://prytimemedical.com/.)

The ER-REBOA™ catheter (see **Fig. 4**) is a new smaller aortic occlusion balloon that is now available (received approval from the US Food and Drug Administration in October 2015). This REBOA catheter allows for percutaneous access through a 7-Fr sheath, can be placed without guidewire, has integrated arterial pressure monitoring, and has distance markings on the catheter to facilitate appropriate length of placement. Arterial repair is not required after removal.

Since 2013, Japan has used 7 Fr REBOA catheters (non–heparin-bonded polyurethane balloon catheter inserted over a 0.025-in guidewire; Rescue Balloon, Tokai Medical Products, Kasugai, Japan) through a 7-Fr sheath for refractory traumatic hemorrhagic shock. A report from January 2014 to June 2015 at 5 hospitals in Japan confirmed that percutaneous arterial access without fluoroscopy was achieved in all 33 patients. Of 33 REBOAs, 20 were performed by emergency medicine practitioners (10 with endovascular training) and 3 by interventional radiologists. No complication related to sheath insertion or removal was identified during the follow-up period, including dissection, pseudoaneurysm, retroperitoneal hematoma, leg ischemia, or distal embolism.[11]

The specific REBOA insertion steps (**Table 1**) are different depending on which REBOA catheter is used. After the aortic occlusion catheter is in place, the subsequent steps are the same for both catheters. Once the REBOA balloon is inflated (**Fig. 5**) and placement is confirmed by portable radiograph, the exact time of aortic balloon inflation is marked, commonly directly on the patient's catheter dressing. The REBOA device must then be stabilized and the patient transported to the appropriate location for definitive hemorrhage control (**Box 1**) depending on institutional resources and trauma team training.

Early aortic occlusion in severe hemorrhagic shock restores increased central aortic pressure, and carotid and brain perfusion. The REBOA balloon ideally should be inflated until definitive hemorrhage control is established. However, sustained aortic occlusion leads to multiple organ ischemia and failure and ultimately death. Intermittent deflation of the REBOA balloon, therefore, is commonly used to provide organ reperfusion.

Table 1
REBOA insertion steps

CODA Balloon Catheter (9 Fr or 10 Fr)	ER-REBOA™ Catheter (7 Fr)

• Micropuncture – common femoral artery (4–5 Fr)
• Advance Guidewire (SuperStiff Amplatz, 0.035 in × 260 cm, Boston Scientific)
• Confirm location of guidewire tip in proximal aorta (portable digital radiology)
• Up-size to 12 Fr or 14 Fr Introducer Sheath
  ○ 12 Fr sheath for 9 Fr CODA
  ○ 14 Fr sheath for 10 Fr CODA
• Advance Coda Balloon over guidewire into introducer sheath
  ○ Zone 1 to above xiphoid, approximately 50 cm
  ○ Zone 3 to just above umbilicus, approximately 40 cm
	• Micropuncture – common femoral artery
	• Terumo pinnacle introducer sheath 7 Fr
	• Slide peel-away sheath toward catheter distal tip to fully enclose/straighten P-tip
	• Connect and flush the arterial line via the 3-way stopcock
	• Insert peel-away sheath and catheter into the 7 Fr introducer sheath approximately 5 mm or until the peel-away sheath hits a stop
	• Advance the catheter 10–20 cm, then slide peel-away sheath away from the catheter
	• Advance catheter to appropriate position
	  ○ Zone 1 to above xiphoid, approximately 50 cm
	  ○ Zone 3 to just above umbilicus, approximately 40 cm

• Obtain digital radiograph to ensure that catheter is within aorta • Inflate REBOA (30 mL syringe, 50/50 contrast/NS) until resistance met • Repeat portable digital radiograph with balloon inflated to ensure proper location • Secure catheter to patient to prevent device migration • Note time of balloon inflation, minimize aortic occlusion time, consider partial occlusion	

Abbreviation: REBOA, resuscitative endovascular balloon occlusion of the aorta.

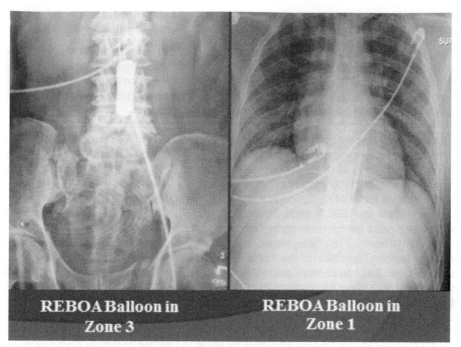

Fig. 5. REBOA balloon inflated in zone 3 (with contrast filling balloon) versus zone 1 (saline filling balloon). REBOA, resuscitative endovascular balloon occlusion of the aorta.

Partial REBOA has been advocated to mitigate the ischemia–reperfusion injury associated with total aortic balloon occlusion.[12] This technique is in common practice in Japan, with intermittent aortic balloon deflation to promote reperfusion or organs when feasible.

Once definitive hemorrhage control is established, the REBOA balloon catheter is removed. The femoral sheath can remain in place as arterial access for arterial blood pressure monitoring and/or for concern that the patient may require additional angiographic evaluation for recurrent hemorrhage. A 7-Fr femoral arterial sheath does not require open arterial repair, and can be removed with use of a closure device or direct pressure for 20 minutes.

Box 1
After REBOA insertion in emergency department

- Definitive hemorrhage control

- Either OR or IR or hybrid suite

- If IR, angioembolization can sometimes be performed via same sheath as REBOA

- After definitive hemorrhage control, REBOA removal must be performed in OR; open repair of femoral artery required if arterial sheath is 12 to 14 Fr, not required if 7 Fr sheath.

Abbreviations: IR, interventional radiology; OR, operating room; REBOA, resuscitative endovascular balloon occlusion of the aorta.

each institution to devise algorithms for REBOA use depending on local institutional and trauma team resources and strengths.

RESUSCITATIVE ENDOVASCULAR BALLOON OCCLUSION OF THE AORTA USE IN PELVIC FRACTURE HEMORRHAGE

Current management of hemorrhage related to severe pelvic fractures is quite variable. The report of the American Association for the Surgery of Trauma multicenter prospective, observational study of patients with pelvic fracture from blunt trauma included 1339 patients from 11 level I trauma centers, with an in-hospital mortality rate of 9.0%. In this study, 178 patients (13.3%) were admitted in shock, 24.7% underwent angiography with contrast extravasation identified in 62%, and 68% were treated with angioembolization. REBOA was used in only 5 patients in shock by only one of the participating centers. Mortality was 32.0% for patients with pelvic fracture admitted in shock.[15]

Angioembolization is the mainstay of treatment for pelvic fracture hemorrhage, but even in mature level I trauma centers there is significant delay in time to angiography and definitive hemostasis for hemorrhage control. The R. Adams Cowley Shock Trauma Center reported their 10-year experience with 344 pelvic hemorrhage patients who underwent pelvic angiography, documenting a median time to hemostasis with embolization was 344 minutes (interquartile range, 262–433). In this trauma center with robust trauma resources, the median procedure time for embolization was 51 minutes (interquartile range, 37–83), confirming that time from admission to angiography took nearly 4 hours. Overall mortality was 18% owing to hemorrhage (16%) and multiple organ failure (43.5%), documenting the high mortality rate.[16]

For exsanguinating pelvic hemorrhage from blunt trauma, REBOA inflated at zone III above the aortic bifurcation is very effective at hemorrhage control (**Box 2**). Once a massive transfusion protocol is initiated in patients with pelvic fracture and severe hemorrhagic shock, REBOA performed in the emergency department and inflated in REBOA zone III is the most efficient method by which to provide early transient control of the source of hemorrhage to transport the patient to the appropriate site for definitive hemorrhage control.

The Western Trauma Association Algorithm for Management of Pelvic Fracture with Hemodynamic Instability (**Fig. 9**) has now incorporated REBOA after initiation of massive transfusion protocol, as an adjunct or alternative to pelvic preperitoneal packing.[17] Similarly, the Denver Health Medical Center incorporated REBOA into the algorithm for management of these patients (**Fig. 10**).[18] These algorithms are useful to review when establishing our own institutional algorithms for severe pelvic hemorrhage management.

Box 2
For exsanguinating pelvic hemorrhage from blunt trauma

- REBOA (zone III, above aortic bifurcation) is less invasive than resuscitative thoracotomy.
- REBOA is more effective at aortic control than thoracotomy with aortic compression.
- REBOA is quicker to perform than resuscitative thoracotomy.
- REBOA is easier to control, that is, intermittent balloon deflation to provide perfusion.

Abbreviation: REBOA, resuscitative endovascular balloon occlusion of the aorta.

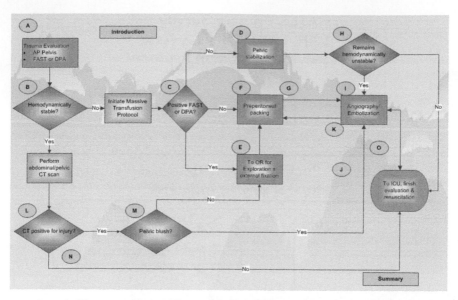

Expanded from zoomed area of Davis algorithm. Decisions will be based on local resources.

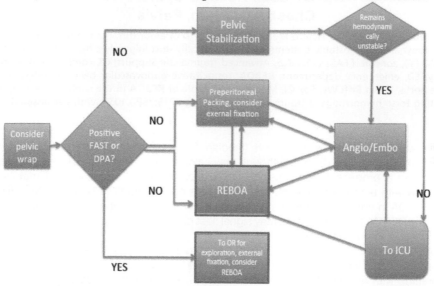

Fig. 9. Western Trauma Association (WTA) algorithm for management of pelvic fracture with hemodynamic instability. AP, anteroposterior; CT, computed tomography; DPA, diagnostic peritoneal aspiration; ICU, intensive care unit; OR, operating room. (*From* Western Trauma Association Algorithms. Available at: http://westerntrauma.org/algorithms/WTAAlgorithms_files/gif_2.htm. Accessed August 25, 2016.)

RESUSCITATIVE ENDOVASCULAR BALLOON OCCLUSION OF THE AORTA OUTCOMES IN TRAUMA

Japan has had the most experience with REBOA in trauma to date. An analysis of the Japan Trauma Data Bank (2004–2011) compared mortality in adult patients who received REBOA with those who did not. Only 1% of trauma patients received REBOA

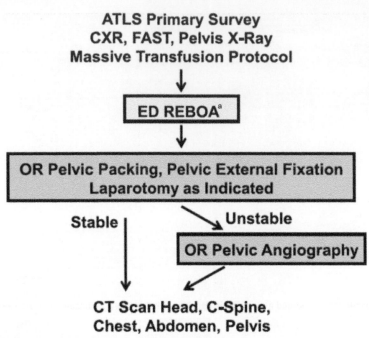

ATLS Primary Survey
CXR, FAST, Pelvis X-Ray
Massive Transfusion Protocol

ED REBOA[a]

OR Pelvic Packing, Pelvic External Fixation
Laparotomy as Indicated

Stable | Unstable

OR Pelvic Angiography

CT Scan Head, C-Spine,
Chest, Abdomen, Pelvis

Fig. 10. Revised Denver Health Medical Center (DHMC) algorithm for the management of hemodynamically unstable patients with mechanically unstable pelvic fractures. [a] Zone I if FAST (+), zone III if FAST (−). ATLS, Advanced Trauma Life Support; CT, computed tomography; ED, emergency department; REBOA, resuscitative endovascular balloon occlusion of the aorta. (*From* Biffl WL, Fox CJ, Moore EE. The role of REBOA in the control of exsanguinating torso hemorrhage. J Trauma Acute Care Surg 2015;78(5):1056; with permission.)

and had higher Injury Severity Score (median, 35 vs 13) and higher mortality (76% vs 16%) than those who did not. Although they calculated the likelihood of REBOA treatment via a propensity score using available pretreatment variables and matched treated with untreated patients, this analysis is not helpful in determining the utility of REBOA in trauma. In fact, the authors stated that, "The higher observed mortality among REBOA treated patients may signal 'last ditch' efforts for severity not otherwise identified in the trauma registry."[19]

A retrospective review of REBOA in 24 blunt trauma patients in Japan over a 6-year period included indications of hemorrhagic shock owing to pelvic fracture or hemoperitoneum, with an overall survival rate of 29.2%. Procedural complications were reported in 3 cases (12.5%) with 1 external iliac artery injury and 2 lower limb ischemia, with lower extremity amputation required in all 3 patients.[20] Similarly, a review of the Japan Trauma Data Bank compared in-hospital mortality in patients who underwent REBOA versus those who did not. In-hospital mortality was significantly greater in patients who underwent REBOA (61.8% vs 45.3%), but the etiology of this excess mortality is not clear.[21]

The first report of patient outcomes with REBOA implementation in 2 US civilian trauma centers was a descriptive case series (December 2012 to March 2013) with 6 patients. Mean SBP at the time of REBOA was 59 mm Hg, and mean base deficit was 13. Arterial access was accomplished using both direct cutdown (n = 3) and percutaneous (n = 3) access to the common femoral artery. Time to aortic occlusion was 4 to 6 minutes in all patients. REBOA resulted in a mean SBP increase of 55 mm Hg, and the mean aortic occlusion time was 18 minutes. There were no REBOA-related complications and no hemorrhage-related mortality. This report confirmed that REBOA was an effective means of traumatic hemorrhage control in mature civilian trauma systems.

A trauma registry report comparing patients undergoing resuscitative thoracotomy (n = 72) or REBOA (n = 24) during an 18-month period from 2 level I trauma centers, documented a significantly greater number of deaths in the emergency department among the resuscitative thoracotomy patients compared with REBOA patients (62.5% vs 16.7%; $P < .001$). Furthermore, REBOA had fewer early deaths and improved overall survival as compared with resuscitative thoracotomy (37.5% vs 9.7%; $P = .003$).[22]

The Aortic Occlusion for Resuscitation in Trauma and Acute Care Surgery (AORTA) Registry provided some data regarding aortic occlusion and REBOA use from 8 American College of Surgeons level I trauma centers. Aortic occlusion patients (n = 114; 46 REBOA, 68 open) most commonly was performed in the emergency department (73.7%) and overall survival was 21.1%. REBOA was inserted by femoral cutdown in 50% of patients. Complications of REBOA were uncommon (pseudoaneurysm, 2.1%; embolism, 4.3%; limb ischemia, 0%). There was no difference in time to successful aortic occlusion between REBOA and open procedures (REBOA, 6.6 ± 5.6 minutes; open occlusion of the aorta, 7.2 ± 15.1; $P = .842$). There was no difference in mortality (REBOA, 28.2% [13 of 46]; open occlusion of the aorta, 16.1% [11 of 68]; $P = .120$).[23]

An interesting report of nonoperative management of hemodynamically unstable abdominal trauma patients with angioembolization and REBOA documented that REBOA can be performed by well-trained physicians in the intensive care unit or the emergency department under ultrasound guidance. These patients were severely injured with an Injury Severity Score ranging from 25 to 75, all hypotensive owing to hemorrhagic shock from trauma, and total aortic occlusion times of 33 to 150 minutes. Only 1 of 7 patients died with an inability to achieve hemorrhage control, and inability to deflate the REBOA balloon.[24]

At present, we do not have high-quality Level I evidence for REBOA efficacy in the treatment of traumatic hemorrhagic shock, and additional research is clearly warranted. But this was true of endovascular aortic repair for blunt traumatic aortic injury as well; a randomized trial has never been performed yet endovascular aortic repair is the current standard of care.[25] Additional advances in REBOA technology and increased use and experience with prospective monitoring of outcomes is necessary.

PREHOSPITAL RESUSCITATIVE ENDOVASCULAR BALLOON OCCLUSION OF THE AORTA

The world's first prehospital REBOA was performed by London's Air Ambulance in June 2014 after 2 years of development with the Royal London Hospital.[26–28] The patient had fallen 15 m and had catastrophic internal hemorrhage owing to pelvic fractures. He was treated by the physician–paramedic team with insertion of a REBOA balloon catheter at the scene to control likely fatal exsanguination. The patient survived transfer to hospital, emergency angioembolization, and subsequent surgery. He was discharged neurologically normal after 52 days and went on to make a full recovery. This group was masterful in establishing the appropriate education and training to safely accomplish prehospital REBOA. There are clearly significant challenges to prehospital REBOA and guidelines will be required to enable safe implementation more widely for the future of trauma patient care.

EDUCATION AND TRAINING

Appropriate education and training for REBOA are required to be able to perform this invasive procedure safely, particularly because it will be performed in patients who are critically ill and hemodynamically unstable owing to hemorrhagic shock.[29] We strongly recommend collaboration with both vascular surgery and interventional radiology at each institution to optimally train trauma surgeons in these endovascular techniques, because it is very important to obtain increased exposure to these techniques in patients commonly managed by these 2 specialty groups.

At present, there is no common standard for competency assessment and credentialing for REBOA insertion and catheter-based hemorrhage control in the United States. We must work toward this goal with inclusion of trauma and acute care surgeons in the provider group for these important skills.

A number of REBOA courses are available for optimal education, including the Endovascular Skills for Trauma and Resuscitative Surgery Course,[30] the BEST course,[31] and others. These courses have confirmed that damage control endovascular procedures can be effectively taught using virtual reality simulation and live animal laboratories.[31,32] By the end of the Endovascular Skills for Trauma and Resuscitative Surgery course, students were able to achieve the first 3 steps of REBOA (vascular access, balloon positioning, balloon inflation) in 2 minutes. Each institution will need to determine optimal training for their trauma team members.

SUMMARY

Exsanguinating torso hemorrhage is a leading killer of trauma patients. The most appropriate means of torso hemorrhage control must be tailored to the clinical situation by the trauma team. Trauma surgeons should have expertise with all approaches for prompt hemorrhage control, including trauma laparotomy, REBOA, and resuscitative thoracotomy. REBOA is an exciting endovascular advancement as an adjunct in traumatic hemorrhage control because it can be deployed quickly, can be placed percutaneously, has a high rate of technical success, balloon inflation/deflation can be varied depending on the patient's physiology, and advances in technology have markedly decreased the size of the aortic balloon catheters. Balloon occlusion of the aorta is equivalent to cross-clamping the aorta. REBOA is effective in hemorrhagic shock as a bridge to definitive hemostasis. REBOA has been used successfully in vascular surgery for the last 20 years and is now expanding to trauma applications. Endovascular training is important for trauma surgeons caring for these critically ill patients at high risk of death from traumatic hemorrhage.

REFERENCES

1. Starnes BW, Quiroga E, Hutter C, et al. Management of ruptured abdominal aortic aneurysm in the endovascular era. J Vasc Surg 2010;51:9–18.
2. Jayarajan S, Napolitano LM, Rectenwald JE, et al. Primary aortoenteric fistula and endovascular repair. Vasc Endovascular Surg 2009;43(6):592–6.
3. Weltz AS, Harris DG, O'Neill NA, et al. The use of resuscitative endovascular balloon occlusion of the aorta to control hemorrhagic shock during video-assisted retroperitoneal debridement or infected necrotizing pancreatitis. Int J Surg Case Rep 2015;13:15–8.
4. Delamare L, Crognier L, Conil JM, et al. Treatment of intra-abdominal haemorrhagic shock by resuscitative endovascular balloon occlusion of the aorta (REBOA). Anaesth Crit Care Pain Med 2015;34(1):53–5.

5. Malina M, Veith F, Ivancev K, et al. Balloon occlusion of the aorta during endovascular repair of ruptured abdominal aortic aneurysm. J Endovasc Ther 2005;12: 556–9.
6. Hughes CW. Use of an intra-aortic balloon catheter tamponade for controlling intra-abdominal hemorrhage in man. Surgery 1954;36(1):65.
7. Low RB, Longmore W, Rubinstein R, et al. Preliminary report on the use of the Percluder occluding aortic balloon in human beings. Ann Emerg Med 1986;15: 1466–9.
8. Gupta BK, Khaneja SC, Flores L, et al. The role of intra-aortic balloon occlusion in penetrating abdominal trauma. J Trauma 1989;29(6):861–5.
9. Morrison JJ, Galgon RE, Jansen JO, et al. A systematic review of the use of resuscitative endovascular balloon occlusion of the aorta in the management of hemorrhagic shock. J Trauma Acute Care Surg 2016;80(2):324–34.
10. Martinelli T, Thony F, Declety P, et al. Intra-aortic balloon occlusion to salvage patients with life-threatening hemorrhagic shock from pelvic fracture. J Trauma 2010;68:942–8.
11. Teeter WA, Matsumoto J, Idoguchi K, et al. Smaller introducer sheaths for REBOA may be associated with fewer complications. J Trauma Acute Care Surg 2016. [Epub ahead of print].
12. Johnson MA, Neff LP, Williams TK, et al, EVAC Study Group. Partial resuscitative balloon occlusion of the aorta (P-REBOA): clinical technique and rationale. J Trauma Acute Care Surg 2016. [Epub ahead of print].
13. Morrison JJ, Ross JD, Rasmussen TE, et al. Resuscitative endovascular balloon occlusion of the aorta: a gap analysis of severely injured UK combat casualties. Shock 2014;41(5):388–93.
14. Available at: http://www.usaisr.amedd.army.mil/assets/cpgs/REBOA_for_Hemorrhagic_Shock_16Jun2014.pdf. Accessed August 25, 2016.
15. Costantini TW, Coimbra R, Holcomb JB, et al, AAST Pelvic Fracture Study Group. Current management of hemorrhage from severe pelvic fractures: results of an American Association for the Surgery of Trauma multi-institutional trial. J Trauma Acute Care Surg 2016;80(5):717–25.
16. Tesoriero R, Bruns B, Narayan M, et al. Angiographic embolization for hemorrhage following pelvic fracture: is it time for a paradigm shift? Oral presentation, Paper 16, AAST Annual Meeting 2015. Las Vegas, NV.
17. Available at: http://westerntrauma.org/algorithms/WTAAlgorithms_files/gif_2.htm. Accessed August 25, 2016.
18. Biffl WL, Fox CJ, Moore EE. The role of REBOA in the control of exsanguinating torso hemorrhage. J Trauma Acute Care Surg 2015;78(5):1054–8.
19. Norii T, Crandall C, Terasaka Y. Survival of severe blunt trauma patients treated with resuscitative endovascular balloon occlusion of the aorta compared with propensity score-adjusted untreated patients. J Trauma Acute Care Surg 2015; 78(4):721–8.
20. Saito N, Matsumoto H, Yagi T, et al. Evaluation of the safety and feasibility of resuscitative endovascular balloon occlusion of the aorta. J Trauma Acute Care Surg 2015;78(5):897–904.
21. Inoue J, Shiraishi A, Yoshiyuki A, et al. Resuscitative endovascular balloon occlusion of the aorta might be dangerous in patients with severe torso trauma: a propensity score analysis. J Trauma Acute Care Surg 2016;80(4):559–66 [discussion: 566–7].
22. Moore LJ, Brenner M, Kozar RA, et al. Implementation of resuscitative endovascular balloon occlusion of the aorta as an alternative to resuscitative thoracotomy

for noncompressible truncal hemorrhage. J Trauma Acute Care Surg 2015;79(4): 523–30 [discussion: 530–2].

23. DuBose JJ, Scalea TM, Brenner M, et al, AAST AORTA Study Group. The AAST prospective Aortic Occlusion for Resuscitation in Trauma and Acute Care Surgery (AORTA) registry: data on contemporary utilization and outcomes of aortic occlusion and resuscitative balloon occlusion of the aorta (REBOA). J Trauma Acute Care Surg 2016;81(3):409–19.

24. Ogura T, Lefor AT, Nakano M, et al. Nonoperative management of hemodynamically unstable abdominal trauma patients with angioembolization and resuscitative endovascular balloon occlusion of the aorta. J Trauma Acute Care Surg 2015;78(1):132–5.

25. Fox N, Schwartz D, Salazar JH, et al. Evaluation and management of blunt traumatic aortic injury: a practice management guideline from the Eastern Association for the Surgery of Trauma. J Trauma Acute Care Surg 2015;78(1):136–46.

26. Sadek S, Lockey DJ, Lendrum RA, et al. Resuscitative endovascular balloon occlusion of the aorta (REBOA) in the pre-hospital setting: an additional resuscitation option for uncontrolled catastrophic haemorrhage. Resuscitation 2016;107: 135–8.

27. London's Air Ambulance. World's first pre-hospital REBOA performed. Available at: https://londonsairambulance.co.uk/our-service/news/2014/06/we-perform-worlds-first-pre-hospital-reboa. Accessed August 25, 2016.

28. EMSWORLD. World's first prehospital REBOA performed in UK. Available at: http://www.emsworld.com/news/11545597/worlds-first-prehospital-reboa-performed-in-uk. Accessed August 25, 2016.

29. Holcomb JB, Fox EE, Scalea TM, et al, Catheter-Based Hemorrhage Control Study Group. Current opinion on catheter-based hemorrhage control in trauma patients. J Trauma Acute Care Surg 2014;76(3):888–93.

30. Villamaria CY, Eliason JL, Napolitano LM, et al. Endovascular Skills for Trauma and Resuscitative Surgery (ESTARS) course: curriculum development, content validation, and program assessment. J Trauma Acute Care Surg 2014;76(4): 929–35 [discussion: 935–6].

31. Brenner M, Hoehn M, Pasley J, et al. Basic endovascular skills for trauma course: bridging the gap between endovascular techniques and the acute care surgeon. J Trauma Acute Care Surg 2014;77(2):286–91.

32. Brenner M, Hoehn M, Teeter W, et al. Trading scalpels for sheaths: catheter-based treatment of vascular injury can be effectively performed by acute care surgeons trained in endovascular techniques. J Trauma Acute Care Surg 2016; 80(5):783–6.

Prediction of Massive Transfusion in Trauma

Paul M. Cantle, MD, MBT, FRCSC, Bryan A. Cotton, MD, MPH, FRCPS(Glasg)*

KEYWORDS

- Massive transfusion • Damage control resuscitation • Coagulopathy • Trauma
- Hemorrhagic shock

KEY POINTS

- Damage control resuscitation with early activation of massive transfusion protocols improves the survival of the 25% or more of trauma patients who arrive with coagulopathy.
- Using the traditional definition of massive transfusion of receiving 10 or more units of red blood cells in 24 hours introduces survival bias to resuscitation studies.
- Use of contemporary concepts of substantial bleeding, resuscitation intensity, and critical administration threshold will improve the analysis of massive transfusion prediction methods in future studies.
- Several highly accurate and validated scores for the prediction of massive transfusion in trauma exist.
- The ABC score is an accurate, rapid, and simple score that can be used widely including in both the rural and the prehospital setting.

INTRODUCTION

Before 2005, reported mortalities for patients receiving a massive transfusion (MT) were 55% to 65%.[1,2] Mortality remained at this level through 2007, dropping to 45% to 50% with increased adoption of MT protocols (MTPs).[3,4] With the transition to damage control resuscitation (DCR) strategies and by making blood available in the emergency department (ED), mortalities continued to decrease to less than 30%.[5,6] Most recently, the Pragmatic Randomized Optimal Platelet and Plasma Ratios (PROPPR) study found that mortality among this patient population continues to decline; 26% for receiving plasma:platelet:red blood cell (RBCs) ratios of 1:1:2 and

Disclaimer: Dr B.A. Cotton has served as a consultant for Haemonetics Corporation, Braintree, MA, makers of Thrombelastograph. Dr P.M. Cantle has no disclosures or conflicts.
Department of Surgery, University of Texas Mcgovern Medical School, 6431 Fannin, Room 4. 286, Houston, TX 77030, USA
* Corresponding author.
E-mail address: Bryan.A.Cotton@uth.tmc.edu

22% for those receiving 1:1:1.[7] Despite these reductions in mortality, hemorrhage remains the leading cause of preventable death in trauma and follows only severe central nervous injury as a cause of mortality in this setting.[8–10]

Although the overwhelming majority (>90%) of injured patients will not receive an MT, in those patients receiving large volume blood resuscitation, a mature and established MTP is critical. MTPs are designed to streamline balanced blood product delivery to bleeding patients and allow DCR to begin before the availability of laboratory results. Rapid identification of these patients and prompt MTP activation has been shown to be an independent predictor of survival.[11,12] However, blood products are both an expensive and a finite resource. The correct implementation of an MTP leads to more efficient use of blood bank resources and less product waste.[4] Therefore, trauma physicians must weigh the risks and benefits of using a precious resource in complex clinical situations. Because early implementation of MTPs improves patient outcomes, identifying which arrival parameters accurately predict the need for an MT is an area of increasing focus.

In this review, the authors discuss the evolving definition of MT and examine various parameters that can be used to predict the need for an MT in the trauma patient. Also evaluated are the role of the clinical gestalt and the predictive value of several MT scores. The article also assesses what role the prediction of MT may have in the prehospital environment, the indications for discontinuing an MT, and how the prediction of MT has performed in trauma trials.

DEFINING MASSIVE TRANSFUSION

Traditionally, MT has been defined as the transfusion of 10 or more units of RBCs within 24 hours of injury (Table 1). The origin of this definition is unclear, and although it is used commonly in both clinical and research realms, it has not been validated as a marker of bleeding severity. For example, a patient who receives 9 units of blood within a few hours who then progresses to either hemorrhage control or death, by this definition, has not had an MT despite clearly being in hemorrhagic shock. In contrast, the patient who receives their 10th RBC unit 23 hours after arrival would be defined as an MT, but is not likely to be the patient one would hope to identify with an MT prediction score.

As such, many have advocated for a change in the definition of MT to 10 units of RBCs within 6 hours, noting the clearly higher mortality of these patients compared with those who received that same amount over 24 hours.[13,14] Unfortunately, neither of these definitions captures the most severely injured patient who may receive only a few units of RBCs before dying. Use of such definitions introduces survival bias. Furthermore, both definitions ignore concomitant plasma and platelet transfusions.

Table 1 Transfusion terminology	
Traditional Massive Transfusion	$\geq$10 RBC units/24 h
Modern MT	$\geq$10 RBC units/6 h
Substantial bleeding[20]	(1) $\geq$1 RBC unit within 2 h AND (2) $\geq$5 RBC units or death from hemorrhage within 4 h
Resuscitation intensity[16]	Number of units[a] infused within 30 min of arrival
CAT positive[17]	$\geq$3 RBC units in any 1 h within 24 h of arrival

[a] 1 unit = 1 L crystalloid, 0.5 L colloid, 1 RBC, 1 plasma, OR 6 platelets.

As a result, contemporary concepts of Substantial Bleeding, Resuscitation Intensity, and Critical Administration Threshold (CAT) are becoming accepted clinical and research terms in the place of MT (see **Table 1**).[15–17]

The term Substantial Bleeding implies a severity of hemorrhage rather than a set volume of transfusion.[15,18–20] It focuses on patients with the greatest physiologic burden and has recently been defined as a patient receiving at least 1 unit of RBCs within the first 2 hours of arrival and 5 or more units of RBCs or dying from hemorrhage within 4 hours of arrival.[20] This definition minimizes survival bias by capturing patients that require early large volume transfusion as well as those that die before reaching a set transfusion volume. Unfortunately, like MT, this term ignores plasma or platelet transfusion amounts.

The Prospective Observational Multicenter Major Trauma Transfusion (PROMMTT) study investigators have proposed the concept of Resuscitation Intensity.[16] Resuscitation Intensity encompasses all fluids used for the initial resuscitation of a patient. Using this definition, each liter of crystalloid, 0.5 L of colloid, unit of RBCs, unit of plasma, and unit of apheresis platelets are all considered equal to 1 unit of resuscitation fluid. Investigators noted a more than 3-fold increase in mortality in patients receiving greater than 3 units of resuscitation fluid within 30 minutes of arrival. Patients exceeding this "Resuscitation Intensity" threshold had a 6-hour mortality of 14.4% versus 4.5% in those receiving 3 or less units. At 24 hours, the group above this threshold had a relative increase in mortality of 76%. The investigators proposed that a Resuscitation Intensity of greater than 3 units within 30 minutes of arrival is a useful marker of hemorrhage severity and is a predictor of early death. The term minimizes the risk of survival bias and accounts for different resuscitation strategies, including balanced resuscitation. It is useful in both the clinical and the research setting when discussing hemorrhage severity and transfusion needs in the trauma population.

The CAT has been proposed as another means of assessing hemorrhage severity.[17] The CAT was developed to minimize survival bias and to create a clinically applicable tool that better reflected resuscitation rate rather than volume alone. Investigators defined a patient as being CAT-positive if they received 3 or more units of blood within any 1-hour time frame during the first 24 hours after injury. CAT-positive patients had a 4-fold higher risk of death compared with CAT-negative patients. CAT identified 75% of all deaths, whereas the MT definition identified only 33%. The developers proposed that a patient becoming CAT-positive should alert the trauma physician to a patient's hemorrhage severity and could act as a trigger for MTP activation and balanced resuscitation initiation.

Using terms such a Resuscitation Intensity and CAT may allow improved analysis of MT prediction methods in the future. They describe a clinically applicable rate of blood loss rather than describing the total volume transfused. Patients meeting these criteria are more likely to be in hemorrhagic shock, are at a higher risk of mortality, and are more likely to benefit from the balanced resuscitation of early MTP activation. From a research standpoint, these concepts are likely to minimize survival bias by capturing moribund patients who may not reach the 10 units needed to be classified as having had an MT.

ISOLATED VARIABLES PREDICTING TRANSFUSION NEEDS

When assessing a severely injured patient, there are numerous physiologic, laboratory, and imaging variables that must be considered. Many of these provide information that can help predict whether a patient has substantial bleeding and requires MTP

Table 2
Commonly used variables in massive transfusion scores

	ABC[33]	TASH[22]	Schreiber et al,[24] 2007	McLaughlin et al,[21] 2008	ETS[a,23]	PWH[36]
Hypotension	X	X	—	X	X	X
Hemoglobin/ hematocrit	—	X	X	X	—	X
Intra-abdominal fluid	X	X	—	—	X	X
Pelvic or long bone fracture	—	X	—	—	X	X
Tachycardia	X	X	—	X	—	X
Base deficit	—	X	—	—	—	X
Gender	—	X	—	—	—	—
Admission from scene	—	—	—	—	X	—
Traffic accident	—	—	—	—	X	—
Fall (>3 m)	—	—	—	—	X	—
Penetrating mechanism	X	—	X	—	—	—
INR	—	—	X	—	—	—
pH	—	—	—	X	—	—
Age	—	—	—	—	X	—
GCS	—	—	—	—	—	X

[a] Score designed to predict the need for any transfusion not only the need for a MT.

which is operator dependent, is the most time-consuming variable to acquire but can usually be obtained within minutes. Furthermore, the score is simple enough to not distract from the management of the severely injured patient and performs with a predictive accuracy similar to other validated yet more complex scores. Although its PPV results in over-triage, you can always send the cooler back. More importantly, its NPV means that less than 5% of patients who will need an MT will not have product delivered early.

The Trauma-Associated Severe Hemorrhage Score

The Trauma-Associated Severe Hemorrhage (TASH) score, described in 2006, relies on 7 different weighted variables used to calculate a score that predicts which patients will require an MT.[22] Using a civilian German trauma database of 4527 patients, investigators identified multiple variables, their associated cut points, and the value of each variable to a composite score useful in predicting MT. The variables included are SBP (<100 mm Hg = 4 points, <120 mm Hg = 1 point), hemoglobin (<7 g/dL = 8 points, <9 g/dL = 6 points, <10 g/dL = 4 points, <11 g/dL = 3 points, and <12 g/dL = 2 points), intra-abdominal fluid (positive = 3 points), complex long bone and/or pelvic fractures (abbreviated injury scale [AIS] 3 and 4 = 3 points and AIS 5 = 6 points), heart rate (>120 bpm = 2 points), base excess (<10 mmol/L = 4 points, <6 mmol/L = 3 points, and <2 mmol/L = 1 point), and gender (male = 1 point). Once each of these 7 variables is given a value, a total score of 0 to 28 is calculated. The probability of requiring an MT is then calculated using a logistic equation where the probability = $1/[1 + exp(4.9 - 0.3 \times TASH)]$. In the initial publication, a score of 16 predicted that a patient had a 50% chance of requiring an MT. The score performed well as a whole, with an AUROC of approximately 0.89.

Nunez and colleagues[33] demonstrated that patients receiving an MT had a significantly higher TASH score (median of 13.4) than the TASH scores of those that did not receive an MT (median of 6.3). However, both Nunez and colleagues[33] and Pommerening and colleagues[32] found the TASH score AUROC to be lower than that published in the original TASH description, at 0.84 and 0.72, respectively. When Pommerening and colleagues compared the TASH score to clinical gestalt, the TASH score was found to be significantly better at predicting the need for an MT.

In 2010, Maegele and colleagues[35] revalidated the TASH score, looking at 5834 new patients from an updated data set. As an overall drop in the precision of the TASH score was noted, the equation for calculation of the logistic function was updated to probability $= 1/[1 + \exp(5.3{-}0.3 \times \text{TASH})]$. The calibration of the score was adjusted based on this change so that a score of 18 now corresponds to a 50% chance of requiring an MT. With this adjustment, the sensitivity of the TASH score dropped from 41% using the old data set to 31% with this updated data set, whereas specificity increased from 89% to 93%. The AUROC increased from 0.89 to 0.90.

When using the TASH score clinically, determining a patient's gender, heart rate, and blood pressure is completed rapidly. Evidence of a pelvic or long bone fracture is often found either during the secondary survey or with basic trauma imaging. A FAST to evaluate for intra-abdominal fluid is readily obtained in most trauma centers, often as part of the primary survey, but is operator dependent. Although hemoglobin and base excess are both usually available within several minutes using point-of-care testing or via a blood gas, the delay in obtaining them may delay the initiation of an MTP. The length of this delay is center dependent but, if using the TASH score, awaiting the return of these values may prolong the decision of implementing an MTP enough to negatively impact patient outcome. Furthermore, the number of variables and the different weighting applicable to each make this score somewhat cumbersome to calculate when simultaneously managing a severely injured patient, which may limit clinical application of the TASH score.

Schreiber Score

In 2007, Schreiber and colleagues[24] described a predictive model for MT that was developed in a combat setting. Comparing 247 patients requiring an MT and 311 patients not requiring an MT, the investigators identified 3 variables that were independent predictors of MT in their multivariate model (hemoglobin of 11 g/dL or less, INR >1.5, and penetrating mechanism). A hemoglobin level of 11 g/dL or less was found to be the single most predictive of MT with an odds ratio of 7.7. The 3 variables together created a predictive model with an AUROC of 0.804, suggesting that together they can accurately predict the need for an MT. Although penetrating mechanism can be determined rapidly, hemoglobin and INR are not as readily available, and the delay in obtaining them may prolong the initiation of an MT, which may, in turn, impact mortality. This delay in determining lab values limits the Schreiber model's clinical usefulness despite it being an accurate score.

McLaughlin Score

In 2008, McLaughlin and colleagues[21] evaluated 302 military trauma patients, 80 of which received an MT. Four independent risk factors for MT were identified: a heart rate greater than 105 bpm, SBP less than 110 mm Hg, pH < 7.25, and hematocrit less than 32%. A predictive equation of $\log (p/[1p]) = 1.576 + (0.825 \times \text{SBP}) + (0.826 \times \text{HR [heart rate]}) + (1.044 \times \text{Hct [hematocrit]}) + (0.462 \times \text{pH})$ was created and found to have an AUROC of 0.839. A patient was found to be 20% likely to require an MT if one variable was positive, but 80% likely to require an MT if all 4 variables were positive. With none of the variables positive, the chance of requiring an MT was still 11%. This model was then validated against an independent data set of 396 patients and found to have an AUROC of 0.747, suggesting that it was an accurate means of predicting the need for an MT. The McLaughlin score was found to have a sensitivity of 59%, a specificity of 77%, a PPV of 66%, and an NPV of 72%.

In a separate population of patients, Pommerening and colleagues[32] assessed the McLaughlin score and found it to have an AUROC of 0.66, which was not statistically significantly different than using clinical gestalt (AUROC 0.62). Nunez and colleagues[33] found the AUROC of the ABC, TASH, and McLaughlin scores were 0.859, 0.842, and 0.767, respectively (**Table 3**). Although heart rate and blood pressure can be rapidly assessed, pH and hematocrit are not immediately available and, as above, the delay in obtaining these laboratory values may delay MTP initiation and negatively impact survival. However, because this score uses fewer variables than TASH and uses dichotomous outcomes that make it easy to score, it may have some clinically utility despite its lower level of accuracy compared with the TASH score.

Emergency Transfusion Score

The Emergency Transfusion Score (ETS) was developed based on a regression analysis of data from 1103 civilian patients and includes 9 variables with a correlation coefficient for the predictive power of each.[23] The variables identified were SBP less than 90 mm Hg (coefficient 2.5), SBP 90 to 120 mm Hg (1.5), free fluid on FAST (2.0), clinically unstable pelvic ring fracture (1.5), age 20 to 60 years (0.5), age less than 60 years (1.5), admission from scene of accident (1.0), traffic accident (1.0), and fall from greater than 3 m (1.0). Each variable was found to be an independent predictor of transfusion need, and the probability of transfusion need increased as the overall score increased. For example, a patient with a score of 3 had a 5% likelihood of requiring a transfusion, whereas with a score of 6 a patient had a 50% likelihood of requiring a transfusion. The ETS had a sensitivity of 97% and a specificity of 68% with a PPV of 22% and an NPV of 99%. As with all scores, there are a few limitations to the ETS. First, it was developed to assess the need for any transfusion (yes, no) and has not been validated in the prediction of MT. Second, the ETS was not designed to evaluate penetrating injury, although it may still have some applicability in this setting. Finally, its reliance on the use of FAST subjects the score to operator variability. However, the ETS does have the advantage of not requiring any laboratory values or a complex calculation and therefore can be determined rapidly thereby minimizing transfusion delay.

Prince of Wales Hospital Score

The Prince of Wales Hospital (PWH) score for the early prediction of MT was developed in Hong Kong in 2011.[36] Included in this study were 1891 patients, of which

Table 3 Performance of transfusion scores to predict massive transfusion					
	Clinical Gestalt[32]	ABC[33,34]	TASH[22,33,35]	McLaughlin[21,33]	PWH[36]
Sensitivity	65.6%	75%	31%	59.4%	31.5%
Specificity	63.8%	86%	93%	77.4%	99.7%
NPV	86.2%	97%	—	71.7%	96.6%
PPV	34.9%	55%	—	66.4%	82.9%
AUROC	0.620	0.859	0.842	0.767	0.889

92 (4.8%) required an MT. Seven independent predictive variables were identified, including heart rate greater than or equal to 120 bpm (score = 1), SBP less than or equal to 90 mm Hg (score = 3), Glasgow Coma Scale (GCS) less than or equal to 8 (score = 1), displaced pelvic fracture (score = 1), abdominal fluid on computed tomography or FAST (score = 2), base deficit greater than 5 mmol/L (score = 1), hemoglobin less than or equal to 7 g/dL (score = 10), or hemoglobin 7.1 to 10 g/dL (score = 1). A cutoff score of 6 or greater yielded a sensitivity of 32%, a specificity of 99%, an NPV of 97%, and a PPV of 83%, with an AUROC of 0.889.

In 2012, Krumrei and colleagues[37] evaluated the ABC, TASH, and McLaughlin scores to determine the ability of each to predict the need for an MT in a rural trauma setting where transport times are longer, penetrating injuries are less common, and patient transfers are frequent. Of the 373 patients included in the study, 38 required an MT and 15 received blood before transfer. The ABC score correctly predicted that 34 patients would require an MT, while the McLaughlin and TASH scores only correctly predicted MT needs for 6 patients and 1 patient, respectively. The ABC score was 89% specific and 85% sensitive. The TASH and McLaughlin scores had sensitivities of 3% and 14% but specificities of 99.7% and 98%, respectively. Overall, this study found that, although the ABC score over-triages patients for the need for an MT, its accurately initiates MTPs in the most severely injured patients. In contrast, both the TASH and the McLaughlin scores were not sensitive enough to be useful predictors of patients requiring an MT in this rural setting.

Several other scores exist for the prediction of MT. These scores include the Vandromme score, the Baker Model, the Larson Model, the Cincinnati Individual Transfusion Trigger study, the Massive Transfusion Score, the Shock Index, and the Trauma Induced Coagulopathy Clinical Score.[38–44] The number of scores that have been developed demonstrates that no one score has proven to be accurate, widely applicable, and easy to use. In general, it appears that as scores increase in the number of variables they include and in their calculation complexity, their prediction accuracy increases. However, with this increase, their clinical utility in the trauma bay decreases, as they become distracting and cumbersome. As a result, complex scores may have the most use in the research setting, whereas simple scores are likely the most clinically useful. As a simple and validated score with proven reliability, the ABC score likely has the greatest utility during the early management of a patient in hemorrhagic shock.

PREHOSPITAL PREDICTION OF MASSIVE TRANSFUSION

Scores used for MT prediction are designed to expedite the initiation of MTPs in DCR in an effort to decrease mortality. The earlier an MTP is initiated, the sooner products may be ordered and delivered to the bedside to be transfused. Can prehospital evaluation accurately predict the need for an MT so that MTPs can be initiated before a patient's arrival? Weaver and colleagues[45] developed a transfusion request policy whereby a caregiver in the prehospital setting can ask that an MT cooler is available when the patient arrives at the trauma center. They studied 3 prehospital criteria: suspicion or evidence of active bleeding, SBP less than 90 mm Hg, and failure to have a blood pressure response to a fluid bolus. Any of these criteria could be used to activate a trauma center MTP before arrival, and they assessed whether these could accurately identify which patients would require an MT. In the study, 91% of patients ended up receiving blood products after arrival, whereas the remaining patients were thought to be hemodynamically stable on arrival and did not get transfused. A mean of 10.4 RBCs was used in the first 24 hours after arrival, and 40% of the transfused patients required an MT. Thus, an experienced prehospital provider can accurately predict which patients will require blood products and an MT. In fact, many air ambulance services now carry blood products and initiate transfusion during transport.[20]

Prehospital FAST (pFAST) has been shown to improve the triage and management of trauma patients.[46] Goodman and colleagues[47] assessed the ability of an ABC Score obtained in the prehospital setting to predict the need for MT. Following formal pFAST training, flight nurses completed pFAST examinations during transport and were able calculate a prehospital ABC (phABC) score, using the standard ABC score variables, before trauma center arrival. Patients found to have a phABC Score of 2 or greater were more likely to receive blood products in the ED, were more likely to have substantial bleeding, were more likely to receive an MT, and were also more likely to die from their injuries. The phABC Score was found to have a sensitivity of 33% and a specificity of 93% for predicting MT, and when used to predict substantial bleeding, had an NPV of 96% and an AUROC of 0.85. The phABC score over-triages patients for an MT but misses very few patients. The study showed that the phABC score is feasible and can help predict which patients require MTP activation even before their arrival at the trauma center.

TURNING OFF MASSIVE TRANSFUSION

Deciding when to turn off an MTP is critical to prevent the misuse of both blood products and the efforts of blood bank staff. MTs account for more than 70% of blood transfused at trauma centers, and turning off these transfusions at an appropriate time minimizes the waste of this expensive and limited resource.[48] The decision to stop an MT should be made jointly among all physicians active in the resuscitation team and should be communicated rapidly to the blood bank.[49] Clearly MT should be stopped when further attempts at patient resuscitation are futile. Otherwise, as discussed in the PROPPR trial, an MT should be stopped when clinically indicated based on anatomic and physiologic criteria.[7,50] The anatomic decision relies on hemorrhage cessation from either operative control or angioembolization, whereas the physiologic decision should be based on a stable or increasing blood pressure and improvement or stability in measures of end organ perfusion. Once anatomic and physiologic confirmation of hemostasis has been obtained, the MTP should be discontinued and, if a patient still requires resuscitation, a switch made to goal-directed transfusion therapy.

THE USE OF MASSIVE TRANSFUSION SCORES IN TRAUMA TRIALS

In order to perform high-quality prospective studies in this area, one must be able to accurately predict which patients will require an MT. Transfusion scores are becoming critical in determining which patients should be included, or excluded, from these trials. In their 2010 revalidation of the TASH score, the creators of the score concluded that although the clinical usefulness of this score remains questionable, it likely has tremendous research value.[35] For example, in 2011, Borgman and colleagues[51] used TASH scores to retrospectively assess plasma:RBC ratios in trauma resuscitation. They found that in patients with TASH scores greater than or equal to 15, receiving a high plasma:RBC ratio was independently associated with survival. In patients with TASH scores less than 15, this high ratio was associated with a greater risk for multiorgan failure. In this study, instead of only including patients that received an MT, TASH scores were used as a marker of patients at risk of needing an MT and performed well in determining the possible benefit and harm of a high plasma:RBC ratio.

In the PROPPR trial, investigators used clinical gestalt or an ABC score greater than or equal to 2 to enroll patients.[7] Of the 680 patients randomized, 438 had an ABC score greater than or equal to 2, whereas the remaining 242 patients were included based on physician judgment. In the 1:1:1 group, 45.3% of patients went on to receive an MT and 83.1% became CAT-positive, whereas in the 1:1:2 group, 46.8% went on to receive an MT and 91.8% became CAT-positive. Its successful use in the PROPPR trial demonstrates that the ABC score is a pragmatic tool that can appropriately capture patients with severe hemorrhage for prospective randomized clinical trials studying resuscitation in trauma.

SUMMARY

The traditional definition of an MT of 10 or more units of RBCs within 24 hours should be considered obsolete. It is now well recognized that the first 6 hours after a trauma are the most important for survival. Contemporary concepts such as Resuscitation Intensity and CAT emphasize the importance of transfusion rates rather than transfusion volumes. These terms allow us to treat, discuss, and study severely hemorrhaging patients with greater accuracy and precision. Their use minimizes survival bias in research and allows one to focus efforts on massively bleeding patients who may not survive to receive their 10th unit of blood.

The ability to determine in which patients one should initiate an MTP has improved with the incorporation of MT scores. These scores should be considered a success if they lead to earlier MTP activation in a patient that needs DCR. For example, a patient that receives only 8 units of RBCs and 8 units of plasma before hemorrhage cessation or a patient that dies after receiving only 4 units of RBCs and 4 units of plasma should not be considered a failure of a transfusion score if use of the score led to earlier MTP initiation. Scores, such as the TASH scores and ABC scores, with high NPVs, are excellent at identifying which patients will not need an MT. Although they may overtriage patients for MTP initiation, they will rarely leave a hemorrhaging patient without needed product (you can always send the product back to blood bank). The ABC score is likely the most clinically useful for aiding the decision of whether to initiate an MTP. It is easily memorized and rapidly calculated. Its key elements are obtained during the primary survey of the patient, and it does not rely on the return of any laboratory values. Furthermore, it has been validated, has a proven applicability in the rural setting, and has potential application in the prehospital setting.

Currently, the American College of Surgeons Trauma Quality Improvement Program Massive Transfusion in Trauma Guidelines (https://www.facs.org/~/media/files/quality%20programs/trauma/tqip/massive%20transfusion%20in%20trauma%20guildelines.ashx) recommend that triggers for the activation of an MT should include an ABC score of 2 or more, blood transfusion in the trauma bay, persistent hemodynamic instability, or active bleeding requiring operation or angioembolization. Ongoing research to determine which patients require MTP initiation, how to predict this need early and accurately, and when to turn off MTPs is likely to further increase the survival of these patients.

REFERENCES

1. Cinat ME, Wallace WC, Nastanski F, et al. Improved survival following massive transfusion in patients who have undergone trauma. Arch Surg 1999;134(9):964–8.
2. Malone DL, Hess JR, Fingerhut A. Massive transfusion practices around the globe and a suggestion for a common massive transfusion protocol. J Trauma 2006;60(6):S91–6.
3. O'Keeffe T, Refaai M, Tchorz K, et al. A massive transfusion protocol to decrease blood component use and costs. Arch Surg 2008;143(7):686–90.

4. Cotton BA, Gunter OL, Isbell J, et al. Damage control hematology: the impact of a trauma exsanguination protocol on survival and blood product utilization. J Trauma 2008;64(5):1177–82.
5. Holcomb JB, del Junco DJ, Fox EE, et al. The prospective, observational, multi-center, major trauma transfusion (PROMMTT) study: comparative effectiveness of a time-varying treatment with competing risks. JAMA Surg 2013;148(2):127–36.
6. Cotton BA, Reddy N, Hatch QM, et al. Damage control resuscitation is associated with a reduction in resuscitation volumes and improvement in survival in 390 damage control laparotomy patients. Ann Surg 2011;254(4):598–605.
7. Holcomb JB, Tilley BC, Baraniuk S, et al. Transfusion of plasma, platelets, and red blood cells in a 1:1:1 vs a 1:1:2 ratio and mortality in patients with severe trauma: the PROPPR randomized clinical trial. JAMA 2015;313(5):471–82.
8. Sauaia A, Moore FA, Moore EE, et al. Epidemiology of trauma deaths: a reassessment. J Trauma 1995;38(2):185–93.
9. Acosta JA, Yang JC, Winchell RJ, et al. Lethal injuries and time to death in a level I trauma center. J Am Coll Surg 1998;186(5):528–33.
10. Rhee P, Joseph B, Pandit V, et al. Increasing trauma deaths in the United States. Ann Surg 2014;260(1):13–21.
11. Cotton BA, Dossett LA, Au BK, et al. Room for (performance) improvement: provider-related factors associated with poor outcomes in massive transfusion. J Trauma 2009;67(5):1004–12.
12. Gunter OL Jr, Au BK, Isbell JM, et al. Optimizing outcomes in damage control resuscitation: identifying blood product ratios associated with improved survival. J Trauma 2008;65(3):527–34.
13. Moore FA, Nelson T, McKinley BA, et al. Massive transfusion in trauma patients: tissue hemoglobin oxygen saturation predicts poor outcome. J Trauma 2008; 64(4):1010–23.
14. Holcomb JB, Jenkins D, Rhee P, et al. Damage control resuscitation: directly addressing the early coagulopathy of trauma. J Trauma 2007;62(2):307–10.
15. Young PP, Cotton BA, Goodnough LT. Massive transfusion protocols for patients with substantial hemorrhage. Transfus Med Rev 2011;25(4):293–303.
16. Rahbar E, Fox EE, del Junco DJ, et al. Early resuscitation intensity as a surrogate for bleeding severity and early mortality in the PROMMTT study. J Trauma Acute Care Surg 2013;75(1):S16–23.
17. Savage SA, Zarzaur BL, Croce MA, et al. Redefining massive transfusion when every second counts. J Trauma Acute Care Surg 2013;74(2):396–400.
18. Holcomb JB, Gumbert S. Potential value of protocols in substantially bleeding trauma patients. Curr Opin Anaesthesiol 2013;26(2):215–20.
19. Liu J, Khitrov MY, Gates JD, et al. Automated analysis of vital signs to identify patients with substantial bleeding before hospital arrival: a feasibility study. Shock 2015;43(5):429–36.
20. Holcomb JB, Donathan DP, Cotton BA, et al. Prehospital transfusion of plasma and red blood cells in trauma patients. Prehosp Emerg Care 2015;19(1):1–9.
21. McLaughlin DF, Niles SE, Salinas J, et al. A predictive model for massive transfusion in combat casualty patients. J Trauma 2008;64(2):S57–63.
22. Yucel N, Lefering R, Maegele M, et al. Trauma Associated Severe Hemorrhage (TASH)-Score: probability of mass transfusion as surrogate for life threatening hemorrhage after multiple trauma. J Trauma 2006;60(6):1228–36.
23. Kuhne CA, Zettl RP, Fischbacher M, et al. Emergency transfusion score (ETS): a useful instrument for prediction of blood transfusion requirement in severely injured patients. World J Surg 2008;32(6):1183–8.

24. Schreiber MA, Perkins J, Kiraly L, et al. Early predictors of massive transfusion in combat casualties. J Am Coll Surg 2007;205(4):541–5.
25. Cotton BA, Faz G, Hatch QM, et al. Rapid thrombelastography delivers real-time results that predict transfusion within 1 hour of admission. J Trauma 2011;71(2): 407–17.
26. Kashuk JL, Moore EE, Sawyer M, et al. Postinjury coagulopathy management: goal directed resuscitation via POC thrombelastography. Ann Surg 2010; 251(4):604–14.
27. Leemann H, Lustenberger T, Talving P, et al. The role of rotation thromboelastometry in early prediction of massive transfusion. J Trauma 2010;69(6):1403–8.
28. Moore HB, Moore EE, Chin TL, et al. Activated clotting time of thrombelastography (T-ACT) predicts early postinjury blood component transfusion beyond plasma. Surgery 2014;156(3):564–9.
29. Holcomb JB, Minei KM, Scerbo ML, et al. Admission rapid thrombelastography can replace conventional coagulation tests in the emergency department: experience with 1974 consecutive trauma patients. Ann Surg 2012;256(3): 476–86.
30. Nunez TC, Dutton WD, May AK, et al. Emergency department blood transfusion predicts early massive transfusion and early blood component requirement. Transfusion 2010;50(9):1914–20.
31. Inaba K, Teixeira PG, Shulman I, et al. The impact of uncross-matched blood transfusion on the need for massive transfusion and mortality: analysis of 5166 uncross-matched units. J Trauma 2008;65(6):1222–6.
32. Pommerening MJ, Goodman MD, Holcomb JB, et al. Clinical gestalt and the prediction of massive transfusion after trauma. Injury 2015;46(5):807–13.
33. Nunez TC, Voskresensky IV, Dossett LA, et al. Early prediction of massive transfusion in trauma: simple as ABC (assessment of blood consumption). J Trauma 2009;66(2):346–52.
34. Cotton BA, Dossett LA, Haut ER, et al. Multicenter validation of a simplified score to predict massive transfusion in trauma. J Trauma 2010;69(1):S33–9.
35. Maegele M, Lefering R, Wafaisade A, et al. Revalidation and update of the TASH-Score: a scoring system to predict the probability for massive transfusion as a surrogate for life-threatening haemorrhage after severe injury. Vox Sang 2011; 100(2):231–8.
36. Rainer T, Ho A, Yeung J, et al. Early risk stratification of patients with major trauma requiring massive blood transfusion. Resuscitation 2011;82(6):724–9.
37. Krumrei NJ, Park MS, Cotton BA, et al. Comparison of massive blood transfusion predictive models in the rural setting. J Trauma 2012;72(1):211–5.
38. Vandromme MJ, Griffin RL, McGwin G Jr, et al. Prospective identification of patients at risk for massive transfusion. Am Surg 2011;77(2):155–61.
39. Baker JB, Korn CS, Robinson K, et al. Type and crossmatch of the trauma patient. J Trauma 2001;50(5):878–81.
40. Larson CR, White CE, Spinella PC, et al. Association of shock, coagulopathy, and initial vital signs with massive transfusion in combat casualties. J Trauma 2010; 69(1):S26–32.
41. Callcut RA, Johannigman JA, Kadon KS, et al. All massive transfusion criteria are not created equal: defining the predictive value of individual transfusion triggers to better determine who benefits from blood. J Trauma 2011;70(4):794–801.
42. Callcut RA, Cotton BA, Muskat P, et al. Defining when to initiate massive transfusion: a validation study of individual massive transfusion triggers in PROMMTT patients. J Trauma 2013;74(1):59–65.

43. Mutschler M, Nienaber U, Brockamp T, et al. Renaissance of base deficit for the initial assessment of trauma patients: a base deficit-based classification for hypovolemic shock developed on data from 16,305 patients derived from the TraumaRegister DGU®. Crit Care 2013;17(2):R42.

44. Tonglet ML, Minon JM, Seidel L, et al. Prehospital identification of trauma patients with early acute coagulopathy and massive bleeding: results of a prospective non-interventional clinical trial evaluating the Trauma Induced Coagulopathy Clinical Score (TICCS). Crit Care 2014;18(6):648.

45. Weaver AE, Hunter-Dunn C, Lyon RM, et al. The effectiveness of a 'Code Red' transfusion request policy initiated by pre-hospital physicians. Injury 2016; 47(1):3–6.

46. Walcher F, Weinlich M, Conrad G, et al. Prehospital ultrasound imaging improves management of abdominal trauma. Br J Surg 2006;93(2):238–42.

47. Goodman MD, Hawes HG, Pommerening MJ, et al. Prehospital ABC score accurately triages patients who will require immediate resource utilization. Presented at the 72nd Annual Meeting of AAST and Clinical Congress of Acute Care Surgery. San Francisco (CA), September 18–21, 2013.

48. Hess JR, Zimrin AB. Massive blood transfusion for trauma. Curr Opin Hematol 2005;12(6):488–92.

49. American College of Surgeons Trauma Quality Improvement Program Massive Transfusion in Trauma Guidelines. Proceedings of the American College of Surgeons, Committee on Trauma.

50. Baraniuk S, Tilley BC, del Junco DJ, et al. Pragmatic randomized optimal platelet and plasma ratios (PROPPR) trial: design, rationale and implementation. Injury 2014;45(9):1287–95.

51. Borgman MA, Spinella PC, Holcomb JB, et al. The effect of FFP:RBC ratio on morbidity and mortality in trauma patients based on transfusion prediction score. Vox Sang 2011;101(1):44–54.

Tranexamic Acid Update in Trauma

Ricardo J. Ramirez, MD[a], Philip C. Spinella, MD[b], Grant V. Bochicchio, MD, MPH[a],*

KEYWORDS

- Tranexamic acid • Trauma • Coagulopathy • Hemorrhage • Antifibrinolytics
- Surgery

KEY POINTS

- Tranexamic acid (TXA), a synthetic lysine derivative, has previously shown efficacy for reducing blood loss in several surgical procedures.
- TXA has shown a mortality benefit in bleeding trauma patients when administered within 3 hours of injury; however, there is no decrease in blood product transfusions.
- Pharmacokinetics and optimal dosing in trauma patients remain unknown.
- Ongoing and future trials are needed to refine current understanding of TXA's mechanisms of action in trauma patients and to optimize drug administration.

INTRODUCTION

Trauma is the leading cause of death and disability worldwide, with an estimated 5.8 million people dying every year as a result of traumatic injury.[1,2] In both military and civilian settings, hemorrhage remains the most common cause of preventable death after traumatic injury.[3–6] In recent years, there has been considerable interest in antifibrinolytic agents for the prevention of hemorrhagic death in severe trauma patients. The Clinical Randomization of an Antifibrinolytic in Significant Hemorrhage (CRASH)-2 and Military Application of Tranexamic Acid in Trauma Emergency Resuscitation (MATTERs) studies were pivotal, landmark studies that brought the antifibrinolytic agent tranexamic acid (TXA) to the forefront of discussion after evidence suggested improved mortality in civilian and military trauma, respectively.[7,8] Based on results

Conflicts of Interest: Drs G.V. Bochicchio and P.C. Spinella are principal investigators of the TAMPITI trial being funded by the United States Department of Defense. Dr R.J. Ramirez has declared no conflicts of interest.

[a] Department of Surgery, Washington University School of Medicine, 660 South Euclid Avenue, St Louis, MO 63110, USA; [b] Department of Pediatrics, Washington University School of Medicine, St Louis, MO, USA
* Corresponding author. Department of Surgery, Washington University School of Medicine, 660 South Euclid Avenue, CB 8109, St Louis, MO 63110.
E-mail address: bochicchiog@wudosis.wustl.edu

from the CRASH-2 trial, in March of 2011, TXA was added to the World Health Organization's list of essential medications. However, widespread adoption by mature trauma systems in the United States has been slow due to concerns about unknown exact mechanism of action, uncertainty surrounding use in patients with concomitant traumatic brain injury (TBI), unknown precise pharmacokinetics in the trauma patient, and safety.[9–11] The results of these landmark studies sparked worldwide debate and prompted funding for several trials to address these and other concerns.[12–18]

This article provides a brief overview of the history of TXA, reviews the known and proposed mechanisms of action, and examines areas of ongoing and future research aimed at addressing unanswered questions.

BACKGROUND

TXA is a synthetic lysine derivative that exerts its action by competitively occupying the lysine binding site of plasminogen, thereby blocking interaction with fibrin and subsequent clot breakdown.[19] TXA has a molecular weight of 157.2 g/mol and its injectable formulation is marketed under the name Cyklokapron. The pharmacokinetics of TXA in healthy individuals after administration of a 10 mg/kg dose demonstrate peak concentrations at 60 minutes postadministration, with a half-life of approximately 2 hours for the terminal elimination phase, and 90% excretion at 24 hours. An antifibrinolytic dose remains in tissues for up to 17 hours and in serum for up to 8 hours. It has also been shown to cross the placental barrier, is excreted in breast milk, and rapidly appears in synovial fluids.[20] The pharmacokinetics in trauma patients may differ, however, and appropriate dosing in this population may not be reflective of clinically effective concentrations previously described in healthy individuals. Pharmacokinetics and effects of TXA on hemostasis and immune systems are currently subjects of large ongoing trials with US government funding.[12,13,15]

In 1986, the Food and Drug Administration (FDA) approved intravenous administration of TXA for the indication of prevention or reduction of bleeding in patients with hemophilia undergoing dental procedures. The oral form of TXA, marketed under the brand name Lysteda, was approved by the FDA in 2009 to control heavy menstrual bleeding.[21] The drug has also been widely studied for the reduction of bleeding in cardiopulmonary bypass (CPB) surgery[22–29] and orthopedic procedures,[30] including its applicability in spine,[31] knee,[32] and shoulder surgery.[33] In the 1990s and early 2000s, the antiinflammatory properties of antifibrinolytics were recognized in patients undergoing CPB surgery. In 2007, Jimenez and colleagues[26] published a paper confirming this observation. The same year, Brohi and colleagues[34] described the protein C pathway and its important role in the development of coagulopathy and hyperfibrinolysis following trauma. This important work gave rise to new interest in antifibrinolytics and their effects on the intimate relationship that exists between inflammatory and coagulation pathways.

A 2012 meta-analysis of surgical studies evaluating TXA included 129 trials (1972 through 2011) with 10,488 subjects mostly in elective surgical procedures, the majority for cardiac surgery. Pooled results from 95 trials evaluating risk of blood product transfusion demonstrated that TXA had a 38% risk reduction of perioperative blood product administration (pooled relative risk [RR] 0.62, 95% confidence interval [CI] 0.58–0.65, $P = .001$). With adequate allocation concealment, 32 trials showed similar results (pooled RR 0.68, 95% CI 0.62–0.74, $P = .001$) and the same was true of 69 trials with adequate blinding (pooled RR 0.63, 95% CI 0.59–0.68, $P = .001$). When analyzing the effect of TXA on death, they found that fewer deaths occurred in the TXA group (RR 0.61, 95% CI 0.38–0.98, $P = .04$). However, when evaluating only those studies with adequate concealment, there was uncertainty (RR 0.67, CI 0.33–1.34, P = .25). Their analysis of TXA's effect on thromboembolic events also yielded inconclusive results.[35]

Clinical Randomization of an Antifibrinolytic in Significant Hemorrhage-2 Trial

The CRASH-2 trial was a randomized placebo controlled trial carried out in 274 hospitals in 40 countries that evaluated the effects of TXA in 20,211 adult trauma subjects who had significant bleeding or were at risk for significant bleeding.[8] The design of the study was pragmatic and enrollment in the study depended on whether a responsible doctor was "substantially uncertain about whether or not to treat with TXA." In other words, those subjects that had either a clear indication or contraindication for administration of antifibrinolytics were excluded. Subjects arriving within 8 hours of injury were randomly assigned to receive a 1 g bolus over 10 minutes followed by a 1 g infusion over 8 hours, or matching placebo. Primary outcome was death in hospital within 4 weeks of injury. The study reported a reduction in all-cause mortality of 14.5% in the treatment group versus 16.0% in the placebo group (RR 0.91, 95% CI 0.85–0.97, P = .0035). A reduction in the risk of death due to bleeding of 4.9% vs 5.7% was also reported (RR 0.85, 95% CI 0.76–0.96, P = .0077). Vascular occlusive events, including myocardial infarction (MI), stroke, deep vein thrombosis, and pulmonary embolism were similar in both groups. There was no significant difference in number of transfusions, need for surgery, or amount of blood products transfused, and baseline demographics for each group were similar.[8] In post hoc analysis, it was confirmed that early treatment with TXA was most effective. Subjects for whom the drug was started within 1 hour of injury had the greatest benefit, with nearly a one-third reduction in risk of death due to bleeding (RR 0.68, 95% CI 0.57–0.82, P<.0001). Treatment started between 1 and 3 hours from time of injury also had reduced risk (RR 0.79, 95% CI 0.64–0.97, P = .03). However, treatment that was started after 3 hours increased the risk of death from bleeding (RR 1.44, 95% CI 1.12–1.84, P = .004).[36] It was estimated that the odds ratio (OR) of TXA on death due to bleeding is multiplied by 1.15 (95% CI 1.08–1.23) for every hour that passes from the time of injury (**Fig. 1**).[36]

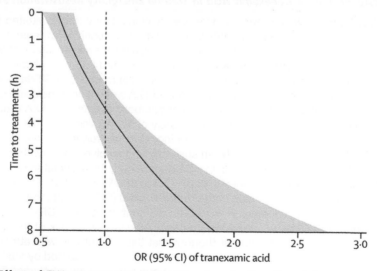

Fig. 1. Effect of TXA on mortality due to bleeding, by time from injury to treatment in hours. (*From* Roberts I, Shakur H, Afolabi A, et al. The importance of early treatment with tranexamic acid in bleeding trauma patients: an exploratory analysis of the CRASH-2 randomised controlled trial. Lancet 2011;377(9771):1101; with permission.)

CRASH-2 is the largest randomized controlled trial ever conducted for trauma and was the first to demonstrate a mortality benefit recommending TXA use in bleeding trauma patients. However, the results of CRASH-2 are controversial and several groups have questioned the applicability in countries with mature trauma networks.[9,10,18] For example, a large number of the subjects were treated in facilities with limited resources, including availability of blood products early on. Furthermore, data concerning burden of injury and quantification of blood loss were lacking, and there was no protocolized approach for the detection and/or diagnosis of thromboembolic events. The trial also left several questions unanswered, such as mechanisms by which the drug reduces mortality in bleeding trauma subjects. CRASH-2 investigators attempted to address some of these concerns by offering several explanations.[37] They argued that large pragmatic study designs are able to yield results that are reflective of everyday clinical practice and that an inherent limitation of such a design is the inability to offer physiologic explanations. Another question arose regarding the seemingly absent effect of TXA on number of blood products transfused. Roberts[38] offered the explanation of survivor bias, meaning that those patients who received TXA were more likely to survive and thus had a greater opportunity to receive more blood products. The investigators admitted that the rate of nonfatal vascular occlusive events was potentially underreported due to limited access and the lack of routine screening.[8] In addition to the controversy in peer-reviewed journals, the study was widely debated online in blogs, medical forums, and other social media.[18]

More recently, several smaller cohort studies integrating TXA in mature trauma systems in the United States have failed to produce favorable results, only further fueling the debate.[39–41] A prospective study in a severely injured civilian cohort within a mature civilian trauma system documented that TXA was not independently associated with any change in outcome for the overall trauma cohort or for nonshock patients. In multivariate analysis, TXA was protective for adjusted all-cause mortality (OR 0.16, CI 0.03–0.86, $P = .03$) in severely injured hemorrhagic shock patients.[11]

Military Application of Tranexamic Acid in Trauma Emergency Resuscitation Study

The MATTERs study was a retrospective observational study that evaluated the effects of TXA in subjects with combat-related injury that received at least 1 unit of packed red blood cells (PRBCs). All subjects were treated in a military surgical hospital at Camp Bastion, in southern Afghanistan. They evaluated 896 consecutive admissions with mortality at 24 and 48 hours, and in-hospital mortality at 30 days as their primary endpoints. Secondary endpoints included TXA's effect on transfusion requirements, measures of coagulopathy, and thromboembolic events. The TXA group was found to have an unadjusted in-hospital mortality of 17.4% versus 23.9% in the no-TXA group ($P = .03$), despite the TXA group being more severely injured (injury severity score [ISS] 25.2 vs 22.5, respectively). In subjects who received massive transfusion, defined as 10 or more units of PRBCs in a 24-hour period, the associated reduction in mortality was even more significant (14.4% in TXA vs 28.1% in no-TXA, $P = .004$). TXA was also independently associated with greater survival (OR = 7.228, 95% CI 3.016–17.322) and less coagulopathy ($P = .003$).[7] In contrast to the CRASH-2 study, however, the MATTERs study reported an associated increased risk of thromboembolic events in the TXA subjects but thought that this greater risk was attributed to the higher injury severity in the TXA subjects. However, when evaluated by multivariate analysis, adjusting for severity of injury, no independent association between TXA use and thromboembolic events was found. The investigators still acknowledged that TXA poses a theoretic increased risk of thromboembolic occurrences and should, therefore, be kept in mind when designing future prospective studies.[7]

PATIENT EVALUATION OVERVIEW
The Role of Fibrinolysis in Trauma

Acute traumatic coagulopathy (ATC) develops in the presence of tissue injury and shock due to bleeding, and has been shown to be present in up to 25% of trauma patients on arrival to the emergency department (ED).[42] ATC is a primary or endogenous cause of coagulopathy associated with increased activated protein C, and is the result of the body's biological response to traumatic injury.[43] It is characterized by dysfibrinogenemia, hyperfibrinolysis, endothelial dysfunction, and impaired platelet activity.[44] Unbalanced resuscitation is an iatrogenic or secondary cause of coagulopathy with hemodilution, hypothermia, and acidosis contributing to exacerbation of hemostatic dysfunction (**Fig. 2**).[43,44]

Fibrinolysis has been shown to be an important pathophysiological component of coagulopathy developing from trauma, and hyperfibrinolysis is a significant contributor to mortality in trauma patients.[34,44–47] Many studies have reaffirmed the integral role of fibrinolysis in the pathogenesis of ATC.[45,48] However, some investigators have cautioned against the generalized use of antifibrinolytic agents such as TXA in all trauma patients due to new evidence that suggests reduced fibrinolytic activity, or fibrinolysis shutdown, in up to 46% of severely injured patients.[49] In a retrospective study, Moore and colleagues[49] very recently published evidence for the possibility of 3 distinct fibrinolytic phenotypes: shutdown, physiologic, and hyperfibrinolysis. Using their thromboelastography (TEG) databank, they evaluated trauma subjects older than 18 years, with an ISS greater than 15, presenting to the ED between 2010 and

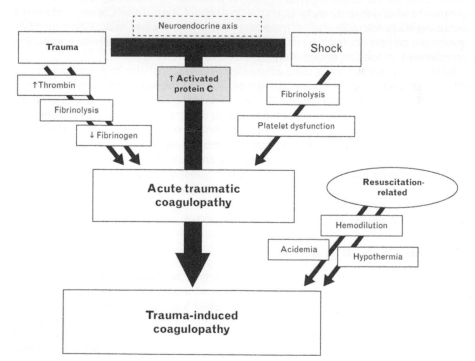

Fig. 2. Pathophysiology of coagulopathy following trauma. (*From* Davenport RA, Brohi K. Cause of trauma-induced coagulopathy. Curr Opin Anaesthesiol 2016;29(2):212–9; with permission.)

2013. A total of 2540 subjects were included. They grouped subjects by lysis measurement 30 minutes after maximum amplitude (LY30, percent) defining shutdown, physiologic, and hyperfibrinolysis with LY30 values of 0.8% or less, 0.9% to 2.9%, and 3% or more, respectively. Fibrinolysis shutdown was the most common phenotype (46%), followed by physiologic (36%) and hyperfibrinolysis (18%). Hyperfibrinolysis accounted for the highest mortality with 34%, shutdown 22%, and physiologic 14%. After adjusting for age, ISS, mechanism, head injury, and blood pressure, risk of mortality remained increased for hyperfibrinolysis (OR 3.3, 95% CI 2.4–4.6, $P<.0001$) and shutdown (OR 1.6, 95% CI 1.3–2.1, $P = .0003$) compared with physiologic (OR 0.82, 95% CI 0.80–0.84). The leading cause of death for the hyperfibrinolysis phenotype was due to acute blood loss, whereas 40% of subjects displaying LY30 consistent with shutdown phenotype died of multiple organ failure. Moore and colleagues[50] have proposed possible mechanisms for microvascular occlusion following fibrinolysis shutdown in severely injured patients. However, their theories have not been demonstrated in vivo and critics of this theory have pointed out that many patients, who might have otherwise benefited from early administration of TXA, might miss out due to wait times for TEG results for lysis.[51]

Proposed Mechanisms of Action in Trauma

The antifibrinolytic effect of TXA is exerted through competitive inhibition of plasmin formation. This occurs when TXA binds to lysine binding domains exposed on plasminogen, resulting in diminished plasmin levels, thereby preventing clot lysis. However, some investigators have suggested that this may not be the sole mechanism of action responsible for increased survival in trauma patients.[9,10] The coagulation cascade, contrary to what was routinely taught in medical school, it is not a simple series of events occurring in a predictable chain of molecular interactions. Rather, coagulation and fibrinolysis are complex pathways influenced by many other complex pathways, including complement, cytokines, endothelium, and cellular immune systems.[52,53]

Before 2007, aprotinin was used extensively in CPB surgery for its antiplasmin properties.[29] Ultimately, aprotinin was withdrawn from the market due to safety concerns after publication of the BART (Blood Conservation Using Antifibrinolytics in a Randomized Trial) study.[54] However, before the drug was withdrawn, investigators took note of its effect on the inflammatory response present in subjects undergoing CPB surgery.[26,55] After 2007, the drug was quickly replaced by TXA, which had previously shown similar efficacy for reducing blood loss and risk of postoperative transfusion, without increased risk in MI, stroke, or death.[56] Subsequent recognition of similar effects of TXA have led to increasing interest in the antiinflammatory and potential immunomodulatory mechanisms of TXA.[26,53] As a result, these parallel mechanisms are the subject of multiple ongoing trials around the world.[12,13,15]

TRANEXAMIC ACID USE IN CHILDREN

TXA use in children has been studied in a variety of surgical settings and has been shown to be effective at reducing blood loss for orthopedic, cardiac, and craniofacial surgeries.[25,57–59] Based on results of the CRASH-2 trial, and that of an observational pediatric study that showed an association with increased survival with TXA use in trauma, some clinicians advocate for its use in children.[60,61] Although TXA has been studied extensively in the adult trauma patient, less evidence exists for children, and its use in the pediatric trauma population is not as widespread. A study using a large administrative dataset from 36 US children's hospitals found that in all instances in which TXA was used (a total of 35,478 records), only 110 encounters (0.31%) were found to have been for trauma. Most patients who received TXA were undergoing cardiac surgery (22,863; 64%).[62] A single retrospective cohort study of 766 injured children in Afghanistan reported that TXA was only used in 10% of pediatric trauma admissions, although its administration was independently associated with a 27% reduction in mortality (P = .03).[60] In a survey study of US and Canadian pediatric hospitals, antifibrinolytics (TXA and/or aminocaproic acid) were reported to be incorporated in 15% of massive transfusion protocols (MTPs).[63] Like adults, early coagulopathy and shock were independent predictors of mortality in children with traumatic injuries who were treated at combat support hospitals in Iraq and Afghanistan. Coagulopathy was present on admission in 27% of the children and a higher ISS predicted increased coagulopathy, shock, and mortality.[64] When TXA is used in pediatric trauma, some centers are using a dose range of 25 to 50 mg/kg IV bolus (maximum 2 g) with or without a 10 mg/kg infusion over 8 hours. Therefore, to the authors' knowledge, there are no data to guide TXA administration in children.

PHARMACOLOGIC TREATMENT OPTIONS
Contraindications

TXA is contraindicated in patients who have hypersensitivity to the drug and ongoing acute vascular occlusion or thrombosis. Relative contraindications include history or risk factors predisposing to thromboembolic events. TXA use in patients with macroscopic hematuria poses risk of development of clot obstructions in the ureters and has been reported to cause acute renal cortical necrosis with oliguria and renal failure.[19] Subarachnoid hemorrhage (SAH) is also considered to be a contraindication by some investigators[65] but others advocate for its use in this population.[66]

Dosing in Trauma

Several TXA dosing regimens for use in traumatic hemorrhage have been described (**Table 1**). The dosing regimen that was selected for the CRASH-2 trial was based on previous studies carried out in surgical subjects.[8] Early studies in this population demonstrated that a dose of 10 mg/kg followed by 1 mg/kg/h decreased bleeding during cardiac surgery and larger doses did not incur greater benefit for preventing blood loss.[67,68] Because TXA has a large therapeutic range, researchers selected the empirical dose of a 1 g bolus followed by a 1 g infusion over 8 hours, to provide adequate plasma levels for patients weighing more than 100 kg while remaining safe for patients weighing less than 50 kg.[19] The meta-analysis by Ker and colleagues[35] also suggested that a dose of 1 g produced a reduction in bleeding in surgical patients with no evidence to support higher doses in this population. However, in trauma patients, it is possible that larger doses could have a greater treatment effect. Ongoing studies will further elucidate pharmacokinetics of TXA in trauma patients and help to determine the appropriate dose.[13]

It has been postulated by some investigators that most of TXA's benefit may come from the initial bolus. If ongoing studies are able to provide evidence for administration of bolus alone, without the use of bolus plus infusion, it may promote wider adoption of TXA protocols. One study found that a barrier to widespread use of TXA at the investigators' institution was the complexity of administration.[70]

Damage Control Resuscitation and Prehospital Management of Hemorrhage

Remote damage control resuscitation (RDCR) is the prehospital application of the basic concepts of RDCR, and has been of recent interest in the military setting in which early intervention is lifesaving.[43,71] Up to 25% of combat-related injuries are considered to be

Table 1
Dosing regimens for traumatic hemorrhage

Study	Dose	Indication
CRASH-2[8]	1 g bolus followed by a 1 g infusion over 8 h	Adult trauma subjects with significant hemorrhage (SBP <90 mm Hg or heart rate >110 beats per minute [bpm], or both), or who were considered to be at risk of significant hemorrhage, and who were within 8 h of injury
MATTERs[7]	1 g bolus repeated at discretion of treating surgeon	Subjects who received at least 1 unit of PRBC within 24 h of admission following combat-related injury
Tranexamic Acid Mechanisms and Pharmacokinetics in Traumatic Injury (TAMPITI)[13]	Ongoing trial: 1-time bolus of 2 or 4 g	Adult trauma subjects ordered to receive at least 1 blood product and/or immediate transfer to operating room to control bleeding, and within 2 h of injury
Study of Tranexamic Acid during Air Medical Prehospital transport (STAAMP)[12]	Ongoing trial: 1-time bolus of 1 g prehospital dose	Adult trauma subjects being transported via air medical services from scene or referring hospital, with SBP <90 mm Hg or heart rate >110 bpm, and within 2 h of injury
Prehospital Antifibrinolytics for Traumatic Coagulopathy and Hemorrhage (PATCH)[69]	Ongoing trial: 1 g prehospital bolus followed by 1 g in-hospital infusion over 8 h	Adult trauma subjects being transported to a trauma center with a coagulopathy of severe trauma (COAST) score of 3 or greater, and within 3 h of injury

Abbreviation: SBP, systolic blood pressure.

potentially survivable, with hemorrhage being the cause of death in 90%.[5,72,73] Currently, TXA may be the best pharmacologic option for prehospital hemostatic interventions, and its administration in the field has been shown to be feasible in both civilian and military settings.[3,74] Prehospital administration of TXA is still controversial, and currently enrolling trials will provide high level evidence regarding its efficacy and safety.

TXA may be considered in the prehospital setting as a single component of care in a "bundle of therapies."[75] In Canada, a team of first responders decided to integrate prehospital TXA as part of their MTP for hemorrhagic shock in civilian, primary, and secondary air medical evacuation.[76] They reported no inflight complications in their cohort of 13 subjects over a 4-month period. The average time to TXA administration was 32 minutes (95% CI 25.76–39.99). Another Canadian group, in a retrospective study, reported on 20 consecutive subjects receiving TXA during helicopter transportation over a 3-year period. The median time in minutes from the time of injury to helicopter arrival, drug administration, and receiving hospital arrival was 90, 114, and 171 minutes, respectively, for calls to the scene.[77] Lipsky and colleagues[78] reported that TXA administration caused no delay in evacuation of 40 consecutive subjects treated in the military setting.

Certain considerations should be made when integrating the use of TXA in the prehospital setting, including pharmacokinetics in trauma patients, storage under field conditions, and potential interactions with other RDCR drugs. Civilian and military personnel administering TXA as part of RDCR should also be trained in management of potential complications, such as seizures or thrombosis, under field conditions.[79] The Study of Tranexamic Acid during Air Medical Prehospital transport (STAAMP) and the Prehospital Antifibrinolytics for Traumatic Coagulopathy and Hemorrhage (PATCH) studies are ongoing randomized controlled trials that will help to address these concerns.[12,15]

ROLE OF VISCOELASTIC TESTING AND MASSIVE TRANSFUSION PROTOCOLS

Some investigators have advocated for viscoelastic testing before administration of TXA due to concern for deleterious effects of TXA in a particular subset of patients.[50,80] Others have argued that viscoelastic tests of coagulation (TEG or ROTEM) may not be sufficiently sensitive, and that delay in drug administration while awaiting these laboratory results will negatively affect patient outcomes.[48,51]

Although TXA use is not universally accepted in the United States, its integration in MTPs is not uncommon. In a national survey of level I and level II trauma centers designated as The American College of Surgeons-Trauma Quality Improvement Program (ACS-TQIP), 50% (65 of 129) of respondents reported incorporation of an antifibrinolytic in their MTPs.[81] The same survey reported low incorporation of point-of-care TEG into MTPs. Identifying the patient in need of MTP activation remains challenging. Although several algorithms have been developed, and in light of less than optimal use of TEG, accurate predictors are still needed for identifying patients who will require MTP.[82]

TREATMENT COMPLICATIONS

There is some concern for seizure with higher doses of TXA and studies demonstrating causal effect have been in subjects who received considerably large amounts. Indeed, up to 10 times higher than the dose used in CRASH-2.[27] Mechanisms of seizure are still poorly understood but past studies have shown cerebral blood flow disturbances and inhibition of gamma-aminobutyric acid receptors.[10] TXA readily crosses the blood brain barrier and has been demonstrated in cerebrospinal fluid in absence of TBI.[22] TXA is structurally similar to glycine and has been shown to be a competitive inhibitor of glycine receptors in mice.[83] It is likely that this leads to neuronal hyperexcitability and diminished seizure threshold.

There have been several studies evaluating TXA in subjects with SAH. In these studies, TXA was shown to reduce bleeding but was also associated with increased cerebral ischemia, hypothetically due to vasospasm or increased microvascular thrombosis.[65] However, because the treatment with TXA in some of the earlier studies was based on the prolonged dosing regimens in patients with hemophilia, these findings may be due in part to the effects of substantially larger doses.[21] A smaller study evaluating outcomes based on short-term treatment produced encouraging results with trends toward improved mortality and no increase of ischemic stroke.[84] The uncertainty currently surrounding the efficacy of TXA for treatment of SAH is the subject of a large multicenter, randomized, placebo-controlled trial currently being conducted in Australia.[66] It is hoped that the results of this trial will shed light on the drug's utility for this indication.

AREAS OF ONGOING RESEARCH

Currently there are 3 ongoing randomized controlled trials in the United States being funded by the US Department of Defense:

- STAAMP is a multicenter, randomized controlled trial to determine the effect of prehospital TXA infusion during air medical transport on 30-day mortality in subjects at risk of traumatic hemorrhage. The trial will also explore the effects of TXA on the coagulation and inflammatory response following injury.[12]

- Tranexamic Acid Mechanisms and Pharmacokinetics in Traumatic Injury (TAM-PITI) is a randomized placebo-controlled trial to evaluate the effects of TXA on the immune system, its pharmacokinetics, as well as safety and efficacy in severely injured trauma subjects.[13]
- Prehospital Tranexamic Acid Use for Traumatic Brain Injury Trial is a randomized control trial to determine the efficacy of 2 dosing regimens of TXA initiated in the prehospital setting in subjects with moderate to severe TBI.[85]

Additionally, there are several other ongoing trials evaluating TXA for other indications. The World Maternal Antifibrinolytic (WOMAN) trial is currently underway to evaluate TXA for the treatment and prevention of postpartum hemorrhage.[16] Haemorrhage Alleviation with Tranexamic Acid-Intestinal System (HALT-IT) is a randomized controlled trial that will determine the effect of TXA in subjects with acute gastrointestinal bleeding.[17] CRASH-3 is an international randomized controlled trial to quantify the effects of the early administration of TXA on death and disability in patients with TBI.[14]

SUMMARY

The positive results of the CRASH-2 trial sparked both enthusiasm and controversy regarding the use of antifibrinolytics for patients with traumatic bleeding. As a result, several high-quality randomized controlled trials are currently underway to help further elucidate the utility of TXA and other antifibrinolytics in traumatic injury, as well as other conditions with severe bleeding. In addition to awaiting the results of ongoing trials addressing the utility of TXA in the prehospital setting, effects on the immune system, and pharmacokinetics in trauma, the new concept of fibrinolysis shutdown has generated much interest and intrigue. This recently introduced theory would have significant implications for the use of TXA in trauma patients if proven in randomized controlled trials. The next few years should lead to a much better understanding of TXA and its utility, indications, and appropriate dosing. Based on the current evidence in the literature, the authors think that TXA is appropriate in massive transfusion situations empirically for patients presenting within 3 hours of injury but should be goal-directed in non-MTP situations. Further trials are needed to refine and optimize TXA dosing regimens.

REFERENCES

1. Ker K, Kiriya J, Perel P, et al. Avoidable mortality from giving tranexamic acid to bleeding trauma patients: an estimation based on WHO mortality data, a systematic literature review and data from the CRASH-2 trial. BMC Emerg Med 2012;12:3.
2. Injuries and violence: the facts. Geneva (Switzerland): World Health Organization; 2010. Available at: http://www.who.int/violence_injury_prevention/key_facts/en/. Accessed April 28, 2016.
3. Nadler R, Gendler S, Benov A, et al. Tranexamic acid at the point of injury: the Israeli combined civilian and military experience. J Trauma Acute Care Surg 2014;77(3 Suppl 2):S146–50.
4. Frith D, Brohi K. The acute coagulopathy of trauma shock: clinical relevance. Surgeon 2010;8(3):159–63.
5. Eastridge BJ, Mabry RL, Seguin P, et al. Death on the battlefield (2001-2011): implications for the future of combat casualty care. J Trauma Acute Care Surg 2012; 73(6 Suppl 5):S431–7.

6. Evans JA, van Wessem KJ, McDougall D, et al. Epidemiology of traumatic deaths: comprehensive population-based assessment. World J Surg 2010; 34(1):158–63.
7. Morrison JJ, Dubose JJ, Rasmussen TE, et al. Military Application of Tranexamic Acid in Trauma Emergency Resuscitation (MATTERs) Study. Arch Surg 2012; 147(2):113–9.
8. Shakur H, Roberts I, Bautista R, et al. Effects of tranexamic acid on death, vascular occlusive events, and blood transfusion in trauma patients with significant haemorrhage (CRASH-2): a randomised, placebo-controlled trial. Lancet 2010;376(9734): 23–32.
9. Napolitano LM, Cohen MJ, Cotton BA, et al. Tranexamic acid in trauma: how should we use it? J Trauma Acute Care Surg 2013;74(6):1575–86.
10. Pusateri AE, Weiskopf RB, Bebarta V, et al. Tranexamic acid and trauma: current status and knowledge gaps with recommended research priorities. Shock 2013; 39(2):121–6.
11. Cole E, Davenport R, Willett K, et al. Tranexamic acid use in severely injured civilian patients and the effects on outcomes: a prospective cohort study. Ann Surg 2015;261(2):390–4.
12. Brown JB, Neal MD, Guyette FX, et al. Design of the Study of Tranexamic Acid during Air Medical Prehospital Transport (STAAMP) Trial: addressing the knowledge gaps. Prehosp Emerg Care 2015;19(1):79–86.
13. Spinella PC, Bochicchio GV. Tranexamic Acid Mechanisms and Pharmacokinetics In Traumatic Injury (TAMPITI Trial). Available at: http://www.tampiti.wustl.edu/. Accessed April 16, 2016.
14. Dewan Y, Komolafe EO, Mejia-Mantilla JH, et al. CRASH-3-tranexamic acid for the treatment of significant traumatic brain injury: study protocol for an international randomized, double-blind, placebo-controlled trial. Trials 2012;13:87.
15. Gruen RL, Jacobs IG, Reade MC. Trauma and tranexamic acid. Med J Aust 2013; 199(5):310–1.
16. Shakur H, Elbourne D, Gulmezoglu M, et al. The WOMAN Trial (World Maternal Antifibrinolytic Trial): tranexamic acid for the treatment of postpartum haemorrhage: an international randomised, double blind placebo controlled trial. Trials 2010;11:40.
17. Roberts I, Coats T, Edwards P, et al. HALT-IT–tranexamic acid for the treatment of gastrointestinal bleeding: study protocol for a randomised controlled trial. Trials 2014;15:450.
18. Binz S, McCollester J, Thomas S, et al. CRASH-2 study of tranexamic acid to treat bleeding in trauma patients: a controversy fueled by science and social media. J Blood Transfus 2015;2015:874920.
19. Tengborn L, Blomback M, Berntorp E. Tranexamic acid–an old drug still going strong and making a revival. Thromb Res 2015;135(2):231–42.
20. CYKLOKAPRON- tranexamic acid injection, solution Pharmacia and Upjohn Company. Available at: http://labeling.pfizer.com/ShowLabeling.aspx?id=556. Accessed April 20, 2016.
21. Cap AP, Baer DG, Orman JA, et al. Tranexamic acid for trauma patients: a critical review of the literature. J Trauma 2011;71(Suppl 1):S9–14.
22. Abou-Diwan C, Sniecinski RM, Szlam F, et al. Plasma and cerebral spinal fluid tranexamic acid quantitation in cardiopulmonary bypass patients. J Chromatogr B Analyt Technol Biomed Life Sci 2011;879(7–8):553–6.
23. Bernet F, Carrel T, Marbet G, et al. Reduction of blood loss and transfusion requirements after coronary artery bypass grafting: similar efficacy of tranexamic acid and aprotinin in aspirin-treated patients. J Card Surg 1999;14(2):92–7.

24. Bokesch PM, Szabo G, Wojdyga R, et al. A phase 2 prospective, randomized, double-blind trial comparing the effects of tranexamic acid with ecallantide on blood loss from high-risk cardiac surgery with cardiopulmonary bypass (CON-SERV-2 Trial). J Thorac Cardiovasc Surg 2012;143(5):1022–9.

25. Couturier R, Rubatti M, Credico C, et al. Continuous or discontinuous tranexamic acid effectively inhibits fibrinolysis in children undergoing cardiac surgery with cardiopulmonary bypass. Blood Coagul Fibrinolysis 2014;25(3):259–65.

26. Jimenez JJ, Iribarren JL, Lorente L, et al. Tranexamic acid attenuates inflammatory response in cardiopulmonary bypass surgery through blockade of fibrinolysis: a case control study followed by a randomized double-blind controlled trial. Crit Care 2007;11(6):R117.

27. Kalavrouziotis D, Voisine P, Mohammadi S, et al. High-dose tranexamic acid is an independent predictor of early seizure after cardiopulmonary bypass. Ann Thorac Surg 2012;93(1):148–54.

28. Karski JM, Teasdale SJ, Norman P, et al. Prevention of bleeding after cardiopulmonary bypass with high-dose tranexamic acid: double-blind, randomized clinical trial. J Thorac Cardiovasc Surg 1995;110(3):835–42.

29. Royston D. The current place of aprotinin in the management of bleeding. Anaesthesia 2015;70(Suppl 1):46–9, e17.

30. Jennings JD, Solarz MK, Haydel C. Application of tranexamic acid in trauma and orthopedic surgery. Orthop Clin North Am 2016;47(1):137–43.

31. Tsutsumimoto T, Shimogata M, Ohta H, et al. Tranexamic acid reduces perioperative blood loss in cervical laminoplasty: a prospective randomized study. Spine (Phila Pa 1976) 2011;36(23):1913–8.

32. Sabatini L, Atzori F, Revello S, et al. Intravenous use of tranexamic acid reduces postoperative blood loss in total knee arthroplasty. Arch Orthop Trauma Surg 2014;134(11):1609–14.

33. Gillespie R, Shishani Y, Joseph S, et al. Neer Award 2015: a randomized, prospective evaluation on the effectiveness of tranexamic acid in reducing blood loss after total shoulder arthroplasty. J Shoulder Elbow Surg 2015;24(11):1679–84.

34. Brohi K, Cohen MJ, Ganter MT, et al. Acute traumatic coagulopathy: initiated by hypoperfusion: modulated through the protein C pathway? Ann Surg 2007; 245(5):812–8.

35. Ker K, Edwards P, Perel P, et al. Effect of tranexamic acid on surgical bleeding: systematic review and cumulative meta-analysis. BMJ 2012;344:e3054.

36. Roberts I, Shakur H, Afolabi A, et al. The importance of early treatment with tranexamic acid in bleeding trauma patients: an exploratory analysis of the CRASH-2 randomised controlled trial. Lancet 2011;377(9771):1096–101, 1101.e1–2.

37. Roberts I, Shakur H, Coats T, et al. The CRASH-2 trial: a randomised controlled trial and economic evaluation of the effects of tranexamic acid on death, vascular occlusive events and transfusion requirement in bleeding trauma patients. Health Technol Assess 2013;17(10):1–79.

38. Roberts I. Tranexamic acid in trauma: how should we use it? J Thromb Haemost 2015;13(Suppl 1):S195–9.

39. Harvin JA, Peirce CA, Mims MM, et al. The impact of tranexamic acid on mortality in injured patients with hyperfibrinolysis. J Trauma Acute Care Surg 2015;78(5): 905–9 [discussion: 909–11].

40. Moore HB, Moore EE, Gonzalez E, et al. Hyperfibrinolysis, physiologic fibrinolysis, and fibrinolysis shutdown: the spectrum of postinjury fibrinolysis and relevance to antifibrinolytic therapy. J Trauma Acute Care Surg 2014;77(6):811–7 [discussion: 817].

41. Valle EJ, Allen CJ, Van Haren RM, et al. Do all trauma patients benefit from tranexamic acid? J Trauma Acute Care Surg 2014;76(6):1373–8.
42. Brohi K, Singh J, Heron M, et al. Acute traumatic coagulopathy. J Trauma 2003; 54(6):1127–30.
43. Jenkins DH, Rappold JF, Badloe JF, et al. Trauma hemostasis and oxygenation research position paper on remote damage control resuscitation: definitions, current practice, and knowledge gaps. Shock 2014;41(Suppl 1):3–12.
44. Davenport RA, Brohi K. Cause of trauma-induced coagulopathy. Curr Opin Anaesthesiol 2016;29(2):212–9.
45. Brohi K, Cohen MJ, Ganter MT, et al. Acute coagulopathy of trauma: hypoperfusion induces systemic anticoagulation and hyperfibrinolysis. J Trauma 2008; 64(5):1211–7 [discussion: 1217].
46. Dirkmann D, Radu-Berlemann J, Gorlinger K, et al. Recombinant tissue-type plasminogen activator-evoked hyperfibrinolysis is enhanced by acidosis and inhibited by hypothermia but still can be blocked by tranexamic acid. J Trauma Acute Care Surg 2013;74(2):482–8.
47. Frith D, Davenport R, Brohi K. Acute traumatic coagulopathy. Curr Opin Anaesthesiol 2012;25(2):229–34.
48. Raza I, Davenport R, Rourke C, et al. The incidence and magnitude of fibrinolytic activation in trauma patients. J Thromb Haemost 2013;11(2):307–14.
49. Moore HB, Moore EE, Liras IN, et al. Acute fibrinolysis shutdown after injury occurs frequently and increases mortality: a multicenter evaluation of 2,540 severely injured patients. J Am Coll Surg 2016;222(4):347–55.
50. Moore EE, Moore HB, Gonzalez E, et al. Rationale for the selective administration of tranexamic acid to inhibit fibrinolysis in the severely injured patient. Transfusion 2016;56(Suppl 2):S110–4.
51. Roberts I. Fibrinolytic shutdown: fascinating theory but randomized controlled trial data are needed. Transfusion 2016;56(Suppl 2):S115–8.
52. Laffey JG, Boylan JF, Cheng DC. The systemic inflammatory response to cardiac surgery: implications for the anesthesiologist. Anesthesiology 2002;97(1):215–52.
53. van der Poll T, Herwald H. The coagulation system and its function in early immune defense. Thromb Haemost 2014;112(4):640–8.
54. Fergusson DA, Hebert PC, Mazer CD, et al. A comparison of aprotinin and lysine analogues in high-risk cardiac surgery. N Engl J Med 2008;358(22):2319–31.
55. Asehnoune K, Dehoux M, Lecon-Malas V, et al. Differential effects of aprotinin and tranexamic acid on endotoxin desensitization of blood cells induced by circulation through an isolated extracorporeal circuit. J Cardiothorac Vasc Anesth 2002;16(4):447–51.
56. Wong BI, McLean RF, Fremes SE, et al. Aprotinin and tranexamic acid for high transfusion risk cardiac surgery. Ann Thorac Surg 2000;69(3):808–16.
57. White N, Bayliss S, Moore D. Systematic review of interventions for minimizing perioperative blood transfusion for surgery for craniosynostosis. J Craniofac Surg 2015;26(1):26–36.
58. Faraoni D, Goobie SM. The efficacy of antifibrinolytic drugs in children undergoing noncardiac surgery: a systematic review of the literature. Anesth Analg 2014; 118(3):628–36.
59. Faraoni D, Willems A, Melot C, et al. Efficacy of tranexamic acid in paediatric cardiac surgery: a systematic review and meta-analysis. Eur J Cardiothorac Surg 2012;42(5):781–6.
60. Eckert MJ, Wertin TM, Tyner SD, et al. Tranexamic acid administration to pediatric trauma patients in a combat setting: the pediatric trauma and tranexamic acid

Coagulopathy of Trauma

 CrossMark

Mitchell J. Cohen, MD*, S. Ariane Christie, MD

KEYWORDS

- Trauma • Hemorrhage • Coagulation • Coagulopathy
- Trauma-induced coagulopathy • Targeted resuscitation • Bleeding

KEY POINTS

- Trauma-induced coagulopathy (TIC) is an endogenous hypocoagulable state distinct from iatrogenic causes.
- Activation of protein C pathway is a key mechanistic mediator of traumatic coagulopathy via downstream effects, including thrombin diversion, deactivation of coagulation factors, and de-repression of fibrinolysis.
- Standard coagulation tests and functional viscoelastic assays are commonly used in the diagnosis and management of TIC.
- Balanced resuscitation is the mainstay of coagulopathy treatment, but precise ratios for empiric resuscitation and optimal monitoring protocols for transfusion practice remain unknown.
- Patients with traumatic coagulopathy have worse outcomes, including increased rates of transfusion, infection, thromboembolism, acute lung injury, multiorgan failure, and death.

INTRODUCTION

Bleeding remains the leading cause of preventable death after injury.[1] Contributing to this problem, coagulopathy develops in approximately one-third of all injured patients,[2–4] resulting in worsened outcomes including higher transfusion requirements; increased multiorgan system failure, increased hospital, intensive care, and ventilator days; and increased mortality.[2,3,5,6]

Grants: Supported by NIH 1UM1HL10877, DOD W911NF-10-1-0384 (M.J. Cohen).
Conflicts of Interest: None declared.
Department of Surgery, San Francisco General Hospital, University of California, San Francisco, School of Medicine, 1001 Potrero Avenue, San Francisco, CA 94110, USA
* Corresponding author. Department of Surgery, San Francisco General Hospital, Ward 3A, 1001 Potrero Avenue, Room 3C-38, San Francisco, CA 94110.
E-mail address: Mitchell.Cohen@ucsf.edu

History of coagulopathy in trauma

Although coagulopathy was known to occur after injury, until recently coagulation was not viewed as a critical driver of postinjury physiology. Instead, injured patients were thought to be coagulopathic owing only to the iatrogenic secondary effects of hemodilution, hypothermia, and acidosis.[7,8] In 2003, 2 independent investigators described admission perturbations of prothrombin time (PT) and partial thromboplastin time (PTT) in newly injured patients before significant fluid administration.[2,3] This phenomenon, which correlated with increasing injury severity and mortality, became known as "acute traumatic coagulopathy" (now "trauma-induced coagulopathy" [TIC]) and effectively changed the paradigm of modern trauma care.[2,3,9] The study of coagulation and inflammation derangements after injury now constitutes one of the most active areas of ongoing trauma research.

This review addresses the current evidence regarding the diagnosis, mechanisms, and management of TIC, highlighting areas of ongoing debate and controversy. Although TIC is emphasized, it is equally important to recognize that coagulopathy after trauma is often caused or compounded by additional contributors of disordered coagulation including hypothermia, acidosis, dilution with large volume of intravenous fluid, or unbalanced blood product, all of which are termed iatrogenic coagulopathy. Management of the injured coagulopathic patient must therefore include a high suspicion for and treatment of multiple different potential etiologies of dysfunctional clotting.

PATIENT EVALUATION AND OVERVIEW
Mechanism and Pathophysiology

Multiple distinct but highly integrated pathways have been implicated as mediators of TIC (**Fig. 1**). Delineating the exact pathophysiology and interplay between disordered coagulation and inflammation mechanisms remains the subject of ongoing research. Herein, we describe the most important known contributors to TIC.

Activated protein C and fibrinolysis

TIC is an endogenous hypocoagulable state that occurs in the setting of tissue hypoperfusion (base deficit) and is primarily mediated by activation of protein C (**Fig. 2**).[10]

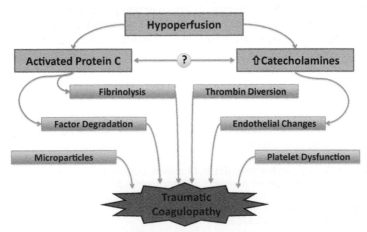

Fig. 1. Pathophysiology of traumatic coagulopathy. Multiple distinct but highly integrated pathways have been implicated as mediators of trauma-induced coagulopathy. Delineation and integration of these pathways remains an area of ongoing research.

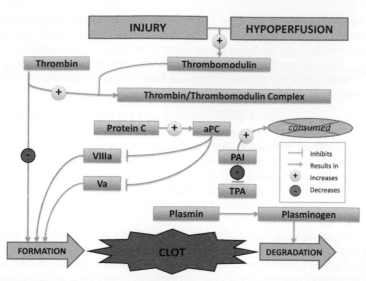

Fig. 2. Critical role of aPC in the pathophysiology of trauma-induced coagulopathy. Severe injury accompanied by tissue hypoperfusion leads to increased endothelial and circulating thrombomodulin, which subsequently binds thrombin. The resultant thrombomodulin-thrombin complex converts protein C into its activated form (aPC). While aPC decreases clot formation via deactivation of factors V and VIII, it is simultaneously consuming plasminogen activator inhibitor-1 (PAI-1), disinhibiting tPA, and leading to unopposed fibrinolysis. APC, activated protein C; PAI, plasminogen activator inhibitor; tPA, tissue plasminogen activator; Va, activated factor V; VIIIa, activated factor VIII.

Multiple prospective clinical studies have linked early coagulopathy in critically injured trauma patients to protein C depletion (activated protein C [aPC] elevation), and increased risk of acute lung injury, ventilator-associated pneumonia, multisystem organ failure, and death.[6,10,11] Protein C is a serine protease with both anticoagulant and inflammomodulatory functions.[12,13] When severe injury is accompanied by shock (tissue hypoperfusion), increased endothelial and circulating thrombomodulin bind thrombin forming thrombomodulin–thrombin complex, which subsequently activates protein C.[10] aPC deactivates factors V and VIII inhibiting clot formation, and depletes plasminogen activator inhibitor-1, leading to unopposed fibrinolysis with increased levels of tissue plasminogen activator and D-dimer.[14]

Fibrinolytic activity is further exacerbated by reduced activation of thrombin-activatable fibrinolysis inhibitor as thrombin is diverted to PC activation.[15] Severe fibrinolysis in TIC portends increased mortality,[16–18] and even low degrees of clot lysis have been associated with poor outcomes.[19] In a murine model, aPC inhibition prevented TIC after trauma and hemorrhagic shock.[12]

Conversely, overinhibition of fibrinolysis, termed "fibrinolysis shutdown," has been demonstrated to be an independent predictor of adverse outcomes after injury, including increased mortality.[20] Furthermore, recent prospective cohort data suggest that more severely injured patients present with fibrinolysis shutdown than either hyperfibrinolysis or physiologic fibrinolysis.[21] These data have important implications with regard to the usefulness of potential fibrinolytic inhibitors, which will need to be carefully targeted to the physiologic range and avoid overinhibition leading to fibrinolysis shutdown.

Platelets
Platelet deficit and dysfunction are also likely to be significant contributors to TIC.[22]

Relative thrombocytopenia Multiple prospective cohort studies have demonstrated that relatively lower admission platelet counts are associated with increased all-cause, hemorrhagic, and central nervous system mortality, and increased blood use after injury, even when the initial platelet count remains well within the normal limits.[23,24] Additionally, the platelet count has been shown to decrease substantially over the course of hospitalization.

Functional platelet impairment Severe injury is also associated with impaired platelet function. In 2001, Jacoby and colleagues[25] used flow cytometery and light aggregrometry first identified decreased admission platelet function in injury nonsurvivors, and, in a separate analysis, in patients with head injury at 24 hours. Thromboelastographic platelet mapping data demonstrated that severely injured trauma patients had impaired platelet stimulation in response to adenosine diphosphate and arachidonic acid stimulation compared with healthy human volunteers, with impairment proportionate to injury severity.[26]

Another prospective clinical study demonstrated that 46% of severely injured patients on admission and 91% of patients at 120 hours had some degree of platelet dysfunction by multiplate impedance aggregometry, despite normal platelet counts.[27] Impaired admission platelet function in response to arachidonic acid, collagen, and thrombin receptor activating peptide were predictive of death. Data from multiple additional animal and clinical studies have corroborated findings of impaired platelet function after severe injury and traumatic brain injury.[28,29]

Endothelial involvement

Recent investigations have also demonstrated evidence that endothelial dysfunction likely plays a role in development of TIC.[30] Admission plasma samples from severely injured patients demonstrate elevated circulating levels of Syndecan-1, a protein normally found in the glycocalyx of the endothelium. Soluble syndecan-1 was associated with increased aPC, prolonged PTT, and increased adrenaline levels, suggesting that tissue hypoperfusion and catecholamine stimulation after injury may result in degradation of the endothelial glycocalyx and contribute to coagulopathy. To date, however, there is no experimental confirmation of this theory, making it possible that the association between catecholamines and coagulopathy is only correlative.

Microparticles

Emerging research suggests that microparticles may also play a role in the mechanism of TIC. Some evidence suggests that systemic release of thrombin-rich microparticles, which likely function normally in local hemostasis after tissue injury, may cause a coagulopathic state similar to DIC. Elevated circulating endothelial-, erythrocyte-, and leukocyte-derived microparticles have been identified in the plasma of injured patients compared with noninjured controls whereas coagulopathic patients demonstrated lower levels of platelet-derived and tissue factor–positive microparticles compared with non-coagulopathic patients.[31] In a single small study, increased circulating microparticles were also found in patients with traumatic brain injury compared with controls.[32]

Diagnosis

Standard clinical and laboratory assessment after severe injury

As with the management of all severely injured patients, diagnosis of TIC should be performed within the context of the Advanced Trauma Life Support evaluation. Obvious sources of active bleeding should be temporized promptly with compression or other hemostatic measures, hypotension should be addressed with administration of packed red blood cells (PRBC), and the patient should be warmed with heated blankets as the patient is exposed. Severe injury and hypotension should prompt a high degree of suspicion for traumatic coagulopathy. Standard trauma laboratory tests should be obtained as soon as intravenous access is secured and can provide indicators of the presence of tissue hypoperfusion and coagulopathy. **Table 1** describes standard admission trauma laboratory tests and their role in the diagnosis of TIC.

Table 1
Standard admission trauma laboratory measures in the evaluation of TIC

Lab	Level	Usefulness in the Diagnosis of TIC
pH	Low	Significant hypoperfusion probable
Base deficit/excess	Negative	Significant hypoperfusion probable
Hemoglobin/hematocrit	Low	Likely significant blood loss
Platelet count	Low	Absolute/relative thrombocytopenia
Partial thromboplastin time	Prolonged	Diagnostic of TIC
Prothrombin time/International Normalized Ratio	Prolonged	Diagnostic of TIC

Abbreviation: TIC, trauma-induced coagulopathy.
We also recommend the standard collection of baseline fibrinogen and D-dimer, which can provide a surrogate estimation of factor consumption and fibrinolysis, respectively.

Diagnostic criteria
Multiple assays currently play a role in the diagnosis of TIC.

Standard assays TIC was initially defined by prolongation of the standard coagulation assays PTT and PT/International Normalized Ratio (INR), and these remain the most widely used method for the diagnosis of TIC. Different cutoffs for these assays have been described in the literature (**Table 2**).

Macleod and colleagues[3] reported that alterations in the cutoffs for PTT and PT did not alter the predictive value of these variables for predicting death in an adjusted regression model. Lower thresholds for INR cutoffs demonstrated improved sensitivity to discriminate patients with higher transfusion requirements in shock in severely injured population (Injury Severity Score >15) in a multicenter retrospective study, but at least 1 prospective study has refuted this finding.[36]

However, concerns have been raised regarding the use of standard coagulation assays as the benchmark for TIC. PTT and INR were designed initially to test heritable coagulopathy, and standard reference ranges were generated using data from healthy volunteers. Additionally, concerns have been raised regarding the length of time required to run standard coagulation tests when rapid and ongoing diagnosis and treatment of the coagulopathic patient are essential to reverse pathophysiology and improve outcomes.

Table 2
Commonly used cutoffs for conventional coagulation assays in trauma-induced coagulopathy

Assay	Cutoff	Or	Any value >1.5× the institutional reference range[33]
Partial thromboplastin time	>34–60 sec[3,30]		
Prothrombin time	>18 sec		
International Normalized Ratio	>1.2–1.5[3,6,34,35]		

Viscoelastic assays There has been increased interest and use of point-of-care functional tests such as thromboelastography (TEG) and rotational thromboelastometry (ROTEM) for the diagnosis and management of patients with TIC. TEG is a modality that assesses multiple real-time viscoelastic properties of coagulation including:

- Time to clot initiation,
- Clot propagation,
- Clot strength, and
- Clot breakdown (fibrinolysis).

The addition of specific clotting activators and inhibitors can be used to assay different contributors to clot formation or breakdown. Multiple studies have demonstrated the capacity of TEG to diagnose hypocoagulability and predict transfusion and mortality in the trauma population.[37–40] TEG has been validated against standard coagulation tests,[40] and assays of both thrombin generation[41] and fibrinolysis.[42] However, there remains ongoing debate regarding the superiority of TEG compared with other assays, in particular with regards to fibrinolysis as plasmin–antiplasmin levels have demonstrated high sensitivity.[43]

Scoring systems Multiple scoring systems have been generated to predict need for massive transfusion, including:

- The Trauma-Associated Severe Hemorrhage score,[44]
- The McLaughlin score,[45] and
- The Assessment of Blood Consumption score.[46]

A retrospective review comparing these 3 scoring systems failed to demonstrate a difference between their capacity to predict massive transfusion.[46] Importantly, the scoring systems do not take into account coagulation parameters and likely reflect significant hemorrhage owing to injury rather than TIC proper. None of these scoring systems have been used widely in the diagnosis of TIC.

Phenotypes of Trauma-Induced Coagulopathy

There is evidence to suggest that traumatic coagulopathy is not a single entity, but rather consists of multiple distinct but related pathophysiologic subtypes. A principle component analysis of a large prospective cohort of injured patients demonstrated 2 such phenotypes.

1. **Coagulation factor deficiency TIC**
   a. Characterized by abnormality of standard coagulation tests and increased mortality.

2. **Fibrinolytic TIC**
   a. Characterized by aPC elevation and is associated with increased end organ failure, infectious complications and mortality.[9]

There are likely even more TIC subtypes that have yet to be identified. By diagnosing and treating specific deficits underlying different coagulopathic phenotypes, it may be possible to streamline individualized care and improved outcomes.

PHARMACOLOGIC TREATMENT OPTIONS

Although balanced product transfusion currently remains the mainstay of treatment for TIC, there are several pharmacologic agents that have the potential to be efficacious based on our mechanistic understanding of traumatic coagulopathy.

Antifibrinolytics

Evidence of hyperfibrinolysis as a critical mechanism underlying traumatic coagulopathy has led to interest antifibrinolytic agents as potential adjuncts for the treatment of TIC. These agents include tranexamic acid (TXA), aminocaproic acid, and aprotinin, of which only TXA has been widely studied in trauma patients.

The CRASH-2 trial (Clinical Randomization of an Antifibrinolytic in Significant Hemorrhage) was a large international randomized trial that reported a 1.5% absolute mortality reduction in patients administered TXA compared with placebo, although there was no difference in blood product transfusion between groups. Furthermore, the subset of patients who received TXA 3 or more hours after injury had increased mortality.[47] Of note, enrollment criteria for this study failed to incorporate coagulation data and included any patients with or at risk for significant hemorrhage limiting the generalizability of these findings.

The MATTERs (Military Application of Tranexamic-acid in Trauma Emergency Resuscitation) study was a retrospective observational study, which identified reduced mortality in patients who received TXA, with greater differences identified in patients requiring massive transfusion.[48] Despite achieving considerable acceptance as an adjunctive treatment for TIC, there has not yet been sufficient evidence to support the routine use of TXA in the trauma setting.[49]

Recombinant Factor Concentrates

Additional pharmaceutical hemostatic agents with potential usefulness in the treatment of TIC include recombinant factor concentrates including recombinant factor VIIa, prothrombin complex concentrate (PCC), and fibrinogen.

Recombinant Factor VII

Fresh frozen plasma (FFP) is often used to reverse coagulopathy, but has limitations including the requirement for thawing and cross-matching, incomplete and variable factor level repletion,[50–52] and coagulation test reversal[53,54] and complications such as transfusion-related acute lung injury and circulatory overload.[55,56]

Physiologically targeted resuscitation could theoretically arrest coagulopathy in a rapid fashion and avoid many of the pitfalls of traditional plasma. There was significant interest in using recombinant factor VIIa to do this; however, key trials failed to show benefit and suggested increased thrombotic complications.[57] It has been pointed out that these trials generally used recombinant factor VIIa late in the resuscitation process, when poor outcomes were relatively certain. It is not known whether recombinant factor VIIa could potentially have a role in trauma resuscitation as part of a more targeted empiric therapy for specific subpopulations of patients with TIC, but at present factor VIIa has not gained widespread support for use in the trauma setting.

Prothrombin Complex Concentrate

PCC comes in several varieties, including 3- and 4-factor formulations. The most common formulation is 4-factor PPC, a human plasma–derived concentrate of vitamin K–dependent clotting factors II, VII, IX, and X that received approval from the US Food and Drug Administration in April 2013 as an alternative to urgent warfarin reversal in the setting of acute bleeding or need for urgent surgery. Since that time, it has developed usage for reversal of nonwarfarin coagulopathy, including coagulopathy induced by new oral anticoagulants and in coagulopathy of nonmedication etiologies.[58–60]

In a porcine trauma models, PCC demonstrated more rapid and effective hemostasis than FFP in the correction of acquired coagulopathy.[61] Multiple retrospective studies have reported decreased time to reversal, decreased product use, and decreased mortality in patients treated with PCC in the setting of traumatic coagulopathy in general and in the population with traumatic brain injury.[62,63] However, there are ongoing concerns regarding the potential for increased thromboembolic complications and cost with 4-factor PPC compared with plasma. At present, the paucity of prospective data limits our ability to draw conclusions regarding the safety and efficacy of 4-factor PPC in severe injury.

Fibrinogen Concentrate

Fibrinogen deficit has been shown to predict TIC,[11] and as described fibrinolysis constitutes an important component of the pathophysiology of TIC. In a prospective cohort study of 517 trauma patients, low fibrinogen levels were independent predictor of mortality at 24 hours and 28 days ($P<.001$), and administration of cryoprecipitate was associated with improved survival.[64] Although the threshold of sufficient fibrinogen to support normal clotting has not been studied rigorously in trauma patients, routine testing and repletion of low admission levels or function may be a reasonable adjunct to the treatment of TIC. FFP does not contain sufficient amounts of fibrinogen for adequate replacement[65] and in the United States cryoprecipitate is commonly used for this purpose. In Europe, retrospective studies in a trauma population have reported good efficacy of fibrinogen concentrate in correcting functional deficits,[66] however, this product is not currently approved in the United States. Current European guidelines for hemorrhage management in trauma patients with fibrinogen levels less than 1.5 to 2.0 g/L or viscoelastic signs of a functional fibrinogen deficit recommend an initial fibrinogen concentrate dose of 3 to 4 g (equivalent to 15–20 single donor units of cryoprecipitate), with further dosing guided by laboratory or viscoelastic testing (**Fig. 3**).[67]

NONPHARMACOLOGIC TREATMENT OPTIONS

Treatment of coagulopathy in the injured patient includes early diagnosis, prompt hemostasis, and early hemorrhage control, prevention of complicating causes of coagulopathy (hypothermia, acidosis, hemodilution), and blood product transfusion with FFP, platelets, and cryoprecipitate. There is ongoing debate regarding the optimal protocol for delivery of blood product resuscitation.

Balanced Resuscitation and Resuscitation Ratios

Although early transfusion was conducted with whole blood, in the last quarter of the 21st century standard practice favored resuscitation of the injured patient with large volumes of crystalloid and PRBC.[68] Then, in the early 2000s, retrospective military data from Afghanistan and Iraq suggested a mortality benefit to trauma resuscitation with a balanced ratio of PRBCs.[69] Civilian retrospective data echoed these findings using a 1:1:1 ratio of PRBCs, FFP, and platelets[70,71] and the trauma community subsequently began to shift toward balanced blood product resuscitation (**Fig. 4**).

The PROMMTT study (Prospective, Observational, Multicenter, Major Trauma Transfusion) demonstrated in a large multicenter cohort that patients who received increased plasma to RBC ratios had reduced 6-hour mortality compared with those who received less plasma.[72] In an attempt to delineate the ideal empiric transfusion ratio, the (PROPPR) trial (Pragmatic, Randomized Optimal Platelet and Plasma Ratios) randomized severely injured patients to 1:1:1 versus 1:1:2 PRBC to FFP to platelet resuscitation, but ultimately failed to demonstrate a difference between resuscitation groups for 24-hour or 28-day mortality,[73] which was likely at least in part owing to poor separation between treatment groups. At present, the precise "ideal" PRBC to plasma

III. Tissue oxygenation, type of fluid and temperature management

R13
Tissue oxygenation
***
A target systolic blood pressure of 80-90 mm Hg should be employed until major bleeding has been stopped in the initial phase following trauma without brain injury. A mean arterial pressure ≥80 mm Hg should be maintained in patients with severe TBI.

R14
Restricted volume replacement
***
A restricted volume replacement strategy should be used to achieve target blood pressure until bleeding can be controlled.

R15
Vasopressors and inotropic agents
***
In addition to fluids, vasopressors should be administered to maintain target blood pressure in the presence of life-threatening hypotension. An inotropic agent should be infused in the presence of myocardial dysfunction.

R16
Type of fluid
***
Use of isotonic crystalloid solutions should be initiated in the hypotensive bleeding trauma patient. Hypotonic solutions such as Ringer's lactate should be avoided in patients with severe head trauma. Excessive use of 0.9% NaCl solution might be avoided and use of colloids might be restricted.

R17
Erythrocytes
***
Treatment should aim to achieve a target Hb of 7-9 g/dl.

R18
Temperature management
***
Early application of measures to reduce heat loss and warm the hypothermic patient should be employed to achieve and maintain normothermia.

IV. Rapid control of bleeding

R19
Damage control surgery
***
Damage control surgery should be employed in the severely injured patient presenting with deep haemorrhagic shock, signs of ongoing bleeding and coagulopathy. Severe coagulopathy, hypothermia, acidosis, inaccessible major anatomic injury, a need for time-consuming procedures or concomitant major injury outside the abdomen should also trigger a damage control approach. Primary definitive surgical management should be employed in the haemodynamically stable patient in the absence of any of these factors.

R20
Pelvic ring closure and stabilisation
***
Patients with pelvic ring disruption in haemorrhagic shock should undergo immediate pelvic ring closure and stabilisation.

R21
Packing, embolisation & surgery
***
Patients with ongoing haemodynamic instability despite adequate pelvic ring stabilisation should undergo early preperitoneal packing, angiographic embolisation and/or surgical bleeding control.

R22
Local haemostatic measures
***
Topical haemostatic agents should be employed in combination with other surgical measures or with packing for venous or moderate arterial bleeding associated with parenchymal injuries.

V. Initial management of bleeding and coagulopathy

R23
Coagulation support
***
Monitoring and measures to support coagulation should be initiated immediately upon hospital admission.

R24
Initial resuscitation
***
Initial management of patients with expected massive haemorrhage should include either plasma (FFP or pathogen-inactivated plasma) and RBC ratio of at least 1:2 as needed or fibrinogen concentrate and RBC according to Hb level.

R25
Antifibrinolytic agents
***
TXA should be administered as early as possible to the trauma patient who is bleeding or at risk of significant haemorrhage at a loading dose of 1 g infused over 10 min, followed by an i.v. infusion of 1 g over 8 h. TXA should be administered to the bleeding trauma patient within 3 h after injury. Protocols for the management of bleeding patients might consider administration of the first dose of TXA en route to the hospital.

VI. Further resuscitation

R26
Goal-directed therapy
***
Resuscitation measures should be continued using a goal-directed strategy guided by standard laboratory coagulation values and/or viscoelastic tests.

R27
Plasma
***
In a plasma-based coagulation strategy plasma (FFP or pathogen-inactivated plasma) should be administered to maintain PT and APTT<1.5 times the normal control. Plasma transfusion should be avoided in patients without substantial bleeding.

R28
Fibrinogen & cryoprecipitate
***
If a concentrate-based strategy is used, fibrinogen concentrate or cryoprecipitate should be administered if significant bleeding is accompanied by viscoelastic signs of a functional fibrinogen deficit or a plasma fibrinogen level of less than 1.5-2.0 g/l. An initial fibrinogen supplementation of 3-4 g, equivalent to 15-20 single donor units of cryoprecipitate or 3-4 g fibrinogen concentrate may be administered. Repeat doses must be guided by viscoelastic monitoring and laboratory assessment of fibrinogen levels.

R29
Platelets
***
Platelets should be administered to maintain a platelet count >50 × 10⁹/l. A platelet count >100 × 10⁹/l in patients with ongoing bleeding and/or TBI may be maintained. If administered, an initial dose of 4-8 single platelet units or one apheresis pack may be used.

R30
Calcium
***
Ionised calcium levels should be monitored and maintained within the normal range during massive transfusion.

R31
Antiplatelet agents
***
Platelets may be administered in patients with substantial bleeding or intracranial haemorrhage who have been treated with APA. Platelet function may be measured in patients treated or suspected of being treated with APA. Platelet concentrates may be used if platelet dysfunction is documented in a patient with continued microvascular bleeding.

R32
Desmopressin
***
Desmopressin (0.3 μg/kg) may be administered in patients treated with platelet-inhibiting drugs or von Willebrand disease. Desmopressin may not be administered routinely in the bleeding trauma patient.

R33
Prothrombin complex concentrate
***
PCC should be used early for the emergency reversal of vitamin K-dependent oral anticoagulants. PCC may be administered to mitigate life-threatening post-traumatic bleeding in patients treated with novel anticoagulants. If fibrinogen levels are normal, PCC or plasma may be administered in the bleeding patient based on evidence of delayed coagulation initiation using viscoelastic monitoring.

R34
Direct oral anticoagulants – FXa inhibitors
***
Plasma levels of oral anti-factor Xa agents such as rivaroxaban, apixaban or edoxaban may be measured in patients treated or suspected of being treated with one of these agents. If measurements are not possible or available advice from an expert haematologist may be sought. Life-threatening bleeding may be treated with i.v. TXA15 mg/kg (or 1 g) and high-dose (25-50 U/kg) PCC/aPCC until specific antidotes are available.

R35
Direct oral anticoagulants – Thrombin inhibitors
***
Dabigatran plasma levels may be measured in patients treated or suspected of being treated with dabigatran. If measurements are not possible or available thrombin time and APTT may be measured to allow a qualitative estimation of the presence of dabigatran. Life-threatening bleeding should be treated with idarucizumab (5 g i.v.) or if unavailable it may be treated with high-dose (25-50 U/kg) PCC / aPCC, in both cases combined with TXA 15 mg/kg (or 1 g) i.v.

R36
Recombinant activated coagulation factor VII
***
Off-label use of rFVIIa may be considered only if major bleeding and traumatic coagulopathy persist despite standard attempts to control bleeding and best practice use of conventional haemostatic measures.

R37
Thromboprophylaxis
***
Pharmacological thromboprophylaxis should be employed within 24 h after bleeding has been controlled. Early mechanical thromboprophylaxis with intermittent pneumatic compression should be applied and early mechanical thromboprophylaxis with anti-embolic stockings may be applied. Inferior vena cava filters as thromboprophylaxis should not be routinely employed.

Fig. 3. Recommendations of European Guideline on management of major bleeding and coagulopathy after trauma, 2016. APA, antiplatelet agents; aPCC, activated prothrombin complex concentrate; APTT, activated partial thromboplastin time; FFP, fresh frozen plasma; Hb, hemoglobin; PCC, prothrombin complex concentrate; PT, prothrombin time; RBC, red blood cells; rFVIIa, recombinant factor VIIa; TBI, traumatic brain injury; TXA, tranexamic acid. (*Adapted from* Rossaint R, Bouillon B, Cerny V, et al. The European guideline on management of major bleeding and coagulopathy following trauma: fourth edition. Crit Care 2016;20:100.)

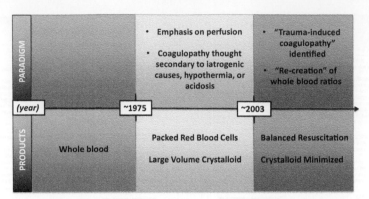

Fig. 4. Evolution of paradigms and resuscitation of injured patients over time. Early transfusion was conducted with whole blood. In the 1970s, resuscitation practice shifted toward an emphasis on perfusion with heavy use of large volumes of crystalloid and packed red blood cells (PRBC). Coagulopathy was understood to occur in severely injured patients but was not recognized as a distinct entity. Rather, it was attributed to iatrogenic dilution, hypothermia, or acidosis. In 2003, trauma-induced coagulopathy was identified as a distinct entity and treatment shifted away from crystalloid and toward balanced hemostatic resuscitation.

to platelet ratio remains undetermined; however, it remains clear that limitation of crystalloid and balanced product transfusion approximating whole blood improve outcomes and should be priorities of trauma resuscitation.

COMBINATION THERAPIES
Targeted Resuscitation Practice

A different paradigm for treatment of the patient with TIC proposes a targeted approach to resuscitation. In this approach, laboratory assays, including point-of-care TEG, are obtained in a serial fashion and used to guide product transfusion and administration of pharmaceutical adjuncts. This allows resuscitation to be tailored to the individual patient in real time, and coordinates the different modalities available for treatment. An additional advantage to this approach is the ability to provide dynamic management as the patient's condition changes. Objections to this approach include the need for infrastructure to support serial and rapid TEG assays, and that these tests depend on and vary by user skill and interpretation.

A recent Cochrane review suggested that there was insufficient evidence to recommend TEG-based transfusion guidelines as superior to established transfusion practice.[74] However, recently published prospective randomized data from the Denver group shows a mortality benefit when viscoelastic functional testing (TEG) was used to guide massive transfusion protocols compared with conventional coagulation assays (CCA).[75] Survival in the TEG group was significantly higher than the CCA group (28-day mortality 36.4% CCA vs 19.6% TEG) and 6-hour mortality was significantly lower in the TEG group (21.7% CCA vs 7.1% TEG; $P = .032$). Importantly, not all centers have access to TEG, and these centers should perform frequent serial measurements of PT/INR, PTT, platelets, hemoglobin/hematocrit, fibrinogen, and D-dimer to help guide resuscitation practice.

SURGICAL TREATMENT OPTIONS

Surgical management of trauma coagulopathy should be directed toward prompt cessation of any anatomic causes of hemorrhage, and thereby avoidance of what has been termed the "lethal triad" of coagulopathy, hypothermia, and acidosis.

TREATMENT RESISTANCE AND COMPLICATIONS
Compounding Coagulopathy

If prompt diagnosis and tailored resuscitation fails to improve TIC, compounding etiologies of coagulopathy should be strongly suspected. These can include hypothermia, acidosis, hemodilution, DIC, and heritable coagulopathies. Treatment includes the approaches described, as well as the following considerations.

Hypothermia

Hypothermia (temperature <36°C) is present in approximately two-thirds of injured patients on admission, and 9% of patients present with severe hypothermia (temperature <33°C) owing to a combination of exposure in the field and during transport and administration of cold intravenous fluids.[76] Patients are at further risk for worsening of hypothermia in the emergency room and operating room, if necessary. Mild to moderate hypothermia (temperature 33°C–36°C) results in impaired platelet aggregation and adhesion and decreased tissue factor activity leading to coagulopathy that is typically not detectable using standard or functional coagulations assays as samples are routinely warmed before testing.[77] Therefore, it is essential to maintain a high level of vigilance against hypothermia with continuous temperature monitoring. All trauma patients should receive passive rewarming with removal of clothing and application warmed blankets, as well as warming of administered fluids. Central warming should be considered in cases of severe or resistant hypothermia.

Acidosis

Severely injured patients frequently present with or develop acidosis during the course of their resuscitation. Assembly of functional coagulation factor complexes are inhibited in acidotic environments (pH <7.2) with increasing dysfunction as acidosis worsens.[78,79] Arterial blood gas should be obtained at admission and repeated at serial time points throughout resuscitation with correction of acidosis as necessary.

Hemodilution

Dilutional coagulopathy, also known as "iatrogenic" or "resuscitation–associated coagulopathy" occurs when coagulation factor proteins are diluted by large volumes of crystalloid, colloid, or PRBCs. Coagulation factor dilution with large volume administration has been demonstrated in multiple laboratory, modeling and healthy control studies.[80–82] Retrospective data have shown admission coagulopathy to be significantly more prevalent among injured patients who received more than 3 L of prehospital fluids compared with those who received little (<500 mL) or no volume.[4] To avoid dilutional coagulopathy, resuscitation should consist primarily of balanced product transfusion with frequent monitoring of ongoing coagulation status. Crystalloid should no longer be considered a resuscitation fluid and only used to facilitate administration of medications and blood products.

Disseminated intravascular coagulation

Disseminated intravascular coagulation (DIC) occurs as a result of systemic microvascular thrombosis causing severe consumptive coagulopathy. Although now understood to be a distinct pathology, some features of DIC overlap with traumatic coagulopathy, making diagnosis challenging. Trauma patient are at increased risk for DIC owing to the potential for embolization of tissue-specific thromboplastin after long bone fractures, amniotic disruption, or brain injury, or later in the clinical course as a result of sepsis. DIC should be considered as an alternate or concomitant etiology of late, recurrent, or treatment-resistant coagulopathy in the severely injured patient, but is not a cause of acute traumatic coagulopathy.

EVALUATION OF OUTCOME AND LONG-TERM RECOMMENDATIONS

Outcomes after treatment of TIC should be assessed by:

1. Improvement in the clinical condition of the injured patient including a trend toward global hemostasis and hemodynamic stability and
2. Reversal of standard and functional laboratory coagulation abnormalities.

Despite advances in the understanding, diagnosis, and resuscitation of injured patients with TIC, patients with traumatic coagulopathy go on to have worse outcomes than noncoagulopathic patients.

Transfusion Requirements

Compared with noncoagulopathic patients, patients with TIC receive substantially increased blood product transfusion,[10] which independently confers a greater risk of complications such as acute respiratory distress syndrome,[83] systemic inflammatory response syndrome,[84] and mortality after injury.[85] As noted, there is no consensus regarding ideal ratios of resuscitation; however, ongoing observational experience from institutions with massive transfusion protocols have described decreased crystalloid and overall product use, and lower PRBC:FFP ratios with concomitant survival benefit.[86]

Hypercoagulability

Multiple investigators have reported an increased incidence of thromboembolic complications in patients with early TIC.[36,87] Given the potential risks of anticoagulation in this patient population, multiple scoring systems including the Trauma Embolic Scoring System and the Risk Assessment Profile have attempted to stratify patients at high risk for venous thromboembolism (VTE), but recent retrospective data suggest that scoring systems often fail to discriminate between patients who go on to develop VTE.[88] It also remains unclear whether standard or functional assays can accurately predict clinically significant hypercoagulability in critically ill trauma patients.[89] Many studies investigating VTE in trauma patients relay on duplex screening, and the significance of these incidentally discovered events remains unknown. Finally, there has not been sufficient evidence to definitively establish whether standard chemoprophylaxis is efficacious in mitigating thromboembolic risk in this population.[90] Further prospective clinical studies are necessary to better delineate the mechanism of VTE in previously coagulopathic trauma patients and to identify potential targets for prevention and treatment.

Acute Lung Injury, Multiorgan Failure, and Death

Despite substantive progress in delineation of the mechanism of TIC and improved outcomes resulting from changes in resuscitation practice, patients with traumatic coagulopathy have vastly increased rates of acute lung injury, multiorgan failure, and death. Unsurprisingly, these patients also have worse hospital metrics, including more days spent on the ventilator, in the intensive care unit, and in the hospital than do noncoagulopathic patients. This highlights the need for continued research efforts and clinical innovation to combat this considerable clinical challenge and improve outcomes. One potential approach is through focus on individualization of diagnosis and resuscitation. As discussed, there is evidence to suggest that traumatic coagulopathy is not a single entity, but rather consists of multiple phenotypes with unique implications for outcomes and management.

SUMMARY

- TIC is an endogenous hypocoagulable state distinct from iatrogenic, dilution, or hypothermic causes.
- Activation of the protein C pathway is a key mechanistic mediator of TIC via multiple downstream effects including thrombin diversion, deactivation of coagulation factors, and de-repression of fibrinolysis.
- Standard coagulation tests and functional viscoelastic assays are commonly used in the diagnosis and management of TIC.
- Balanced resuscitation is the mainstay of TIC treatment, but precise ratios for empiric resuscitation and optimal monitoring protocols for transfusion practice remain hotly debated.
- Patients with TIC have worse outcomes including increased rates of transfusion, infection, thromboembolism, acute lung injury, multiorgan failure, and death.

REFERENCES

1. Sauaia A, Moore FA, Moore EE, et al. Epidemiology of trauma deaths: a reassessment. J Trauma 1995;38(2):185–93.
2. Brohi K, Singh J, Heron M, et al. Acute traumatic coagulopathy. J Trauma 2003; 54(6):1127–30.
3. MacLeod JB, Lynn M, McKenney MG, et al. Early coagulopathy predicts mortality in trauma. J Trauma 2003;55(1):39–44.
4. Maegele M, Lefering R, Yucel N, et al. Early coagulopathy in multiple injury: an analysis from the German Trauma Registry on 8724 patients. Injury 2007;38(3): 298–304.
5. Cohen MJ, Bir N, Rahn P, et al. Protein C depletion early after trauma increases the risk of ventilator-associated pneumonia. J Trauma 2009;67(6):1176–81.
6. Cohen MJ, Call M, Nelson M, et al. Critical role of activated protein C in early coagulopathy and later organ failure, infection and death in trauma patients. Ann Surg 2012;255(2):379–85.
7. Hess JR, Brohi K, Dutton RP, et al. The coagulopathy of trauma: a review of mechanisms. J Trauma 2008;65(4):748–54.
8. Kirkpatrick AW, Chun R, Brown R, et al. Hypothermia and the trauma patient. Can J Surg 1999;42(5):333–43.
9. Kutcher ME, Ferguson AR, Cohen MJ. A principal component analysis of coagulation after trauma. J Trauma Acute Care Surg 2013;74(5):1223–9 [discussion: 1229–30].
10. Brohi K, Cohen MJ, Ganter MT, et al. Acute traumatic coagulopathy: initiated by hypoperfusion: modulated through the protein C pathway? Ann Surg 2007; 245(5):812–8.
11. Cohen MJ, Kutcher M, Redick B, et al. Clinical and mechanistic drivers of acute traumatic coagulopathy. J Trauma Acute Care Surg 2013;75(1 Suppl 1):S40–7.
12. Chesebro BB, Rahn P, Carles M, et al. Increase in activated protein C mediates acute traumatic coagulopathy in mice. Shock 2009;32(6):659–65.
13. Esmon CT. Protein C pathway in sepsis. Ann Med 2002;34(7–8):598–605.

14. Rezaie AR. Vitronectin functions as a cofactor for rapid inhibition of activated protein C by plasminogen activator inhibitor-1. Implications for the mechanism of profibrinolytic action of activated protein C. J Biol Chem 2001;276(19):15567–70.

15. Bajzar L, Jain N, Wang P, et al. Thrombin activatable fibrinolysis inhibitor: not just an inhibitor of fibrinolysis. Crit Care Med 2004;32(5 Suppl):S320–4.

16. Schochl H, Frietsch T, Pavelka M, et al. Hyperfibrinolysis after major trauma: differential diagnosis of lysis patterns and prognostic value of thrombelastometry. J Trauma 2009;67(1):125–31.

17. Kashuk JL, Moore EE, Sawyer M, et al. Primary fibrinolysis is integral in the pathogenesis of the acute coagulopathy of trauma. Ann Surg 2010;252(3):434–42 [discussion: 443–4].

18. Cotton BA, Harvin JA, Kostousouv V, et al. Hyperfibrinolysis at admission is an uncommon but highly lethal event associated with shock and prehospital fluid administration. J Trauma Acute Care Surg 2012;73(2):365–70 [discussion: 370].

19. Chapman MP, Moore EE, Ramos CR, et al. Fibrinolysis greater than 3% is the critical value for initiation of antifibrinolytic therapy. J Trauma Acute Care Surg 2013; 75(6):961–7 [discussion: 967].

20. Moore HB, Moore EE, Gonzalez E, et al. Hyperfibrinolysis, physiologic fibrinolysis, and fibrinolysis shutdown: the spectrum of postinjury fibrinolysis and relevance to antifibrinolytic therapy. J Trauma Acute Care Surg 2014;77(6):811–7 [discussion: 817].

21. Moore HB, Moore EE, Liras IN, et al. Acute fibrinolysis shutdown after injury occurs frequently and increases mortality: a multicenter evaluation of 2,540 severely injured patients. J Am Coll Surg 2016;222(4):347–55.

22. Davenport RA, Brohi K. Coagulopathy in trauma patients: importance of thrombocyte function? Curr Opin Anaesthesiol 2009;22(2):261–6.

23. Brown LM, Call MS, Margaret Knudson M, et al. A normal platelet count may not be enough: the impact of admission platelet count on mortality and transfusion in severely injured trauma patients. J Trauma 2011;71(2 Suppl 3):S337–42.

24. Stansbury LG, Hess AS, Thompson K, et al. The clinical significance of platelet counts in the first 24 hours after severe injury. Transfusion 2013;53(4):783–9.

25. Jacoby RC, Owings JT, Holmes J, et al. Platelet activation and function after trauma. J Trauma 2001;51(4):639–47.

26. Wohlauer MV, Moore EE, Thomas S, et al. Early platelet dysfunction: an unrecognized role in the acute coagulopathy of trauma. J Am Coll Surg 2012;214(5): 739–46.

27. Kutcher ME, Redick BJ, McCreery RC, et al. Characterization of platelet dysfunction after trauma. J Trauma Acute Care Surg 2012;73(1):13–9.

28. Sillesen M, Johansson PI, Rasmussen LS, et al. Platelet activation and dysfunction in a large-animal model of traumatic brain injury and hemorrhage. J Trauma Acute Care Surg 2013;74(5):1252–9.

29. Solomon C, Traintinger S, Ziegler B, et al. Platelet function following trauma. A multiple electrode aggregometry study. Thromb Haemost 2011;106(2):322–30.

30. Johansson PI, Stensballe J, Rasmussen LS, et al. A high admission syndecan-1 level, a marker of endothelial glycocalyx degradation, is associated with inflammation, protein C depletion, fibrinolysis, and increased mortality in trauma patients. Ann Surg 2011;254(2):194–200.

31. Matijevic N, Wang YW, Wade CE, et al. Cellular microparticle and thrombogram phenotypes in the Prospective Observational Multicenter Major Trauma Transfusion (PROMMTT) study: correlation with coagulopathy. Thromb Res 2014; 134(3):652–8.

32. Nekludov M, Mobarrez F, Gryth D, et al. Formation of microparticles in the injured brain of patients with severe isolated traumatic brain injury. J Neurotrauma 2014; 31(23):1927–33.

33. Hoyt DB, Dutton RP, Hauser CJ, et al. Management of coagulopathy in the patients with multiple injuries: results from an international survey of clinical practice. J Trauma 2008;65(4):755–64 [discussion: 764–5].

34. Brohi K, Cohen MJ, Davenport RA. Acute coagulopathy of trauma: mechanism, identification and effect. Curr Opin Crit Care 2007;13(6):680–5.

35. Kashuk JL, Moore EE, Johnson JL, et al. Postinjury life threatening coagulopathy: is 1:1 fresh frozen plasma:packed red blood cells the answer? J Trauma 2008; 65(2):261–70 [discussion: 270–1].

36. Peltan ID, Vande Vusse LK, Maier RV, et al. An International normalized ratio-based definition of acute traumatic coagulopathy is associated with mortality, venous thromboembolism, and multiple organ failure after injury. Crit Care Med 2015;43(7):1429–38.

37. Kaufmann CR, Dwyer KM, Crews JD, et al. Usefulness of thrombelastography in assessment of trauma patient coagulation. J Trauma 1997;42(4):716–20 [discussion: 720–2].

38. Carroll RC, Craft RM, Langdon RJ, et al. Early evaluation of acute traumatic coagulopathy by thrombelastography. Transl Res 2009;154(1):34–9.

39. Rugeri L, Levrat A, David JS, et al. Diagnosis of early coagulation abnormalities in trauma patients by rotation thrombelastography. J Thromb Haemost 2007;5(2): 289–95.

40. Cotton BA, Faz G, Hatch QM, et al. Rapid thrombelastography delivers real-time results that predict transfusion within 1 hour of admission. J Trauma 2011;71(2): 407–14 [discussion: 414–7].

41. Rivard GE, Brummel-Ziedins KE, Mann KG, et al. Evaluation of the profile of thrombin generation during the process of whole blood clotting as assessed by thrombelastography. J Thromb Haemost 2005;3(9):2039–43.

42. Levrat A, Gros A, Rugeri L, et al. Evaluation of rotation thrombelastography for the diagnosis of hyperfibrinolysis in trauma patients. Br J Anaesth 2008;100(6): 792–7.

43. Raza I, Davenport R, Rourke C, et al. The incidence and magnitude of fibrinolytic activation in trauma patients. J Thromb Haemost 2013;11(2):307–14.

44. Yucel N, Lefering R, Maegele M, et al. Trauma Associated Severe Hemorrhage (TASH)-Score: probability of mass transfusion as surrogate for life threatening hemorrhage after multiple trauma. J Trauma 2006;60(6):1228–36 [discussion: 1236–7].

45. McLaughlin DF, Niles SE, Salinas J, et al. A predictive model for massive transfusion in combat casualty patients. J Trauma 2008;64(2 Suppl):S57–63 [discussion: S63].

46. Nunez TC, Voskresensky IV, Dossett LA, et al. Early prediction of massive transfusion in trauma: simple as ABC (assessment of blood consumption)? J Trauma 2009;66(2):346–52.

47. CRASH-2 trial collaborators, Shakur H, Roberts I, Bautista R, et al. Effects of tranexamic acid on death, vascular occlusive events, and blood transfusion in trauma patients with significant haemorrhage (CRASH-2): a randomised, placebo-controlled trial. Lancet 2010;376(9734):23–32.

48. Morrison JJ, Dubose JJ, Rasmussen TE, et al. Military Application of Tranexamic Acid in Trauma Emergency Resuscitation (MATTERs) Study. Arch Surg 2012; 147(2):113–9.

49. Napolitano LM, Cohen MJ, Cotton BA, et al. Tranexamic acid in trauma: how should we use it? J Trauma Acute Care Surg 2013;74(6):1575–86.
50. Chowdary P, Saayman AG, Paulus U, et al. Efficacy of standard dose and 30 ml/kg fresh frozen plasma in correcting laboratory parameters of haemostasis in critically ill patients. Br J Haematol 2004;125(1):69–73.
51. Cardigan R, Lawrie AS, Mackie IJ, et al. The quality of fresh-frozen plasma produced from whole blood stored at 4 degrees C overnight. Transfusion 2005; 45(8):1342–8.
52. Stanworth SJ. The evidence-based use of FFP and cryoprecipitate for abnormalities of coagulation tests and clinical coagulopathy. Hematology Am Soc Hematol Educ Program 2007;179–86.
53. Abdel-Wahab OI, Healy B, Dzik WH. Effect of fresh-frozen plasma transfusion on prothrombin time and bleeding in patients with mild coagulation abnormalities. Transfusion 2006;46(8):1279–85.
54. Holland LL, Brooks JP. Toward rational fresh frozen plasma transfusion: the effect of plasma transfusion on coagulation test results. Am J Clin Pathol 2006;126(1): 133–9.
55. Kor DJ, Stubbs JR, Gajic O. Perioperative coagulation management–fresh frozen plasma. Best Pract Res Clin Anaesthesiol 2010;24(1):51–64.
56. Toy P, Gajic O, Bacchetti P, et al. Transfusion-related acute lung injury: incidence and risk factors. Blood 2012;119(7):1757–67.
57. Levi M, Levy JH, Andersen HF, et al. Safety of recombinant activated factor VII in randomized clinical trials. N Engl J Med 2010;363(19):1791–800.
58. Marlu R, Hodaj E, Paris A, et al. Effect of non-specific reversal agents on anticoagulant activity of dabigatran and rivaroxaban: a randomised crossover ex vivo study in healthy volunteers. Thromb Haemost 2012;108(2):217–24.
59. Gorlinger K, Dirkmann D, Hanke AA, et al. First-line therapy with coagulation factor concentrates combined with point-of-care coagulation testing is associated with decreased allogeneic blood transfusion in cardiovascular surgery: a retrospective, single-center cohort study. Anesthesiology 2011;115(6):1179–91.
60. Tanaka KA, Mazzeffi M, Durila M. Role of prothrombin complex concentrate in perioperative coagulation therapy. J Intensive Care 2014;2(1):60.
61. Dickneite G, Pragst I. Prothrombin complex concentrate vs fresh frozen plasma for reversal of dilutional coagulopathy in a porcine trauma model. Br J Anaesth 2009;102(3):345–54.
62. Schochl H, Nienaber U, Hofer G, et al. Goal-directed coagulation management of major trauma patients using thromboelastometry (ROTEM)-guided administration of fibrinogen concentrate and prothrombin complex concentrate. Crit Care 2010; 14(2):R55.
63. Joseph B, Pandit V, Khalil M, et al. Use of prothrombin complex concentrate as an adjunct to fresh frozen plasma shortens time to craniotomy in traumatic brain injury patients. Neurosurgery 2015;76(5):601–7 [discussion: 607].
64. Rourke C, Curry N, Khan S, et al. Fibrinogen levels during trauma hemorrhage, response to replacement therapy, and association with patient outcomes. J Thromb Haemost 2012;10:1342–51.
65. Theusinger OM, Baulig W, Seifert B, et al. Relative concentrations of haemostatic factors and cytokines in solvent/detergent-treated and fresh-frozen plasma. Br J Anaesth 2011;106(4):505–11.
66. Schlimp CJ, Voelckel W, Inaba K, et al. Impact of fibrinogen concentrate alone or with prothrombin complex concentrate (+/- fresh frozen plasma) on plasma

fibrinogen level and fibrin-based clot strength (FIBTEM) in major trauma: a retrospective study. Scand J Trauma Resusc Emerg Med 2013;21:74.

67. Rossaint R, Bouillon B, Cerny V, et al. The European Guideline on management of major bleeding and coagulopathy following trauma: fourth edition. Crit Care 2016;20:100.

68. Duchesne JC, Kimonis K, Marr AB, et al. Damage control resuscitation in combination with damage control laparotomy: a survival advantage. J Trauma 2010; 69(1):46–52.

69. Borgman MA, Spinella PC, Perkins JG, et al. The ratio of blood products transfused affects mortality in patients receiving massive transfusions at a combat support hospital. J Trauma 2007;63(4):805–13.

70. de Biasi AR, Stansbury LG, Dutton RP, et al. Blood product use in trauma resuscitation: plasma deficit versus plasma ratio as predictors of mortality in trauma (CME). Transfusion 2011;51(9):1925–32.

71. Brown LM, Aro SO, Cohen MJ, et al. A high fresh frozen plasma: packed red blood cell transfusion ratio decreases mortality in all massively transfused trauma patients regardless of admission international normalized ratio. J Trauma 2011; 71(2 Suppl 3):S358–63.

72. Holcomb JB, del Junco DJ, Fox EE, et al. The prospective, observational, multicenter, major trauma transfusion (PROMMTT) study: comparative effectiveness of a time-varying treatment with competing risks. JAMA Surg 2013;148(2): 127–36.

73. Holcomb JB, Tilley BC, Baraniuk S, et al. Transfusion of plasma, platelets, and red blood cells in a 1:1:1 vs a 1:1:2 ratio and mortality in patients with severe trauma: the PROPPR randomized clinical trial. JAMA 2015;313(5):471–82.

74. Hunt H, Stanworth S, Curry N, et al. Thromboelastography (TEG) and rotational thromboelastometry (ROTEM) for trauma induced coagulopathy in adult trauma patients with bleeding. Cochrane Database Syst Rev 2015;(2):CD010438.

75. Gonzalez E, Moore EE, Moore HB, et al. Goal-directed hemostatic resuscitation of trauma-induced coagulopathy: a pragmatic randomized clinical trial comparing a viscoelastic assay to conventional coagulation assays. Ann Surg 2016;263(6): 1051–9.

76. Tsuei BJ, Kearney PA. Hypothermia in the trauma patient. Injury 2004;35(1):7–15.

77. Wolberg AS, Meng ZH, Monroe DM 3rd, et al. A systematic evaluation of the effect of temperature on coagulation enzyme activity and platelet function. J Trauma 2004;56(6):1221–8.

78. Martini WZ. Coagulopathy by hypothermia and acidosis: mechanisms of thrombin generation and fibrinogen availability. J Trauma 2009;67(1):202–8 [discussion: 208–9].

79. Engstrom M, Schott U, Romner B, et al. Acidosis impairs the coagulation: a thromboelastographic study. J Trauma 2006;61(3):624–8.

80. Hirshberg A, Dugas M, Banez EI, et al. Minimizing dilutional coagulopathy in exsanguinating hemorrhage: a computer simulation. J Trauma 2003;54(3):454–63.

81. Coats TJ, Brazil E, Heron M. The effects of commonly used resuscitation fluids on whole blood coagulation. Emerg Med J 2006;23(7):546–9.

82. Brazil EV, Coats TJ. Sonoclot coagulation analysis of in-vitro haemodilution with resuscitation solutions. J R Soc Med 2000;93(10):507–10.

83. Silverboard H, Aisiku I, Martin GS, et al. The role of acute blood transfusion in the development of acute respiratory distress syndrome in patients with severe trauma. J Trauma 2005;59(3):717–23.

84. Dunne JR, Malone DL, Tracy JK, et al. Allogenic blood transfusion in the first 24 hours after trauma is associated with increased systemic inflammatory response syndrome (SIRS) and death. Surg Infect (Larchmt) 2004;5(4):395–404.
85. Charles A, Shaikh AA, Walters M, et al. Blood transfusion is an independent predictor of mortality after blunt trauma. Am Surg 2007;73(1):1–5.
86. Kutcher ME, Kornblith LZ, Narayan R, et al. A paradigm shift in trauma resuscitation: evaluation of evolving massive transfusion practices. JAMA Surg 2013; 148(9):834–40.
87. Knudson MM, Collins JA, Goodman SB, et al. Thromboembolism following multiple trauma. J Trauma 1992;32(1):2–11.
88. Zander AL, Van Gent JM, Olson EJ, et al. Venous thromboembolic risk assessment models should not solely guide prophylaxis and surveillance in trauma patients. J Trauma Acute Care Surg 2015;79(2):194–8.
89. Van Haren RM, Valle EJ, Thorson CM, et al. Hypercoagulability and other risk factors in trauma intensive care unit patients with venous thromboembolism. J Trauma Acute Care Surg 2014;76(2):443–9.
90. Allen CJ, Murray CR, Meizoso JP, et al. Coagulation profile changes due to thromboprophylaxis and platelets in trauma patients at high-risk for venous thromboembolism. Am Surg 2015;81(7):663–8.

Management of Trauma-Induced Coagulopathy with Thrombelastography

Eduardo Gonzalez, MD[a], Ernest E. Moore, MD[a,b,c],*,
Hunter B. Moore, MD[a]

KEYWORDS

- Coagulopathy • Resuscitation • Thrombelastography • TEG • Fibrinolysis
- Transfusion

KEY POINTS

- Thrombelastography characterizes the life-span of a clot; from initial fibrin formation, to incorporation of platelets, to fibrinolysis.
- Thrombelastography yields the following real-time coagulation variables: reaction time (R-time), activated clotting time (ACT), rate of clot formation angle (angle), maximum amplitude (MA), and clot lysis at 30 minutes (LY30).
- These point-of-care variables enable the clinician with "live" management-driving data in the trauma bay, allowing for goal-directed hemostatic resuscitation of bleeding injured patients.
- A recent clinical trial demonstrated that the use of thrombelastography to guide massive transfusion in trauma patients, compared with conventional coagulation assays, resulted in a decrease in mortality while using less blood products.
- Thrombelastography is currently used for patient-personalized administration of antifibrinolytics (eg, tranexamic acid) based on LY30 parameters.

The authors E. Gonzalez, E.E. Moore, and H.B. Moore report support from Haemonetics Inc and TEM International GmbH in the way of laboratory reagents, which had no role in the conception or preparation of this article. The authors' work is funded by grant support from National Institute of General Medical Sciences (P50 GM049222 and T32 GM008315-21); National Heart, Lung, and Blood Institute (UM1 HL120877); Department of Defense (W81XWH 12-2-0028).
^a Department of Surgery, University of Colorado, 12700 East 19th Avenue, Denver, CO 80045, USA; ^b Department of Surgery, Denver Health Medical Center, 77 Bannock Street, Denver, CO 80204, USA; ^c Editorial office, Journal of Trauma and Acute Care Surgery, 655 Broadway, Suite 365, Denver, CO 80203, USA
* Corresponding author. Journal of Trauma and Acute Care Surgery, 655 Broadway, Suite 365, Denver, CO 80203.
E-mail address: ernest.moore@dhha.org

INTRODUCTION

Contemporary trauma care comprises advanced prehospital care, regionalized trauma systems, damage control operative techniques, advanced critical care, rehabilitation with reintegration into society, and injury prevention.[1,2] Despite these efforts, deaths from injury have increased in the United States over the last decade relative to other causes of mortality.[3,4] To make strides in trauma outcomes this high mortality of severe injuries must be mitigated.

Injury mortality was classically described as having a trimodal distribution with immediate deaths at the scene, early deaths caused by hemorrhage, and late deaths caused by organ dysfunction.[5] Damage control surgery and advances in critical care have decreased the incidence and severity of organ dysfunction after injury,[6,7] although it is arguable that immediate deaths at the scene can only be addressed through injury prevention. Thus, deaths caused by hemorrhage continue to represent a target for intervention to mitigate mortality from severe injuries. Recent studies analyzing the time course of hemorrhage-related mortality report that these deaths occur despite ongoing therapies of resuscitation.[8] Such data call for a paradigm shift in the resuscitation of patients with injury-related hemorrhage.

Resuscitation from hemorrhage is compounded by dysfunctional hemostasis seen in severely injured patients,[9,10] hindering the effectiveness of resuscitation and damage and bleeding control surgery if patients are not resuscitated from this coagulopathy. Thus, in the severely injured patient hemodynamic and hemostatic resuscitation go hand in hand. Furthermore, experimental and clinical data exist to suggest that some current resuscitation strategies, particularly the use of crystalloid and colloid fluids, may in fact exacerbate coagulopathy and further worsen bleeding.[11–15]

In this context, viscoelastic assays, such as thrombelastography (TEG) and rotational thrombelastometry (ROTEM), have emerged as point-of-care tools that can guide the hemostatic resuscitation of bleeding injured patients.[16] These assays provide information about patients' coagulation status, which paired with other point-of-care available assays, such as hemoglobin and blood gas, enable the clinician with early management-driving data in the trauma bay. Furthermore, TEG and ROTEM assessments can be continued in the point-of-care mode into patients' anesthesia course in the operating room and during resuscitation and recovery in the critical care unit. Recently, a randomized clinical trial demonstrated that the use of TEG to guide a massive transfusion protocol (MTP) in trauma patients, compared with conventional coagulation assays (CCA) (ie, international normalized ratio of prothrombin time [PT/INR], partial thromboplastin time [PTT], fibrinogen level, platelet count), resulted in a statistically significant decrease in mortality while using less plasma and platelet blood products.[17]

This article describes the role of TEG in contemporary trauma care by explaining this assay' methodology, clinical applications, and result interpretation through description of supporting studies to provide the reader with an evidence-based user's guide. Although TEG and ROTEM are assays based on the same viscoelastic principle, this article is focused on data supporting the use of TEG in trauma, because it is available in trauma centers in North America; ROTEM is mostly available in Europe.

HISTORICAL CONTEXT

Hartert[18] conceived TEG in Germany, at the Heidelberg University School of Medicine in 1948. TEG was applied increasingly throughout Europe during the 1950s, validating its use for assessment of anticoagulant effect, effect of thrombocytopenia, fibrinolysis, and monitoring of coagulation during liver transplantation.[19,20] The first report on the use of TEG outside of Europe came from Henry Swan at the University of Colorado, who in 1958 published on the use of TEG to characterize the effects of hypothermia and cardiopulmonary bypass during cardiac surgery.[21] Subsequently, Thomas Starzl used TEG to detect fibrinolysis during the anhepatic phase of liver transplantation.[22,23] It gained further applicability for monitoring heparinization during cardiopulmonary bypass and was also found beneficial for predicting postoperative bleeding.[24] TEG gained additional acceptance as a tool for assessment of coagulation in the general surgical patient, permitting differentiation of coagulopathy from surgical bleeding.[25]

ASSAY METHODOLOGY

The first descriptions on the methodology of this assay refer to TEG as "Hartert's instrument."[20] The principles on which TEG is currently based remain the same since that time. In the current TEG system (Analyzer 5000, Haemonetics, Braintree, MA), a cylindrical plastic cup containing a 360 µL whole blood sample oscillates through 4°45' (0.1 Hz) and a pin on a torsion wire is suspended in the blood (**Fig. 1**). Initially, movement of the cuvette does not affect the pin, but as the clot develops, resistance from the developing fibrin strands couples the pin to the motion of the cuvette. As the viscoelastic strength of the clot increases more rotation torque is transmitted to the torsion wire and detected by an electromagnetic transducer. The transducer signal is then interpreted by TEG software, which represents such changes as the characteristic TEG tracing. The first iteration of TEG used a light beam paired to the pin in motion; movement of the light beam was optically recorded through a visible scale on a roll film. The distance between the lines represents the degree of firmness with which the cup is bound to the pin. If the clot subsequently undergoes lysis, this is recorded as a decrease in amplitude, consequently decreasing the distance between the lines. These changes in amplitude are plotted as a function of time. The current instrument allows near real time data gathering with most results available between 10 and 30 minutes after blood draw. Most institutions transmit a "live" TEG tracing to the emergency department trauma bay and operating room via computer, enabling prompt interpretation for goal-directed therapy.

TEG analysis is performed on whole blood with no anticoagulant (native), whole blood collected into sodium citrate 3.2% (0.109 mol/L; nine volumes blood to one volume anticoagulant), and whole blood collected into heparin (>14.5 IU heparin/mL of blood sample). There has been growing interest in the effects of citrate on

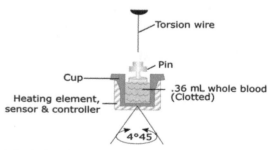

Fig. 1. TEG cup and pin design. (TEG Hemostasis Analyzer Operating Principle image is used by permission of Haemonetics Corporation. TEG® and Thromboelastograph® are registered trademarks of Haemonetics Corporation in the US, other countries or both.)

thrombelastographic profiles, and whether citrate can introduce variation to interpretation of results. Studies on healthy volunteers performing serial TEG assays at different time points from collection show that citrated samples produce variable results when the assay is performed within 5 minutes from sample collection but stabilize thereafter for up to 2 hours.[26–29]

The first step in preparing a sample to execute a TEG assay is to identify the method of collection; that is, whether or not the sample is anticoagulated. For samples collected with no anticoagulant, the assay must be performed as soon as possible, and recommended within 4 minutes from sample collection. For samples collected in citrate, the assay must be performed between 5 minutes and 2 hours from collection. Most centers adopt a 30-minute time from collection for citrated samples; this standardizes practice and allows for logistics of transportation and quality control of instruments. However, data have demonstrated no changes in coagulation profiles when performed as early as 5 minutes from collection,[26,30] allowing for the use of citrated samples when TEG is performed at point-of-care in trauma settings. Citrated samples are recalcified immediately before assay initiation. This is done by placing 20 µL of calcium chloride (0.2 M) into the plastic TEG cup followed by addition of the whole blood sample. The instrument is adjusted to match the patient's core temperature, which is useful during cardiopulmonary bypass and intraoperative protective hypothermia. Some clinicians, in such situations as trauma, prefer to run the assay at the ideal temperature of 37°C to assess the hemostasis at the goal temperature to which the patient will be resuscitated.

ASSAY INTERPRETATION

Based on time-resistance associations, the following TEG variables are obtained: reaction time (R-time), activated clotting time (ACT), coagulation time (K-time), angle, maximum amplitude (MA), and lysis at 30 minutes (LY30). Of note, the TEG variables that have been clinically validated and are routinely used in clinical practice are R-time, ACT, angle, MA, and LY30; other variables are mostly used for research purposes. A characteristic TEG tracing is shown in **Fig. 2**. A summary of the most commonly used TEG variables is shown in **Table 1**.

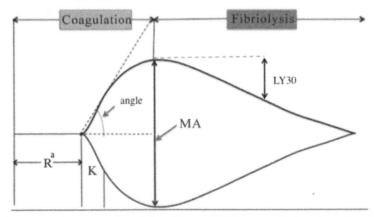

Fig. 2. Characteristic TEG tracing. [a] For the rapid-TEG assay, R-time is replaced by ACT. (*Adapted from* Trapani L. Thromboelastography: current applications, future directions. Open J Anesthesiol 2013;3(1):23–7; with permission.)

Table 1
TEG variables most commonly used in clinical practice

TEG Variable	Significance	Unit of Measure
R-time	Time elapsed from the initiation of the test until the point where the onset of clotting provides enough resistance to produce a 2-mm amplitude reading on the TEG tracing.	Minutes
ACT	Used as a surrogate of R-time in the rapid-TEG assay, which uses tissue factor to obtain a quicker reading.	Seconds
Angle	Angle of a tangent line between the initial split point of the tracing and the growing curve. Reflects potentiation phase of enzymatic factors yielding clot strengthening mostly derived from fibrinogen cleavage and fibrin polymerization.	Degrees
MA	Point at which clot strength reaches its maximum measure in millimeters on the TEG tracing; reflects the end result of maximal platelet-fibrin interactions.	Millimeters
LY30	Percentage of clot strength amplitude lost 30 min after reaching maximal amplitude; reflects amount of fibrinolysis.	Percent

Reaction Time

R-time (or gelation time) represents the latent period from the beginning of the TEG assay to the establishment of a three-dimensional fibrin gel network with measurable rigidity of amplitude of 2 mm. This variable has also been referred to as the clot initiation time. R-time is measured in minutes and has been suggested to be analogous to PT/INR and PTT, although results are not interchangeable. R-time reflects coagulation factor activity. Nielsen and colleagues[31] undertook a study performing TEG on plasma with specific coagulation factor deficiencies (II, VII, X, XII). Of all TEG variables analyzed, R-time was the most affected by these deficiencies. In a study performed in severe hemophiliacs receiving recombinant factor VIII prophylaxis for bleeding, TEG and a thrombin generation assay were performed to characterize the viscoelastic response of hemophiliac blood to factor VIII. Both TEG R-time and log thrombin generation velocity demonstrated a strong correlation with factor VIII activity (R = −0.81, P = .001; and R = −0.90, P = .001, respectively). R-time is currently used in clinical algorithms and protocols to trigger plasma transfusion.[32]

Activated Clotting Time

ACT is a variable that is exclusive to the rapid-TEG assay. Because of the rapidity of clotting in rapid-TEG, the R-time (expressed in minutes) is extremely small, and the range is narrow. Because of this, an ACT time is derived in seconds, providing a broader range that allows for defining normal and abnormal values.[33] ACT and R-time are thought to represent the same phase of hemostasis. Cotton and colleagues[34] performed a prospective observational study in 583 consecutive trauma patients (median injury severity score [ISS], 14) using rapid-TEG on arrival. ACT had a significant correlation with INR and PTT (R = 0.71 and 0.75, respectively). Linear regression demonstrated that ACT predicted red blood cell, plasma, and platelet transfusions within the first 2 hours of arrival. Controlling for demographics and arrival vital signs, an ACT greater than 128 seconds predicted massive transfusion (≥10 blood product units in the first 6 hours; odds ratio, 5.1; 95% confidence interval, 1.3–19.4). In addition, an ACT less than 105 seconds predicted patients who did not require any transfusions in the first 24 hours (odds ratio, 2.80; 95% confidence interval, 1.02–7.07). A recent study from our group has demonstrated that in trauma patients, an ACT greater than 140 seconds can predict the angle and MA being abnormal.[33] Correspondingly, patients with an ACT greater than 140 seconds required more cryoprecipitate and platelet transfusions. Thus, an ACT being available within 5 minutes allows for early delivery of cryoprecipitate and platelets units to the bedside based solely on ACT, before angle and MA are reported. This strategy has been adopted at our institution. ACT is currently used in clinical algorithms and protocols to trigger plasma transfusion.

Coagulation Time

The K time is a measurement of the time interval from the R-time (2-mm tracing amplitude) to the point where fibrin cross-linking provides enough clot resistance to produce a 20-mm amplitude reading. It is thought to represent the propagation phase of enzymatic factors resulting in clot strengthening, which in this phase of clotting is mostly achieved by fibrinogen cleavage and fibrin polymerization. K-time occurs in the same time interval as angle (described next), which has replaced K-time in clinical practice. One of the reasons for this is that the calculation of K-time requires the TEG tracing to reach 20 mm of amplitude; in cases of severe coagulopathy this amplitude may not be reached and a K-time cannot be calculated. Consequently, most clinical algorithms and protocols do not use K-time to guide therapy.

Angle

This variable is the amount of degrees of the angle of a tangent line drawn between the initial split point of the tracing and the growing TEG curve. It is thought to represent the propagation phase of enzymatic factors resulting in clot strengthening, which in this phase of clotting is mostly achieved by fibrinogen cleavage and fibrin polymerization. A lower angle represents a decreased rate of clot strength growth, whereas a higher angle represents a greater rate of clot strength growth. Clinically, angle is used as a marker of fibrinogen concentration and function and correlates well with the specialized TEG assay functional fibrinogen TEG ($R = 0.7$; $P<.0001$).[35] Angle is currently used in clinical algorithms and protocols to trigger fibrinogen replacement in the way of cryoprecipitate or fibrinogen concentrate.[36]

Maximal Amplitude

Maximal amplitude is the greatest strength achieved by the clot, which on the TEG tracing is represented as the width in millimeters of the widest gap in TEG tracing. MA assesses the combination of platelet count and function and fibrinogen activity (cleavage to fibrin and polymerization). Kang and colleagues[22] studied patients undergoing liver transplantation and used linear regression to evaluate the relationship between TEG variables and PT; PTT; platelet count; and factors I, II, V, VII, VIII, IX, X, XI, and XII. In this study, MA correlated with platelet count ($r = 0.59$; $P<.001$) and fibrinogen level ($r = 0.64$; $P<.001$). The relationship of platelet count and MA was further investigated by measuring the MA and platelet count following infusion of platelets. Ten units of platelets led to an increment of 40 (±31) $\times$ 10^9/L in platelet count and an increase in MA of 13.2 mm. Interestingly, another study reported that the association between MA and platelet count becomes linear when the platelet count was less than 100×10^9/L.[37] However, it is important to underscore that platelet count does not necessarily correlate with platelet function, particularly in pathologic conditions, such as hemorrhagic shock. As a measure of the maximal amplitude of strength reached by the clot, MA reflects all factors that contribute to clot strength, which is mostly represented by fibrin-platelet interactions. Functional fibrinogen TEG studies in healthy volunteers have demonstrated that approximately 20% of the clot strength (MA) is determined by fibrin, with the remaining 80% attributable to platelets. In trauma, studied on admission, the contribution of fibrinogen to total clot strength is approximately 30%.[35,38] Thus, MA should be interpreted as a function of interactions between these two factors, and not a sole reflection of platelet function.[39] MA is currently used in clinical algorithms and protocols to trigger platelet transfusion.

Shear Elastic Modulus Strength

Because MA reflects the modulus of clot strength, yet it is expressed as the amplitude of the tracing, a physical translation into an output of viscoelastic strength has been derived from MA. This variable is known as G, represents the shear elastic modulus strength, and is expressed in dynes per square centimeter. G is calculated as follows:

$$G = (5000 \times MA)/(100 - MA)$$

G is a parametric measure of clot strength. The relationship between MA and G is not linear but curvilinear; MA can vary from 0 to 100, whereas G varies from 0 to infinity. Because it is expressed in units of strength, G facilitates interpreting clot strength as a viscoelastic variable. This relationship has led investigators to believe that compared with G, MA may underestimate the changes in thrombus resistance characteristics. For example, when a clot with an MA of 35 mm is compared with another with amplitude of 70 mm, the difference in strength between the clots in terms of dynes per square centimeter (G) is not two-fold but rather four-fold. The G variable is used mostly for research.

Lysis at 30 Minutes

LY30 is the standard measure of fibrinolysis by TEG. LY30 is determined by calculating the percent reduction of clot strength (amplitude) 30 minutes after reaching MA. Per the manufacturer, an LY30 greater than 7.5% (ie, 7.5% clot strength reduction between MA and amplitude 30 minutes after reaching MA) is considered abnormal. Two recent studies have investigated the ideal threshold of LY30 in trauma patients. Our group prospectively studied 73 trauma patients meeting criteria for MTP activation with citrated kaolin-TEG on admission. Those patients with an LY30 greater than or equal to 3% were more likely to require a massive transfusion (90.9% vs 30.5%; P = .0008) and to die from hemorrhage (45.5% vs 4.8%; P = .0014) compared with those with an LY30 less than 3%. In a similar study performed using citrated rapid-TEG, Cotton and colleagues[12] found that the LY30 value associated with a significant increase in mortality was greater than or equal to 3%. The odds of mortality increased 10-fold when an LY30 greater than or equal to 3% was reached. These authors called for reconsideration of the LY30 threshold given that the normal reference range had been considered to be 0.0% to 7.5%.

It has been speculated that the use of a citrated sample and an activator (kaolin or tissue factor) can yield different LY30 sensitivities among TEG assays. Our group investigated this by performing a study on healthy control blood samples in which tissue plasminogen activator was used to induce fibrinolysis in vitro and head-to-head citrated kaolin, native rapid, and native TEG (noncitrated) were performed.[40] Citrated native TEG detected fibrinolysis by LY30 earlier and to a greater degree. This finding remains to be validated in trauma patients with coagulopathy with fibrinolysis;

however, a citrated native TEG should be considered the assay of choice for detecting fibrinolysis in experimental models and is the assay modality currently used in the newly developed tissue plasminogen activator challenge TEG. Furthermore, our group has recently reported data demonstrating that in trauma patients, an LY30 approximating 0 is abnormal. We studied trauma patients with an ISS greater than 15 by stratifying this cohort by the degree of fibrinolysis (LY30) evident on arrival.[41] A total of 64% of patients had an LY30 less than 0.8 (referred to as fibrinolysis shutdown), which was associated with a greater mortality rate (26%) compared with patients with an intermediate degree (LY30 0.8%–3.0%) of fibrinolysis (5% mortality; $P = .001$). These data suggest that in trauma patients, the degree of normal fibrinolysis (ie, physiologic fibrinolysis associated with the least mortality) is in the range of 0.8% to 3.0% LY30, in contrast to the 0% to 7.5% range reported by the manufacturer.

Reference Ranges

Although reference ranges based on multi-institutional studies have been published for TEG, recent proficiency data indicate large interinstitutional variation in results, with coefficients of variation of up to 80%.[42] This is thought to be caused by age-related changes and variations in phenotypes of hemostasis seen across populations, and instrument operator variability. Thus, generic reference ranges may not be applicable to individual centers and should be locally produced. Reference ranges for the most commonly used TEG assays, rapid-TEG and kaolin-TEG, are shown in **Table 2** as reported by the manufacturer. Our group recently conducted a comprehensive analysis of TEG in 160 healthy volunteers in Denver to validate and standardize normal ranges of TEG. Results from this study are summarized in **Table 3**.

Given that these reference ranges represent coagulation in a healthy state and may not reflect unique pathophysiologic aspects only seen once trauma-induced coagulopathy (TIC) ensues, our group recently studied 190 severely injured patients at risk for TIC on presentation to clinically validate parameters for goal-directed treatment.[43] By performing an optimal cut-point analysis on these data the parameters for the TEG variables depicted in **Fig. 3** were derived.

Rotational Thrombelastometry

ROTEM is another viscoelastic coagulation test that provides a more comprehensive and dynamic overview of individual patient coagulation compared with standard coagulation testing. ROTEM, like TEG, also provides information on the speed of coagulation initiation, kinetics of clot growth, clot strength, and breakdown of the clot. The ROTEM device uses a plastic pin immersed vertically into a cup containing the patient blood sample. The pin is rotated slowly through an angle of 4.75°. Four tests are performed simultaneously: intrinsic activation, extrinsic activation, fibrin

Table 2
Manufacturer reference ranges of TEG variables for the two most commonly used TEG assays in clinical practice: rapid-TEG and kaolin-TEG

		TEG Variable				
TEG Assay	Sample Collection	ACT (s)	R-time (min)	Angle (Degrees)	MA (Millimeters)	LY30 (%)
Kaolin	Noncitrated	N/A	4–9	59–74	55–74	0–7.5
	Citrated		5–10	53–72	50–70	0–7.5
Rapid	Noncitrated	78–110	N/A	66–82	54–72	0–7.5
	Citrated	86–118		64–80	52–71	0–7.5

Table 3
Range of TEG variables from healthy control study (N = 160) performed in Denver

TEG Assay	Sample Collection	TEG Parameter				
		ACT (s)	R-time (min)	Angle (Degrees)	MA (Millimeters)	LY30 (%)
Native	Noncitrated	N/A	8–12	12–34	39–60	1.6–5
	Citrated		9–17	26–61	44–67	1.8–5
Kaolin	Noncitrated	N/A	4–11	53–75	56–75	0.7–5
	Citrated		6–12	49–69	54–71	0.9–5
Rapid	Noncitrated	78–146	N/A	66–81	56–74	0.2–5
	Citrated	91–140		62–81	53–71	0.1–5

Range determined by ± 2 standard deviations from the mean.

component of the clot, and aprotinin (fibrinolysis inhibitor used with extrinsic activation). ROTEM, like TEG, has also been used to guide early and individualized goal-directed therapy for TIC. Several institutions have ROTEM-based algorithms (**Fig. 4**) for management of acute hemorrhage and coagulation disorders in trauma patients.

LIMITATIONS OF VISCOELASTIC ASSAYS

Understanding the limitations of viscoelastic assays is essential for adequate clinical implementation and therapy guidance. First, these assays do not reflect most

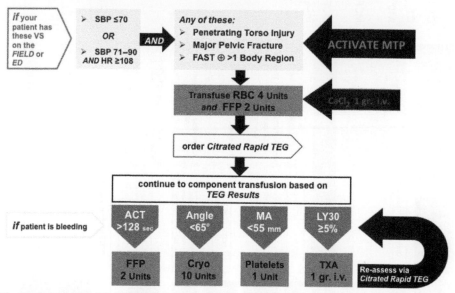

Fig. 3. Denver Health Medical Center goal-directed massive transfusion protocol. CaCl₂, calcium chloride; cryo, cryoprecipitate; ED, emergency department; FAST, focused assessment with sonography for trauma; FFP, fresh frozen plasma; gr, gram; HR, heart rate; i.v., intravenous; mm, millimeter; RBC, red blood cells; SBP, systolic blood pressure; sec, seconds; TXA, tranexamic acid; VS, vital signs. (*From* Einersen PM, Moore EE, Chapman MP, et al. Rapid-thromboelastography (r-TEG) thresholds for goal-directed resuscitation of patients at risk for massive transfusion. J Trauma Acute Care Surg 2016. [Epub ahead of print].)

Algorithm for treating bleeding in patients with trauma-induced coagulopathy

ROTEM® Results in Clinically Significant Bleeding

CT_{IN} — *Prolonged* — Suggests Heparin influence or intrinsic factor deficiency

CT_{EX} — *Prolonged* — Suggests extrinsic factor deficiency

$A10_{IN, EX}$ — *Reduced* — Suggests poor clot firmness as a result of decreased: Platelets, fibrinogen and/or FXIII

$MCF_{IN, EX}$ — *Reduced* — Suggests poor clot firmness as a result of decreased: Platelets, fibrinogen and/or FXIII

MCF_{FIB} — *Reduced* — Suggests poor fibrin contribution to clot firmness

$ML_{IN, EX, FIB}$ — *>15%* — Suggests hyperfibrinolysis

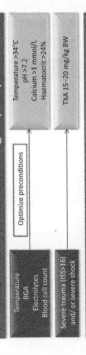
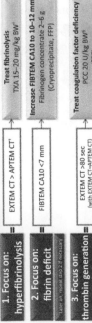
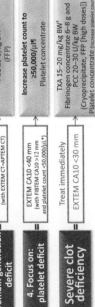
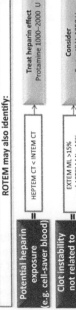

Temperature
BGA
Electrolytes
Blood cell count → Optimize preconditions → Temperature >34°C, pH >7.2, Calcium >1 mmol/L, Haematocrit >24%

Severe trauma (ISS>16) and/ or severe shock → TXA 15–20 mg/kg BW

Run ROTEM (EXTEM, INTEM, FIBTEM, APTEM)*

1. Focus on: hyperfibrinolysis = EXTEM CT > APTEM CT† → **Treat fibrinolysis** TXA 15–20 mg/kg BW†

2. Focus on: fibrin deficit (Later on, repeat step 2, if necessary) = FIBTEM CA10 <7 mm → **Increase FIBTEM CA10 to 10–12 mm** Fibrinogen concentrate 2–6 g (Cryoprecipitate, FFP)

3. Focus on: thrombin generation deficit = EXTEM CT >80 sec (with EXTEM CT>APTEM CT) → **Treat coagulation factor deficiency** PCC 20 U/kg BW§ (FFP)

4. Focus on: platelet deficit = EXTEM CA10 <40 mm (with FIBTEM CA10 >12 mm and platelet count <50,000/µL*) → **Increase platelet count to ≥50,000/µl** Platelet concentrate

Severe clot deficiency = Treat immediately EXTEM CA10 <30 mm → TXA 15–20 mg/kg BW‡ Fibrinogen concentrate 6–8 g and PCC 20–30 U/kg BW Platelet concentrate (increase platelet count to ≥50,000/µL*) (Cryoprecipitate, FFP [high doses])

ROTEM may also identify:

Potential heparin exposure (e.g. cell-saver blood) = HEPTEM CT < INTEM CT → **Treat heparin effect** Protamine 1000–2000 U

Clot instability not related to hyperfibrinolysis = EXTEM ML >15% and APTEM ML >15% → **Consider** Factor XLLL 1250 U interactions occurring between the fluid phase of coagulation and the endothelial cell surface. This dynamic is clearly present in the patient with coagulopathy; however, it remains to be understood. Second, platelet inhibition/dysfunction may not be evident with the standard assays, unless thrombin is inhibited and platelet agonists are used in the specialized TEG platelet mapping assay.[16] Third, TEG and results are currently operator dependent and subject to sampling and/or processing errors, and intersampling variability. A newer generation of the TEG analyzer currently in development may obviate these issues.

THROMBELASTOGRAPHY IN TRAUMA-INDUCED COAGULOPATHY

Until a decade ago, the diagnosis of TIC was made with conventional coagulation tests, such as PT/INR. It is important to recognize that PT/INR and PTT were initially developed for the screening of heritable coagulopathies, such as hemophilia, and subsequently used to monitor anticoagulant therapy.[44] The end point for these tests is the time, in seconds, until the earliest formation of fibrin is detected. These assays do not assess the evolution of the clot beyond the formation of the first strands of fibrin. Furthermore, they have shown to correlate poorly with bleeding risk in elective general and vascular surgeries.[45] Because classic coagulation tests have shortcomings when used to diagnose and monitor coagulopathy in the trauma patient, viscoelastic assays, such as TEG, have emerged in the last decade as a novel application of a well-established technology.

TEG was first used in trauma patients during the late 1990s as a research tool to characterize changes in the different stages of hemostasis during TIC.[46] It was not until a decade after that the first reports on standardized management strategies of TIC using TEG were published by our group and others.[47–49]

The greatest clinical application of TEG in trauma is in the guidance of MTP. Until recently, the ideal strategy to guide MTP in injured patients remained elusive. In 2013 Tapia and coworkers[50] published a study comparing their TEG-guided MTP with a historical cohort in which MTP was carried out using a fixed transfusion ratio of 1:1:1 red blood cell to plasma to platelet units. Patients studied were transfused six or more units of red blood cells in the first 24 hours from arrival. The median ISS of patients ranged from 23 to 29 and was not significantly different between the groups compared. These authors found that patients with penetrating trauma that had an MTP guided by TEG had improved mortality compared with the fixed-ratio MTP

Fig. 4. ROTEM-guided treatment algorithm for managing trauma-induced coagulopathy and diffuse microvascular bleeding (AUVA Trauma Hospital, Salzburg, Austria). The algorithm represents standard operating procedure for ROTEM-guided hemostatic therapy on admission of trauma patients to the emergency room. APTEM, aprotinin (fibrinolysis inhibitor used with EXTEM); ATIII, anti-thrombin; BGA, blood gas arterial; BW, body weight; EXTEM, extrinsic activation; FFP, fresh frozen plasma; FIBTEM, fibrin component of the clot; g, gram; INTEM, intrinsic activation; ISS, injury severity score; kg, kilogram; mg, milligram; mm, millimeter; mmol/L, millimol per liter; PCC, pro-thrombin complex concentrate; s, seconds; TXA, tranexamic acid; U, units; μl, microliter. *For patients who are unconscious or known to be taking platelet inhibitor medication. §If ATIII deficiency suspected or known, consider co-administration of ATIII. †Any major improvement in APTEM parameters compared to corresponding EXTEM parameters may be interpreted as a sign of hyperfibrinolysis. ‡Only for patients not receiving TXA at an earlier stage of the algorithm. (From Schöchl H, Maegele M, Solomon C, et al. Early and individualized goal-directed therapy for trauma-induced coagulopathy. Scand J Trauma Resusc Emerg Med 2012;20:15; with permission.)

historic cohort. Our group recently published a randomized clinical trial in which patients were randomized to either an MTP guided by TEG or CCA (eg, INR, PTT, platelet count, fibrinogen, D dimer).[17] A total of 111 patients were enrolled with median ISS of 30, and 27% had a penetrating injury mechanism. The TEG-guided MTP group had a survival advantage over the CCA group; mortality of 19% in the TEG group compared with 36% in the CCA group ($P = .04$; hazards ratio of mortality in the CCA group of 2.1; 95% confidence interval, 1.02–4.45). The difference in mortality was attributed to less early hemorrhagic deaths in the TEG group. More plasma and platelet units were transfused to the CCA group in the first 2 hours from arrival, whereas more cryoprecipitate was transfused overall to the CCA group. There were no differences in the timing and amount of crystalloid and red blood cell units administered. This finding suggests that TEG allows for more appropriate hemostatic blood product use. Patients in the TEG group also had more ventilator-free and intensive care unit–free days, which is potentially related to appropriateness of blood product administration. Our institution's goal-directed TEG-guided MTP is shown in **Fig. 3**.

TEG has also allowed for characterization of distinct phenotypes of TIC, indicating that the pathophysiologic mechanisms of TIC may be different based on patient characteristics, comorbidities, and injury patterns. Our group performed a principal component analysis on TEG variables of severely injured patients (median ISS of 31).[51] Principal component analysis identified three principal components that together explained 93% of the overall variance. The first phenotype reflected global coagulopathy with depletion of platelets and fibrinogen, a second group consisted of fibrinolysis as the main driver of TIC. Kutcher and colleagues[52] from the San Francisco group performed a similar study applying principal component analysis to coagulation factor activity. These authors also reported two principal component groups; the first one consisting of global clotting factor depletion and a second one characterized by activation of protein C and hyperfibrinolysis. These data suggest that trauma patients present with different pathophysiologic drivers of coagulopathy and underscore the importance of personalized resuscitation of TIC.

Clinical studies have identified that in those patients with coagulopathy with the highest hemorrhage-related mortality fibrinolysis is a conspicuous factor.[41,53,54] Thus, treating fibrinolysis with antifibrinolytic medication poses a potential strategy to improve outcomes of trauma patients. However, controversy exists regarding the threshold for administering this medication and potential adverse effects. Although the CRASH-2 trial reported a 1.5% benefit in mortality when the antifibrinolytic tranexamic acid was administered empirically to all trauma patients,[55] there has been significant criticism regarding the clinical applicability of this study's findings.[56] This trial did not perform any coagulation assays to either demonstrate the patients' degree of coagulopathy and fibrinolysis or to characterize the effect of the drug. Importantly, this study also found that administration of tranexamic acid greater than 3 hours after injury was associated with increased mortality; the study did not report any causality or mechanism to explain this finding. It seems intuitive that an antifibrinolytic medication (eg, tranexamic acid) should only be administered to those who have demonstrable hyperfibrinolysis; however, advocates for its empiric administration to all trauma patients still exist. TEG is the only clinically available assay that can detect fibrinolysis accurately and in a point-of-care setting. Several studies have demonstrated an association of hyperfibrinolysis detected by TEG with increased mortality and need for massive transfusion.[12,41,57] Furthermore, with the recent characterization of fibrinolysis shutdown,[41] present in 63% of severely injured patients on arrival, administration of an antifibrinolytic to these patients should be avoided. Our institution's approach to hyperfibrinolysis is goal-directed,[32] just as it is for transfusion of hemostatic blood products, administering tranexamic acid only to those patients who have an LY30 greater than 3% to 5%.

SUMMARY

Viscoelastic assays, such as TEG, are the coagulation tests that better represent TIC and enable the clinician with data for critical decision making. TEG's greatest application in trauma care is in the guidance of MTP. In summary, the insights into TIC that TEG has provided, from the clinical and biologic mechanism standpoint, are substantial, and pose an opportunity for further investigations.

REFERENCES

1. Norton R, Kobusingye O. Injuries. N Engl J Med 2013;368(18):1723–30.
2. MacKenzie EJ, Rivara FP, Jurkovich GJ, et al. A national evaluation of the effect of trauma-center care on mortality. N Engl J Med 2006;354(4):366–78.
3. Rhee P, Joseph B, Pandit V, et al. Increasing trauma deaths in the United States. Ann Surg 2014;260(1):13–21.
4. Sauaia A, Gonzalez E, Moore HB, et al. Fatality and severity of firearm injuries in a Denver Trauma Center, 2000-2013. JAMA 2016;315(22):2465–7.
5. Trunkey DD. Trauma. Accidental and intentional injuries account for more years of life lost in the U.S. than cancer and heart disease. Among the prescribed remedies are improved preventive efforts, speedier surgery and further research. Sci Am 1983;249(2):28–35.
6. Zambon M, Vincent JL. Mortality rates for patients with acute lung injury/ARDS have decreased over time. Chest 2008;133(5):1120–7.
7. Ciesla DJ, Moore EE, Johnson JL, et al. Decreased progression of postinjury lung dysfunction to the acute respiratory distress syndrome and multiple organ failure. Surgery 2006;140(4):640–7 [discussion: 647–8].
8. Tisherman SA, Schmicker RH, Brasel KJ, et al. Detailed description of all deaths in both the shock and traumatic brain injury hypertonic saline trials of the resuscitation outcomes consortium. Ann Surg 2015;261(3):586–90.
9. Brohi K, Singh J, Heron M, et al. Acute traumatic coagulopathy. J Trauma 2003; 54(6):1127–30.
10. MacLeod JB, Lynn M, McKenney MG, et al. Early coagulopathy predicts mortality in trauma. J Trauma 2003;55(1):39–44.
11. Torres LN, Sondeen JL, Ji L, et al. Evaluation of resuscitation fluids on endothelial glycocalyx, venular blood flow, and coagulation function after hemorrhagic shock in rats. J Trauma Acute Care Surg 2013;75(5):759–66.
12. Cotton BA, Harvin JA, Kostousouv V, et al. Hyperfibrinolysis at admission is an uncommon but highly lethal event associated with shock and prehospital fluid administration. J Trauma Acute Care Surg 2012;73(2):365–70 [discussion: 370].
13. Nielsen VG. Hemodilution with lactated Ringer's solution causes hypocoagulability in rabbits. Blood Coagul Fibrinolysis 2004;15(1):55–9.
14. Nielsen VG, Lyerly RT 3rd, Gurley WQ. The effect of dilution on plasma coagulation kinetics determined by thrombelastography is dependent on antithrombin activity and mode of activation. Anesth Analg 2004;99(6):1587–92.
15. Moore HB, Moore EE, Gonzalez E, et al. Plasma is the physiologic buffer of tissue plasminogen activator-mediated fibrinolysis: rationale for plasma-first resuscitation after life-threatening hemorrhage. J Am Coll Surg 2015;220(5):872–9.
16. Gonzalez E, Moore H, Moore EE. Trauma Induced Coagulopathy. Switzerland: Springer International Publishing AG; 2016.

17. Gonzalez E, Moore EE, Moore HB, et al. Goal-directed hemostatic resuscitation of trauma-induced coagulopathy: a pragmatic randomized clinical trial comparing a viscoelastic assay to conventional coagulation assays. Ann Surg 2016;263(6): 1051–9.

18. Hartert H. Blutgerinnungsstudien mit der Thrombelastographie; einem neuen Untersuchungs verfahren. Klin Wochenschr 1948;26(37–38):577–83.

19. De Nicola P, Mazzetti GM. Evaluation of thrombelastography. Am J Clin Pathol 1955;23(4):447–52.

20. Von Kaulla KN, Weiner M. Studies of coagulation and fibrinolysis by new technic of continuous recording. Blood 1955;10(4):362–9.

21. Von Kaulla KN, Swan H. Clotting deviations in man during cardiac bypass: fibrinolysis and circulating anticoagulant. J Thorac Surg 1958;36(4):519–30.

22. Kang YG, Martin DJ, Marquez J, et al. Intraoperative changes in blood coagulation and thrombelastographic monitoring in liver transplantation. Anesth Analg 1985;64(9):888–96.

23. Von Kaulla KN, Kaye H, von Kaulla E, et al. Changes in blood coagulation. Arch Surg 1966;92(1):71–9.

24. Tuman KJ, Spiess BD, McCarthy RJ, et al. Comparison of viscoelastic measures of coagulation after cardiopulmonary bypass. Anesth Analg 1989;69(1):69–75.

25. Gibbs NM, Crawford GP, Michalopoulos N. Thrombelastographic patterns following abdominal aortic surgery. Anaesth Intensive Care 1994;22(5):534–8.

26. Wasowicz M, Srinivas C, Meineri M, et al. Technical report: analysis of citrated blood with thromboelastography: comparison with fresh blood samples. Can J Anaesth 2008;55(5):284–9.

27. Vig S, Chitolie A, Bevan DH, et al. Thromboelastography: a reliable test? Blood Coagul Fibrinolysis 2001;12(7):555–61.

28. Bowbrick VA, Mikhailidis DP, Stansby G. The use of citrated whole blood in thromboelastography. Anesth Analg 2000;90(5):1086–8.

29. Zambruni A, Thalheimer U, Leandro G, et al. Thromboelastography with citrated blood: comparability with native blood, stability of citrate storage and effect of repeated sampling. Blood Coagul Fibrinolysis 2004;15(1):103–7.

30. Johansson PI, Bochsen L, Andersen S, et al. Investigation of the effect of kaolin and tissue-factor-activated citrated whole blood, on clot-forming variables, as evaluated by thromboelastography. Transfusion 2008;48(11):2377–83.

31. Nielsen VG, Cohen BM, Cohen E. Effects of coagulation factor deficiency on plasma coagulation kinetics determined via thrombelastography: critical roles of fibrinogen and factors II, VII, X and XII. Acta Anaesthesiol Scand 2005; 49(2):222–31.

32. Gonzalez E, Moore EE, Moore HB, et al. Trauma-induced coagulopathy: an institution's 35 year perspective on practice and research. Scand J Surg 2014;103(2): 89–103.

33. Moore HB, Moore EE, Chin TL, et al. Activated clotting time of thrombelastography (T-ACT) predicts early postinjury blood component transfusion beyond plasma. Surgery 2014;156(3):564–9.

34. Cotton BA, Faz G, Hatch QM, et al. Rapid thrombelastography delivers real-time results that predict transfusion within 1 hour of admission. J Trauma 2011;71(2): 407–14 [discussion: 414–7].

35. Harr JN, Moore EE, Ghasabyan A, et al. Functional fibrinogen assay indicates that fibrinogen is critical in correcting abnormal clot strength following trauma. Shock (Augusta, Ga) 2013;39(1):45–9.

36. Montupil J, Carlier C, Van der Linden P. Use of fibrinogen concentrate in bleeding patients. Anaesthesia 2015;70(11):1323–4.
37. Bowbrick VA, Mikhailidis DP, Stansby G. Influence of platelet count and activity on thromboelastography parameters. Platelets 2003;14(4):219–24.
38. Kornblith LZ, Kutcher ME, Redick BJ, et al. Fibrinogen and platelet contributions to clot formation: implications for trauma resuscitation and thromboprophylaxis. J Trauma Acute Care Surg 2014;76(2):255–6 [discussion: 262–3].
39. Galanakis DK, Neerman-Arbez M, Brennan S, et al. Thromboelastographic phenotypes of fibrinogen and its variants: clinical and non-clinical implications. Thromb Res 2014;133(6):1115–23.
40. Quinn B, Gonzalez E, Moore EE, et al. Defining the optimal thrombelastography assay to detect tissue plasminogen induced fibrinolysis. Surgery 2016, in press.
41. Moore HB, Moore EE, Gonzalez E, et al. Hyperfibrinolysis, physiologic fibrinolysis, and fibrinolysis shutdown: the spectrum of postinjury fibrinolysis and relevance to antifibrinolytic therapy. J Trauma Acute Care Surg 2014;77(6):811–7.
42. Quarterman C, Shaw M, Johnson I, et al. Intra- and inter-centre standardisation of thromboelastography (TEG(R)). Anaesthesia 2014;69(8):883–90.
43. Einersen PM, Moore EE, Chapman MP, et al. Rapid-thromboelastography (r-TEG) thresholds for goal-directed resuscitation of patients at risk for massive transfusion. J Trauma Acute Care Surg 2016. [Epub ahead of print].
44. Owen CA Jr. Historical account of tests of hemostasis. Am J Clin Pathol 1990;93(4 Suppl 1):S3–8.
45. Eckman MH, Erban JK, Singh SK, et al. Screening for the risk for bleeding or thrombosis. Ann Intern Med 2003;138(3):W15–24.
46. Kaufmann CR, Dwyer KM, Crews JD, et al. Usefulness of thrombelastography in assessment of trauma patient coagulation. J Trauma 1997;42(4):716–20 [discussion: 720–2].
47. Kashuk JL, Moore EE. The emerging role of rapid thromboelastography in trauma care. J Trauma 2009;67(2):417–8.
48. Kashuk JL, Moore EE, Sawyer M, et al. Postinjury coagulopathy management: goal directed resuscitation via POC thrombelastography. Ann Surg 2010; 251(4):604–14.
49. Gonzalez E, Pieracci FM, Moore EE, et al. Coagulation abnormalities in the trauma patient: the role of point-of-care thromboelastography. Semin Thromb Hemost 2010;36(7):723–37.
50. Tapia NM, Chang A, Norman M, et al. TEG-guided resuscitation is superior to standardized MTP resuscitation in massively transfused penetrating trauma patients. J Trauma Acute Care Surg 2013;74(2):378–85 [discussion: 385–6].
51. Chin TL, Moore EE, Moore HB, et al. A principal component analysis of postinjury viscoelastic assays: clotting factor depletion versus fibrinolysis. Surgery 2014; 156(3):570–7.
52. Kutcher ME, Ferguson AR, Cohen MJ. A principal component analysis of coagulation after trauma. J Trauma Acute Care Surg 2013;74(5):1223–9 [discussion: 1229–30].
53. Schochl H, Frietsch T, Pavelka M, et al. Hyperfibrinolysis after major trauma: differential diagnosis of lysis patterns and prognostic value of thrombelastometry. J Trauma 2009;67(1):125–31.
54. Kashuk JL, Moore EE, Sawyer M, et al. Primary fibrinolysis is integral in the pathogenesis of the acute coagulopathy of trauma. Ann Surg 2010;252(3):434–42 [discussion: 443–4].

55. Shakur H, Roberts I, Bautista R, et al. Effects of tranexamic acid on death, vascular occlusive events, and blood transfusion in trauma patients with significant haemorrhage (CRASH-2): a randomised, placebo-controlled trial. Lancet 2010;376(9734):23–32.
56. Napolitano LM, Cohen MJ, Cotton BA, et al. Tranexamic acid in trauma: how should we use it? J Trauma Acute Care Surg 2013;74(6):1575–86.
57. Chapman MP, Moore EE, Ghasabyan A, et al. TEG fibrinolysis above 3% is the critical value for initiation of antifibrinolytic therapy. J Trauma Acute Care Surg 2013;75(6):961–7.

Optimal Reversal of Novel Anticoagulants in Trauma

 CrossMark

Jason Weinberger, DO[a], Mark Cipolle, MD, PhD, FCCM[b],*

KEYWORDS

- Novel anticoagulants • NOACs • Coagulopathy of trauma • Reversal agents
- Anticoagulants in trauma

KEY POINTS

- Patients are increasingly using novel oral anticoagulants such as dabigatran, rivaroxaban, apixaban, and edoxaban for both the prophylaxis and treatment of a wide spectrum of diseases, including atrial fibrillation, stroke, myocardial infarction, valvular disease, deep venous thrombosis, and pulmonary embolism.
- Urgent or immediate reversal of anticoagulants in patients with trauma with major or critical bleeding can predispose to catastrophic thrombotic complications such as stroke, myocardial infarction, and pulmonary embolism. The risk versus benefit balance of reversal should therefore be individualized and based on the severity of the hemorrhage or need to perform an emergent procedure and the patient's underlying thromboembolic risk.
- Target-specific antidotes are currently being evaluated, and some just recently approved, for the reversal of these novel oral anticoagulants. Meanwhile, evidence supporting advanced therapies such as antifibrinolytics, prothrombin complex concentrates, and these new target-specific antidotes is largely limited to healthy human volunteers, animal models, and in vitro studies.
- It is important to address resumption of anticoagulation before patient discharge so as not to expose the patient to an extended period of thromboembolic risk after traumatic bleeding has been stopped.

INTRODUCTION

Trauma is the third leading cause of death in the United States and accounts for 30% of all life-years lost.[1] Recent trends suggest that trauma centers are seeing an increasing number of severely injured elderly patients. Falls, head injuries, and

Conflicts of Interest: The authors have no financial or commercial conflicts of interest.
Human and animal rights and informed consent: This article does not contain any studies with human or animal subjects performed by either of the authors.
[a] Department of Surgical Critical Care, R Adams Cowley Shock Trauma Center, University of Maryland Medical Center, 22 South Greene Street, T1R53, Baltimore, MD 21201, USA; [b] Department of Surgery, Christiana Care Health System, Sidney Kimmel School of Medicine, Thomas Jefferson University, 4755 Ogletown-Stanton Road, Suite 1320, Wilmington, DE 19718, USA
* Corresponding author.
E-mail address: MCipolle@christianacare.org

hemorrhagic complications account for a substantial proportion of these fatalities.[2] Coagulopathy and associated bleeding have always beset patients with trauma, but in the elderly trauma population the incidence of pharmacologically induced coagulopathy poses a new and substantial risk for worsening hemorrhage.

Anticoagulants have long been the mainstay of therapy for the acute and long-term prevention or treatment of numerous thromboembolic disorders. For years, warfarin (vitamin K antagonist [VKA]) was the only available oral anticoagulant. Its usage was often plagued by unpredictable pharmacokinetics, narrow therapeutic windows, multiple food and medication interactions, need for frequent monitoring, and a high complication rate. In North Americans taking warfarin for atrial fibrillation who present to an emergency department, only about 59% are in the therapeutic range.[3]

Over the last decade, the pharmaceutical industry has focused on developing novel oral anticoagulants (NOACs) by means of direct thrombin or factor Xa inhibitors for patients requiring treatment or prevention of thromboembolic disorders. These novel direct and indirect inhibitors of coagulation are being increasingly used for both the prophylaxis and treatment of a wide spectrum of diseases: atrial fibrillation, stroke, myocardial infarction, valvular disease, deep venous thrombosis, and pulmonary embolism (**Table 1**).

Compared with warfarin, these NOACs have far more reliable pharmacokinetics, an ability to quickly achieve therapeutic levels in the blood stream, reliable drug elimination rates, and are largely unaffected by food or other medications. NOAC efficacy has been best studied in the setting of atrial fibrillation. A large systematic review and meta-analysis of 44,563 patients across 3 randomized controlled trials (RCTs) that compared NOACs (dabigatran, rivaroxaban, or apixaban) with warfarin in patients with atrial fibrillation reported a decreased risk of all-cause stroke and systemic embolism, ischemic stroke, hemorrhagic stroke, all-cause mortality, and vascular mortality with NOAC use.[4]

Patients and clinicians alike must be cognizant of the NOACs' adverse effects as well. Individual results from these 3 large RCTs (RE-LY,[5] ROCKET-AF,[6] ARISTOTLE[7]) documented that the rates of major bleeding in patients receiving NOACs were 2.13% to 3.6% per year versus 3.09% to 3.4% in those taking warfarin. Similarly, rates of hemorrhagic stroke were lower for NOACs (NOACs 0.1%–0.5% vs warfarin 0.38%–0.70%). Both the incidence and outcomes of NOAC-associated bleeding seem favorable compared with warfarin.

A recent meta-analysis of 13 RCTs, which included 102,707 patients being treated with a NOAC or warfarin for atrial fibrillation or venous thromboembolism,[8] confirmed a reduced mortality for major bleeding in patients on NOACs (7.6% NOAC vs 11% warfarin). Additional analysis favored NOACs, compared with warfarin, with reductions in the relative risk (RR) of fatal bleeding (RR, 0.53; 95% confidence interval [CI], 0.43–0.64), cardiovascular mortality (RR, 0.88; 95% CI, 0.82–0.94), and all-cause mortality (RR, 0.91; 95% CI, 0.87–0.96).

Albeit justified, the initial high enthusiasm for these NOACs must be tempered by 3 notable concerns: there is often no readily available means for assessing the degree of pharmacologic coagulopathy in patients on these agents, the optimal reversal strategy for many of these NOACs is still in development, and there is a threat of life-threatening bleeding complications after any injury in patients taking these new agents. Therefore, it is important to have clarity for optimal reversal strategies and proper management when treating critically ill patients with trauma on NOACs.

PATIENT EVALUATION OVERVIEW

The initial evaluation and management of critically ill patients with trauma must always include the establishment of an effective airway, rapid and continuous hemodynamic

Table 1
Pharmacokinetics and characteristics of common NOACs and warfarin

Drug	Trade Name	FDA Indication	Mechanism of Action	Plasma Peak Level (h)	Half-life (h)	Metabolism
Warfarin	Coumadin	Prophylaxis and treatment of VTE Atrial fibrillation Valvular heart disease Thromboembolic events such as MI, CVA	Vitamin K Antagonist	4 (5–7 d for full therapeutic effect)	40	Hepatic metabolism
Dabigatran	Pradaxa	Prophylaxis and treatment of VTE Nonvalvular atrial fibrillation	Direct thrombin inhibitor	2	14 Prolonged with renal impairment[a]	Hepatic metabolism 85% renal clearance
Apixaban	Eliquis	Prophylaxis and treatment of VTE Nonvalvular atrial fibrillation	Factor Xa inhibitor	3–4	12	Hepatic metabolism 27% renal clearance
Edoxaban	Savaysa	Prophylaxis and treatment of VTE Nonvalvular atrial fibrillation	Factor Xa inhibitor	1–2	12	Hepatic metabolism 50% renal clearance
Rivaroxaban	Xarelto	Prophylaxis and treatment of VTE Nonvalvular atrial fibrillation	Factor Xa inhibitor	2–4	7	Hepatic metabolism 66% renal clearance

Abbreviations: CVA, cardiovascular accident; MI, myocardial infarction; VTE, venous thromboembolism.
[a] Indicates that half-life of dabigatran can be prolonged with renal impairment.
Adapted from Lexicomp online, pediatric and neonatal Lexi-Drugs online. Hudson (OH): Lexi-Comp. Available at: http://online.lexi.com/action/home. Accessed April 1, 2016.

assessment, large-bore intravenous access, and transfusions for treatment of hemorrhagic shock, ongoing blood loss, severe anemia, and thrombocytopenia, or correction of trauma-associated coagulopathies. Rapid correction of body temperature, blood pH, and electrolyte balance (notably calcium) ensures optimal function of the natural coagulation cascade. Management of patients with trauma with an added complexity of existing pharmacologic coagulopathy from NOAC use requires diligent history taking and thorough assessment for active bleeding.

Proper management of patients with trauma on NOACs requires first an accurate medical history and detailed reconciliation of all their medications that includes the last time doses of each were taken. Patients on NOACs frequently take other medications that could affect hemostasis as well (eg, aspirin, clopidogrel). Clinicians must also consider the possibility that a patient may have taken an intentional or unintentional overdose of these anticoagulants. Underlying patient comorbidities, such as chronic renal disease or hepatic dysfunction, must be taken into consideration as well because they could promote additional bleeding and delay standard drug elimination of NOACs already ingested.

The most critical part in the assessment of patients with trauma on NOACs is the determination of their last dose ingestion. The degree or status of anticoagulation based on the ingestion of the last NOAC dose is important both for predicting the course of current bleeding and which interventions will be required. When treating patients anticoagulated with dabigatran, rivaroxaban, or apixaban, clinicians must remember that the physiologic effect of these NOACs is much shorter in duration than that of warfarin. The half-life of warfarin is 40 hours on average and the drug can remain effective in terms of anticoagulation for up to 4 or 5 days. In comparison, the direct thrombin inhibitor, dabigatran, has an average half-life of 14 hours and the factor Xa inhibitors, rivaroxaban (7 hours) and apixaban (12 hours), have considerably shorter half-lives as well, which contributes to quicker drug elimination (see **Table 1**).[9] Metabolism and elimination of NOACs depends on renal and hepatic function and therefore clearance of NOACs may be delayed in patients with underlying renal or hepatic dysfunction. With proper understanding of the specific NOAC agent, dose, time since last ingestion, and underlying renal or hepatic function, the optimal reversal strategy can then be undertaken.

Urgent or immediate reversal of anticoagulants can predispose to catastrophic thrombotic complications such as stroke, myocardial infarction, venous thromboembolism, and pulmonary embolism. Accurate assessment of current traumatic bleeding and the need for emergent procedures for cessation of hemorrhage are critically important when deciding to emergently reverse anticoagulants. Clinicians must first determine and take into consideration where the bleeding is located and whether it is active or has stopped. Bleeding, like many things, occurs on a spectrum, but bleeding that is initially minor or mundane can sometimes become much more significant or even life threatening, especially when patients are pharmacologically anticoagulated (**Fig. 1**).

Major bleeding associated with significant blood loss (eg, vascular injuries, gastrointestinal [GI]) or bleeding critically into a closed space (eg, intracranial, thoracic, compartment syndrome) are examples of hemorrhage that may require emergent reversal of anticoagulation. Often, these major or critical bleeding episodes require an interventional procedure in their course of management. Thus, swift clinical judgment is required in all patients with trauma on NOACs to determine their current bleeding risk and the urgency of their anticoagulation reversal. Given the short half-lives of the NOACs, it may be possible to delay an intervention long enough to allow the anticoagulant effect to dissipate naturally in select patients with trauma with minor

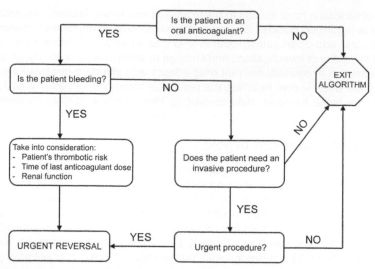

Fig. 1. Management algorithm of patients with trauma on oral anticoagulants, showing the assessment of bleeding and the need for a potentially urgent, invasive procedure.

bleeding. In contrast, if urgent or emergent intervention is deemed necessary, optimal reversal strategies may be most appropriate. These critical decisions regarding the need for reversal are individualized based on the urgency and bleeding risk of the patient and procedure at hand.

LABORATORY EVALUATION OVERVIEW

Much of the fervor for NOACs compared with the traditional use of warfarin as oral anticoagulants is caused by the conception that anticoagulation monitoring is not required and patients therefore do not require frequent blood sampling for titration of dosages to a narrow therapeutic prothrombin time (PT)/International Normalized Ratio (INR) window, as is required with warfarin. The predictable pharmacokinetics of NOACs have obviated routine laboratory monitoring. Caution is needed when interpreting standard coagulation tests during emergent settings, such as the evaluation of patients with trauma, because all NOACs may alter common coagulation laboratory tests. Standard coagulation assays, such as PT/INR, activated partial thromboplastin time (aPTT), thrombin time (TT), and anti-factor Xa activity, are of limited utility in measuring NOAC activity. A true caveat to the statement that anticoagulation monitoring is not required is that there is no reliable, timely, objective test to monitor them.

In patients on dabigatran, there is some evidence that an aPTT may be useful in determining continued anticoagulant activity. Lindahl and colleagues[10] showed that a prolonged aPTT of greater than 90 seconds indicates a continued anticoagulation effect from dabigatran. However, the most sensitive test for dabigatran is TT, because a normal value in a bleeding patient on dabigatran can assure the clinician that there is no significant anticoagulant effect present. In contrast, an increased TT is not helpful in determining the amount of anticoagulant effect present.[11] Dilute TT and ecarin clotting times may be best for monitoring the anticoagulant effect of dabigatran, but most institutions do not have these routinely available.[11]

With regard to the assessment of rivaroxaban, apixaban, or edoxaban, specific assays for factor Xa activity are available in many institutions, although only a small number of clinicians have access to these assays in a timely fashion. Systematic reviews have published detailed laboratory measurements of dabigatran, rivaroxaban, apixaban, and edoxaban activity both in vivo and ex vivo.[12,13] **Table 2** provides an adapted summary of investigations and findings to determine appropriate screenings for the presence of clinically relevant drug effects with standard coagulation assays. NOACs have been shown to affect the results of thromboelastography and similar point-of-care tests; however, data correlating these tests with drug concentration, major bleeding, and/or clinically significant anticoagulant effect are lacking.[14–18]

PHARMACOLOGIC TREATMENT OPTIONS

Emergent reversal of NOACs may be required in patients with trauma with serious or life-threatening bleeding who are anticoagulated, actively bleeding, and/or about to undergo a surgical intervention. An antidote or direct reversal agent for many of these NOACs is currently unavailable (except dabigatran [idarucizumab]). Strategies for optimal reversal are then derived from limited clinical experience and combinations of prohemostatic therapies such as vitamin K, blood component transfusions, recombinant activated factor VIIa, desmopressin, prothrombin complex concentrates (PCCs), antifibrinolytic agents, and target-specific antidotes. Each therapy is discussed individually later, along with a summary of reversal strategy for each individual NOAC.

Vitamin K

Vitamin K (phytonadione) can be used to normalize the PT/INR by providing necessary substrate to synthesize coagulation factors eliminated by warfarin (II, VII, IX, X) and proteins C and S. Intravenous administration of vitamin K is more effective at INR reversal than the same dose of vitamin K administered subcutaneously and should be given in a protocol-driven reversal algorithm along with fresh frozen plasma (FFP) or PCC to improve functional outcomes.[19,20] Increase in PT/INR in patients on

Table 2
NOAC effects on common coagulation tests

Test	Dabigatran	Apixaban	Rivaroxaban	Edoxaban
aPTT	Normal aPTT excludes excess drug levels			
PT			Normal PT/INR excludes significant drug levels	Sensitive if calibrated
TT	Normal TT excludes significant drug levels			
Activated factor Xa activity		Normal anti-Xa excludes significant drug levels	Normal anti-Xa excludes significant drug levels	Sensitive if calibrated
Recommended screening test	*TT*	*Anti-Xa*	*Anti-Xa*	*Anti-Xa*

Data from Refs.[11–13]

other NOACs is misleading and not representative of clotting factor deficit. Administration of vitamin K for reversal of NOACs is therefore not recommended.

Blood Product Transfusions

Blood product transfusions are often a necessary component of supportive care for patients with trauma with severe bleeding. Packed red blood cell transfusion may be required, depending on the rate of bleeding and amount of blood loss. Typically, platelet transfusion is not used to reverse the anticoagulant effect of NOACs in patients with a normal platelet count; however, thrombocytopenic patients with bleeding should be treated for the underlying cause of thrombocytopenia and receive platelets if the bleeding is major or life threatening. FFP may be given as part of a massive transfusion protocol to replace coagulation factors lost by severe bleeding. In 2012, the American College of Chest Physicians (ACCP) revised the CHEST guidelines and made a recommendation for treatment of VKA-associated major bleeding that suggests rapid reversal of anticoagulation with 4-factor PCC rather than with FFP.[21] There is no evidence to support the individual use of FFP as a reversal strategy in NOAC-associated bleeding.

Antifibrinolytics

Antifibrinolytic agents, including tranexamic acid, have been used in the treatment of severe or life-threatening bleeding. Although clinical data are lacking, adjunctive tranexamic acid should be considered in patients with life-threatening bleeding associated with NOACs. The CRASH-2 analysis revealed early treatment (<3 hours from time of injury) with tranexamic acid (1g intravenous [IV] bolus followed by 1g infused over 8 hours) significantly reduced the risk of death caused by bleeding after trauma.[22] The dose of ϵ-aminocaproic acid, another antifibrinolytic agent, depends on the urgency with which the bleeding needs to be reversed, although studies in patients with trauma are lacking.

Desmopressin

DDAVP can be used for treatment of impaired platelet function, as occurs in the setting of uremia, von Willebrand disease, or antiplatelet agents. Typical dosing is 0.3 µg/kg given intravenously 15 to 30 minutes before an anticipated procedure to improve platelet function by the release of von Willebrand factor from endothelium.[9] High-quality data are lacking regarding the efficacy of DDAVP in the setting of NOAC-associated bleeding; however, given its low risk of thrombosis, low cost, and widespread availability, it may be an appropriate adjunct in treatment of patients with severe or life-threatening bleeding.

Recombinant Activated Factor VIIa

Recombinant activated factor VIIa (rFVIIa; NovoSeven) aids hemostasis in the presence of tissue factor from injured endothelium to propagate clot formation as well as directly binding to platelets and improving clot stability. The drug is US Food and Drug Administration (FDA) indicated for treatment of congenital hemophilia but it has also been used off label for hemostasis in acute bleeding, surgical bleeding, trauma, and management of intracerebral hemorrhage. Results of the CONTROL trial revealed that rFVIIa reduced the total amount of blood products transfused but did not affect mortality compared with placebo.[23]

Several retrospective studies suggest that rFVIIa rapidly reverses some coagulation parameters in patients on NOACs, but there are limited data to support clinically improved hemostasis, mortality, or functional outcomes with the sole use of rFVIIa compared with other reversal strategies.[24–30] The high risk of complications with administration of rFVIIa administered for off-label use of severe bleeding was best shown by Levy and colleagues[31] in a study showing that the rates of arterial thromboembolic events among 4468 subjects was significantly higher among those who received rFVIIa compared with patients who received placebo (5.5% vs 3.2%; $P = .003$). Thromboembolic complications were even higher among subjects 75 years of age or older (10.8% vs 4.1%; $P = .02$).

Prothrombin Complex Concentrates

PCCs contain multiple coagulation factors, proteins, and heparin purified from plasma. They contain high levels of 3 or 4 coagulation factors based on their formulary (II, IX, and X in 3-factor PCCs; II, VII, IX, and X in 4-factor PCCs). Activated PCCs (aPCCs) are PCCs that contain at least 1 factor in the activated form. Benefits of PCCs include their fast preparation time, rapid INR reversal, small volume, and lower risk of infection compared with standard coagulation factor replacement with FFP.[32] Limitations of PCCs include cost and availability.

Kcentra is currently the only 4-factor PCC available in the United States and its FDA indication is for the urgent reversal of vitamin K antagonist–related bleeding, although it has also been used off label for reversal of NOACs. Likewise, factor VIII inhibitor activity bypassing agent (FEIBA) is the only aPCC available in the United States and its FDA indication is for the management of severe bleeding in patients with hemophilia.

A 4-factor PCC corrected thrombin generation previously impaired by rivaroxaban in 10 healthy, nonbleeding volunteers in a dose-dependent manner.[25] Again, in 12 nonbleeding volunteers, a European 4-factor PCC (Cofact), was able to reverse rivaroxaban-associated PT prolongation and normalize the endogenous thrombin potential, but failed to correct clotting times in these volunteers on dabigatran.[33] All 4-factor PCCs are not equivalent in reversing the anticoagulant effect of rivaroxaban. Note that a similar study using the US 4-factor PCC (Kcentra) at a dose of 50 units/kg was only slightly effective in correcting clotting times in healthy volunteers administered rivaroxaban.[34] Studied in a rabbit hemorrhagic model, 4-factor PCC had no effect on blood loss and partially corrected clotting times for rivaroxaban-induced bleeding.[28]

With regard to PCC reversal of dabigatran, a rodent study by Zhou and colleagues[24] compared hemostatic therapy for management of intracranial hemorrhage (ICH) with 4-factor PCC, rFVIIa, and FFP. There was no significant difference in ICH volume among 4-factor PCC, rFVIIa, and FFP treatments; however, mortality was dramatically reduced with treatment of 4-factor PCC compared with rFVIIa and FFP. In this same model, venous bleeding after transection of the rodent's tail was reduced with 4-factor PCC but only at a dose of 100 units/kg, but doses of 25 to 50 units/kg were not effective.[24] A small clinical case series of 6 patients using FEIBA (50 units/kg) for reversal of ICH associated with rivaroxaban, apixaban, and dabigatran found no subsequent ICH expansion or any thrombotic or hemorrhagic complications after treatment.[35]

Most studies examining PCC efficacy in reversal of NOACs are based on animal or in vitro models or healthy human volunteers.[24–30,33–36] The authors extrapolated from these results, but the extent to which ex vivo or in vitro evidence from healthy human volunteers or animal models correlates with in vivo efficacy for the management of severely bleeding patients with trauma is still not known.

Antidotes

In general, none of the prohemostatic agents are true antidotes to NOACs because they do not reverse the ongoing inhibitory effects of these drugs on thrombin or factor X.

Idarucizumab (Praxbind), a human antibody fragment, was developed to reverse the specific anticoagulant effects of dabigatran. The RE-VERSE AD study included 90 patients with serious bleeding or the need for an urgent invasive procedure (<8 hours) while receiving dabigatran who subsequently received idarucizumab (2 doses of 2.5 g given 15 minutes apart). Reversal was assessed using a dilute TT and ecarin clotting time and anticoagulation effect was reversed in more than 90% of patients within the first 10 to 30 minutes of drug administration.[37]

A reversal agent for all factor Xa inhibitors is in development and expected to receive FDA approval soon (andexanet alfa). This agent works as a decoy and binds the factor Xa inhibitors to render them inert. In a series of 101 healthy volunteers aged 50 to 75 years who were given apixaban or rivaroxaban at therapeutic doses, intravenous bolus of andexanet alfa (400 mg for apixaban or 800 mg for rivaroxaban) was given and was effective at reversing anticoagulant activity within minutes.[38] It is not yet approved, but a small molecule antidote (PER977, Perosphere) has been shown in preliminary studies to bind directly and reverse the anticoagulation properties of direct thrombin inhibitors, factor Xa inhibitors, and heparins (including enoxaparin).[39] Future data and clinical experience with these proposed NOAC antidotes is required, but thus far there have been no major adverse effects cited.

NONPHARMACOLOGIC TREATMENT OPTIONS

Optimal reversal of NOACs for patients with trauma includes other nonpharmacologic treatment options as well. When possible, drug removal from the circulation and/or GI tract aids in the prevention of further coagulopathy.

Activated Charcoal

Activated charcoal (Actidose) is designed to bind certain drugs and toxins, facilitating elimination before absorption from the GI tract. In terms of its studied use with NOACs, activated charcoal has been found to bind dabigatran in vitro and may be effective in decreasing drug absorption following recent ingestion.[40] Although no data show that activated charcoal binds the selective factor Xa inhibitors, this strategy is a reasonable option to attempt to decrease absorption in cases of recent ingestions and need for reversal. If ingestion has occurred in the last 1 to 2 hours, activated charcoal in the form of an oral suspension may be given as a single dose of 25 to 100 g and administered via the oral or nasogastric route.[9]

Hemodialysis

For the urgent reversal of dabigatran, hemodialysis remains an option because the drug is not plasma bound and renally excreted to decrease the duration of the drug's anticoagulant effect. Hemodialysis for 2 hours is able to decrease dabigatran drug levels by roughly 65% in patients with end-stage renal disease but the drug's high volume of distribution leads to eventual rebound in drug levels.[41] Because of pharmacokinetic differences, hemodialysis is unlikely to be effective in the removal of rivaroxaban and apixaban and is not indicated to reverse these agents.

COMPLICATIONS

It must be remembered that bleeding patients are taking these medications for a reason: to reduce thromboembolic risk. In general, clinicians are very good at stopping the NOAC when a patient presents with bleeding. Rapidly reversing the anticoagulant is associated with exposing the patient to the same thromboembolic risk for which they are taking the medication in the first place. If the question is posed to well-informed patients, most patients choose to have some bleeding, which could be more easily treated than a debilitating stroke. Understanding the balance between the thromboembolic risk and the bleeding risk is critical in effectively managing these patients. The decision to urgently reverse the anticoagulant is a multifactorial decision that must take into account the magnitude of the thromboembolic risk versus the severity of the bleeding (**Fig. 2**).

Basic calculations of the CHADS$_2$ (congestive heart failure, hypertension, age>75 years, diabetes mellitus, history of stroke/transient ischemic attack [TIA]) or CHADS$_2$-VASc (CHADS$_2$–vascular disease, age 65–74 years, sex category [female]) score for patients with atrial fibrillation can quickly define a patient's thromboembolic risk for stroke (**Table 3**).[42] Further stratification into low, medium, or high risk for thrombotic complications can be based on the indication for therapeutic anticoagulation and past medical history (**Table 4**).[43] For example, the authors would not recommend rapid reversal for a patient in a high-risk thromboembolic complication stratification who is not experiencing a life-threatening hemorrhage, such as noncompressible torso hemorrhage or severe central nervous system hemorrhage in a closed space.

RESUMING ANTICOAGULATION

Failing to resume anticoagulation in a timely fashion is associated with poor outcomes. Patients do not die of recurrent hemorrhage, but die of thromboembolic complications by failing to resume anticoagulation in a timely fashion after hemorrhage.

Although there are certain patients who clearly should not have their anticoagulation resumed after a hemorrhage, these patients are in the minority. The most common patients in whom clinicians need to make this resumption decision are elderly patients who had bleeding as a result of a fall.[44] A study using Markov decision analysis of data obtained from a MEDLINE review concluded that a patient with an annual stroke risk of 5% from AF would need to fall 295 times in 1 year for the calculated risk of subdural hematoma from falling to outweigh the stroke reduction benefit of anticoagulation.[45]

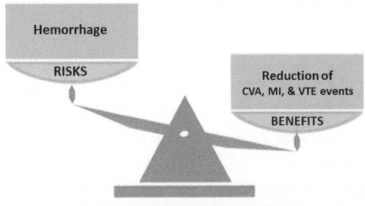

Resumption of Anticoagulation

Fig. 2. Risks versus benefits in resumption of anticoagulation after reversal for bleeding. CVA, cerebrovascular accident; MI, myocardial infarction; VTE, venous thromboembolism.

Table 3
Stroke risk stratification for patients with atrial fibrillation

$CHADS_2$ Risk

Risk Factor	Score
Congestive heart failure	1
Hypertension	1
Age>75 y	1
Diabetes mellitus	1
History of stroke/TIA	2

Stroke Risk According to $CHADS_2$ Score in Patients with Atrial Fibrillation

$CHADS_2$ Score	Nonperioperative Setting: Annual Stroke Rate (95% CI)	Perioperative Setting: 30-d Postoperative Stroke Rate (95% CI)
0	1.9 (1.2–3)	1.01 (0.83–1.21)
1	2.8 (2–3.8)	1.62 (1.46–1.79)
2	4 (3.1–5.1)	2.05 (1.87–2.24)
3	5.9 (4.6–7.3)	2.63 (2.26–3.04)
4	8.5 (6.3–11.1)	3.62 (2.66–4.8)
5	12.5 (8.2–17.5)	3.65 (1.83–6.45)
6	18.2 (10.5–27.4)	7.35 (2.42–16.3)

CHA_2DS_2-VASc

Risk Factor	Score
Congestive Heart Failure	1
Hypertension	1
Age ≥75 y	2
Diabetes mellitus	1
Stroke/TIA/thromboembolism	2
Vascular disease	1
Age 65–74 y	1
Sex category (female)	1

Stroke Risk According to CHA_2DS_2-VASC Score in Patients with Atrial Fibrillation

CHA_2DS_2-VASC Score	Adjusted Stroke Rate (%/y)
0	0
1	1.3
2	2.2
3	3.2
4	4
5	6.7
6	9.8
7	9.6
8	6.7
9	15.2

The $CHADS_2$ and CHA_2D_2-VASc risk criteria are well-validated tools for the assessment of risk for stroke in patients with atrial fibrillation. These tools can also be used to determine whether aspirin or oral anticoagulation is warranted based on the score.

Adapted from Fuster V, Ryden LE, Cannom DS, et al. ACC/AHA/ESC 2006 guidelines for the management of patients with atrial fibrillation. Circulation 2006;114:e257–354; and Camm AJ, Kirchhof P, Lip GYH, et al. Guidelines for the management of atrial fibrillation. Eur Heart J 2010;31:2369–429.

Table 4
Thrombotic risk stratification for patients requiring therapeutic anticoagulation

Thrombotic Risk Stratification	Indication for Therapeutic Anticoagulation		
	Mechanical Heart Valve	Atrial Fibrillation	VTE
High risk	Any mitral prosthesis Any caged-ball or tilting disc aortic valve prosthesis Recent (within 6 mo) stroke or TIA	CHADS$_2$ score of 5 or 6 Recent (within 3 mo) stroke or TIA Rheumatic valvular heart disease	Recent (within 3 mo) VTE Severe thrombophilia[a]
Moderate risk	Bileaflet aortic valve prosthesis and ≥1 of the following risk factors: atrial fibrillation, prior stroke or TIA, hypertension, diabetes, CHF, age >75 y	CHADS$_2$ score of 3 or 4	VTE within past 3–12 mo Recurrent VTE Active cancer (treated within 6 mo or palliative) Nonsevere thrombophilia[b]
Low risk	Bileaflet aortic valve prosthesis without atrial fibrillation and no other risk factors for stroke	CHADS$_2$ score of 0–2	VTE >12 mo previous and no other risk factors

Patients who require therapeutic anticoagulation must have their underlying thrombotic risk taken into consideration when deciding the risks versus benefits of urgent reversal from their pharmacologic coagulopathy.

Abbreviation: CHF, congestive heart failure.

[a] Severe thrombophilia: deficiency of protein C, protein S, or antithrombin; antiphospholipid syndrome; or multiple abnormalities.

[b] Nonsevere thrombophilia: heterozygous factor V or factor II mutation.

Adapted from Douketis JD, Spyropoulos AC, Spencer FA. Perioperative management of antithrombotic therapy: antithrombotic therapy and prevention of thrombosis, 9th ed: American College of Chest Physicians evidence-based clinical practice guidelines. Chest 2012;141(2 Suppl):e330S; with permission.

A retrospective trial showed that failing to resume warfarin in patients with GI hemorrhage resulted in a more than 10-fold increase in recurrent thrombotic events at 90 days (0.4% warfarin resumed vs 5.5% warfarin not resumed). More importantly, resumption of warfarin decreased the risk of death by 68% in these patients after GI hemorrhage, and no deaths in the 90-day follow-up were attributed to recurrent GI hemorrhage. The lowest risk of death was achieved when warfarin was resumed between 15 and 90 days after the GI bleed.[46]

A recent study from Denmark examined 1-year outcomes in patients with ICH related to oral anticoagulation (OAC). Three nationwide registries were used and there were 1752 patients with a 1-year follow-up. The combined primary outcome was ischemic stroke/systemic embolism/all-cause mortality. Three groups were compared: OAC was resumed, antiplatelet therapy was substituted for OAC, and no resumption of OAC or antiplatelet therapy. The primary outcome was only reduced in the patients who had their OAC resumed. Occurrence of primary outcome: OAC resumed, 13.6 (10.1–18.3); antiplatelet, 25.7 (20.7–31.9); no treatment resumed, 27.3 (23.6–31.6). Importantly, there was not a significant difference in recurrent ICH among the 3 groups. Mortality over 5 years was greatly reduced in the patients who had their OAC resumed compared with the other two groups.[47]

A recent multicenter retrospective cohort study conducted in 19 German centers assessed the effects of rapid anticoagulation reversal, blood pressure control, and anticoagulation resumption in patients with OAC-related ICH. Several important findings were reported in this large study. Achieving an INR less than 1.3 within 4 hours combined with a reduction of systolic blood pressure to less than 160 mm Hg within 4 hours was successful in reducing hemorrhage growth more effectively than either therapy alone. The investigators also showed that ischemic events occurred significantly more frequently in patients who did not have an OAC resumed in the 1 year after the index ICH. However, there was no difference in hemorrhagic events over the first year between groups. One-year survival was greatly improved in patients who had their OAC resumed compared with patients who had no OAC resumption. The only parameter significantly associated with a decreased risk reduction for an unfavorable functional long-term neurologic outcome was resumption of OAC based on modified Rankin scoring at discharge, 3 months, and 1 year.[48]

Table 5
Resumption of therapeutic anticoagulation and antiplatelets after traumatic injury

| Type of Bleed | Resuming Therapeutic Anticoagulation[a,b] | |
	Anticoagulant	Antiplatelet
Extremity, thoracic, or abdominal trauma	Full anticoagulation should be resumed after bleeding stopped based on thrombotic risk High risk: within 4 d Moderate risk: within 1–2 wk Low risk: consider within 2–4 wk	Withhold DAPT for 24 h to assess bleed For all patients on aspirin the authors recommend resuming aspirin (81 mg) 24 h after bleeding stops For patients with a DES<12 mo, BMS <3 mo, or intracranial stent <12 mo, restart second agent within 1–2 wk
Traumatic intracranial or intraspinal hemorrhage	Reevaluate reason for anticoagulation: antithrombotics vs antiplatelets Anticoagulation should be resumed after bleeding stopped based on thrombotic risk: High risk: resume 7–10 d after bleeding event Moderate risk: resume within 2–3 wk Low risk: resume within 3–4 wk	Withhold DAPT for 24 h to assess bleed For all patients on aspirin the authors recommend resuming aspirin (81 mg) 24 h after bleeding stops For patients with a DES<12 mo, BMS <3 mo, or intracranial stent <12 mo, restart second agent within 1–2 wk Small bleeds: within 48 h if neurologic examination and CT stable improved for small bleeds Large bleeds: hold aspirin for 5 d

Our institutional recommendations for resumption of therapeutic anticoagulation and antiplatelets after traumatic injury are based on expert consensus.

Abbreviations: BMS, bare metal stent; CT, computed tomography; DAPT, dual antiplatelet therapy; DES, drug eluting stent.

[a] Need to assess indication for use, risk for thrombosis, and risk of clinically significant rebleeding.

[b] If patients are on aspirin only for primary prevention of atherosclerotic events, it is reasonable to stop aspirin until the bleeding event is completely treated.

Resumption of anticoagulation should be addressed before discharge and carefully communicated with the patient, and/or surrogate, and the patient's primary care provider and/or specialist who had been prescribing the anticoagulant before it being stopped. It is a multidisciplinary decision that should include all the key stakeholders. Our institution has developed a guideline based on some evidence, but mostly based on expert opinion from a multidisciplinary group that included representation from trauma surgery, cardiology, neurointerventional surgery, GI medicine, and vascular surgery. The decision when, and whether, to resume anticoagulation is based primarily on the patient's thromboembolic risk (ie, why were they placed on the drug in the first place, and the type of hemorrhage they had). **Table 5** provides example of our recommendation for a patient who sustained a hemorrhage caused by trauma.

SUMMARY

Treatment of severely injured patients with trauma on NOACs is becoming more common. It is imperative that clinicians understand the appropriate management of NOAC-induced coagulopathy in trauma.

For patients who are at imminent risk of death from bleeding associated with direct factor Xa inhibitor anticoagulation (rivaroxaban, apixaban, edoxaban), the authors suggest administering a 4-factor PCC (Kcentra) at a dose of 50 units/kg IV or aPCC

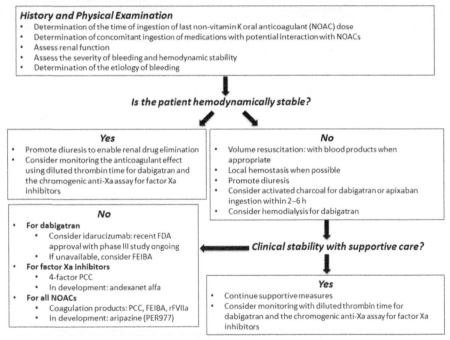

Fig. 3. Strategy for management of acute bleeding on NOACs. A clinical approach to the management of bleeding on NOACs using available data. In light of current trials of targeted reversal agents for this clinical use, algorithms for the management of bleeding are likely to evolve in the near future. (*From* Sarma A. Update on reversal agents for novel oral anticoagulant. Available at: http://www.acc.org/latest-in-cardiology/articles/2015/12/11/08/20/update-on-reversal-agents-for-novel-oral-anticoagulants#sthash.tzash12j.dpuf. Accessed May 1, 2016. Used with permission of the American College of Cardiology.)

(FEIBA) at a dose of 50 units/kg IV. If a 4-factor PCC is unavailable, a 3-factor PCC supplemented with FFP or rFVIIa may be considered. If ingestion of the last dose of the NOAC was within 2 hours, activated charcoal at a dose of ~50 g should be administered orally or via nasogastric route. Once approved and available, the anti–factor Xa antidote (andexanet alfa) should be strongly considered as the first-line agent for emergent reversal of direct factor Xa inhibitor anticoagulation.

In patients with trauma with severe or critical bleeding and imminent risk of death from hemorrhage associated with direct thrombin inhibitor anticoagulation (dabigatran), the authors suggest the new antidote idarucizumab (Praxbind) as the first-line agent for reversal at 2 doses of 2.5 g IV given 15 minutes apart. If this antidote is unavailable, consider administering a FEIBA at a dose of 50 units/kg IV. The 4-factor PCC, Kcentra, is the last choice based on the literature. These PCCs (activated and unactivated) should not be thought of as the standard of care for reversal of dabigatran-associated bleeding because the quality of evidence is low. It is often

Table 6
Summary of reversal strategies for NOACs

| | Optimal Reversal Strategy | |
Drug	Emergent Need (Reversal Needed in <1 h)	Nonurgent
Warfarin	5 mg IV vitamin K 4-factor PCC (Kcentra) INR Dose 2–4 25 units/kg (max = 2500 units) 4–6 35 units/kg (max = 3500 units) >6 50 units/kg (max = 5000 units) Can build 4-factor PCC with PCC3 + rFVIIa	Withhold drug May consider FFP Consider 1–5 mg PO vitamin K Trend PT/INR until INR ≤1.7

Dabigatran	Consider activated charcoal if last
	  dose was ingested within 2 h
	Idarucizumab (Praxbind)
	2.5 g IV q 15 min × 2 doses
	If antidote unavailable, consider
	aPCC (FEIBA) 50 units/kg
	max = 200 units/kg/d
	Or
	4-factor PCC (Kcentra) 50units/kg
	max = 5000 units
	Consider urgent hemodialysis
		Withhold drug
		Consider activated charcoal if last
		  dose was ingested within 2 h
		Consider prolonged dialysis (up to
		  60% of drug removed)
		If CrCl ≤30 mL/min consider holding
		  drug before invasive procedure for
		  ≥48 h caused by/because of
		  prolonged half-life

Rivaroxaban
Apixaban
Edoxaban
	Consider activated charcoal if last
	  dose was ingested within 2 h
	Andexanet alfa antidote when
	  available
	If antidote unavailable, consider
	4-factor PCC (Kcentra) 50 units/kg
	max = 5000 units
	or
	aPCC (FEIBA) 50 units/kg
	max = 200 units/kg/d
		Withhold drug
		Consider activated charcoal if last
		  dose was ingested within 2 h
		If CrCl ≤30 mL/min consider holding
		  drug before invasive procedure for
		  ≥36 h because of prolonged half-
		  life

Our institutional recommendations for resumption of therapeutic anticoagulation and antiplatelets after traumatic injury based on expert consensus and available evidence.
Abbreviations: CrCl, creatinine clearance; max, maximum; PO, by mouth; q, every.

logistically difficulty, but urgent hemodialysis should be considered to reduce the anti-coagulant effects of dabigatran. Similarly, if ingestion of the last dose was within 2 hours, activated charcoal should be administered to limit further drug absorption and pharmacologic coagulopathy.

Clinicians must always remember that treatment with PCCs or any other prohemostatic agents carries a substantial thrombotic risk. Therefore, clinical judgment is required in determining the individual bleeding and thrombotic risks of each patient on a case-by-case basis. Evolving anticoagulants require equally complex and evolving care plans to manage these patients with critical trauma and their injuries. A summary of recommendations and the strategy for optimal reversal of major bleeding in patients with trauma on NOACs is presented in **Fig. 3** and **Table 6**.

REFERENCES

1. Centers for Disease Control and Prevention. Trauma statistics. 2014. Available at: http://www.nationaltraumainstitute.org/home/trauma_statistics.html. Accessed April 1, 2016.
2. Adams SD, Cotton BA, McGuire MF, et al. The unique pattern of complications in elderly trauma patients at a level I trauma center. J Trauma Acute Care Surg 2012; 72(1):112–8.
3. Pokorney SD, Simon DN, Thomas L, et al. Patients' time in therapeutic range on warfarin among US patients with atrial fibrillation: results from ORBIT-AF registry. Am Heart J 2015;170(1):141–8.
4. Miller CS, Grandi S, Shimony A, et al. The efficacy and safety of new oral anticoagulants versus warfarin in patients with atrial fibrillation: a systematic review and meta-analysis. J Am Coll Cardiol 2012;59(13s1):E604.
5. Granger CB, Alexander JH, McMurray JJ, et al. Apixaban versus warfarin in patients with atrial fibrillation. N Engl J Med 2011;365:981–92.
6. Connolly SJ, Ezekowitz MD, Yusuf S, et al. Dabigatran versus warfarin in patients with atrial fibrillation. N Engl J Med 2009;361:1139–51.
7. Patel MR, Mahaffey KW, Garg J, et al. Rivaroxaban versus warfarin in nonvalvular atrial fibrillation. N Engl J Med 2011;365:883–91.
8. Chai-Adisaksopha C, Hillis C, Isayama T, et al. Mortality outcomes in patients receiving direct oral anticoagulants: a systematic review and meta-analysis of randomized controlled trials. J Thromb Haemost 2015;13(11):2012–20.
9. Lexi-Comp online. Pediatric and neonatal Lexi-drugs online. Hudson (OH): Lexi-Comp. Available at: http://online.lexi.com/action/home. Accessed April 1, 2016.
10. Lindahl T, Baghaei F, Fagerberg Blixter I, et al. Effects of the oral, direct thrombin inhibitor dabigatran on five common coagulation assays. Thromb Haemost 2011; 105(2):371–8.
11. Nutescu E, Dager W, Cipolle M, et al. Management of bleeding and reversal strategies for oral anticoagulants: clinical practice considerations. Am J Health Syst Pharm 2013;70:e82–97.
12. Cuker A, Siegal DM, Crowther MA, et al. Laboratory measurement of the anticoagulant activity of the non-vitamin K oral anticoagulants. J Am Coll Cardiol 2014; 64:1128–39.
13. Cuker A, Husseinzadeh H. Laboratory measurement of the anticoagulant activity of edoxaban: a systemic review. J Thromb Thrombolysis 2015;39:288–94.
14. Eller T, Busse J, Dittrich M, et al. Dabigatran, rivaroxaban, apixaban, argatroban and fondaparinux and their effects on coagulation POC and platelet function tests. Clin Chem Lab Med 2014;52:835.

15. Herrmann R, Thom J, Wood A, et al. Thrombin generation using the calibrated automated thrombinoscope to assess reversibility of dabigatran and rivaroxaban. Thromb Haemost 2014;111:989.

16. Neyens R, Bohm N, Cearley M, et al. Dabigatran-associated subdural hemorrhage: using thromboelastography (TEG®) to guide decision-making. J Thromb Thrombolysis 2014;37:80.

17. Xu Y, Wu W, Wang L, et al. Differential profiles of thrombin inhibitors (heparin, hirudin, bivalirudin, and dabigatran) in the thrombin generation assay and thromboelastography in vitro. Blood Coagul Fibrinolysis 2013;24:332.

18. Casutt M, Konrad C, Schuepfer G. Effect of rivaroxaban on blood coagulation using the viscoelastic coagulation test ROTEM™. Anaesthesist 2012;61:948.

19. Watson HG, Baglin T, Laidlaw SL, et al. A comparison of the efficacy and rate of response to oral and intravenous vitamin K in reversal of over-anticoagulation with warfarin. Br J Haematol 2001;115:145–9.

20. Frontera JA, Gordon E, Zach V, et al. Reversal of coagulopathy using prothrombin complex concentrates is associated with improved outcome compared to fresh frozen plasma in warfarin-associated intracranial hemorrhage. Neurocrit Care 2014;21:397–406.

21. Holbrook A, Schulman S, Witt DM, et al. Evidence-based management of anticoagulant therapy: antithrombotic therapy and prevention of thrombosis, 9th ed: American College of Chest Physicians evidence-based clinical practice guidelines. Chest 2012;141:e152S–84S.

22. Crash-2 Collaborators, Roberts I, Shakur H, Afolabi A, et al. The importance of early treatment with tranexamic acid in bleeding trauma patients: an exploratory analysis of the CRASH-2 randomized controlled trial. Lancet 2011;377(9771): 1096–101.

23. Hauser CJ, Boffard K, Dutton R, et al. Results of the CONTROL trial: efficacy and safety of recombinant activated factor VII in the management of refractory traumatic hemorrhage. J Trauma Acute Care Surg 2010;69(3):489–500.

24. Zhou W, Schwarting S, Illanes S, et al. Hemostatic therapy in experimental intracerebral hemorrhage associated with the direct thrombin inhibitor dabigatran. Stroke 2011;42:3594–9.

25. Marlu R, Hodaj E, Paris A, et al. Effect of non-specific reversal agents on anticoagulant activity of dabigatran and rivaroxaban: a randomised crossover ex vivo study in healthy volunteers. Thromb Haemost 2012;108:217–24.

26. van Ryn J, Stangier J, Haertter S, et al. Dabigatran etexilate–a novel, reversible, oral direct thrombin inhibitor: interpretation of coagulation assays and reversal of anticoagulant activity. Thromb Haemost 2010;103:1116–27.

27. Halim AB, Li Y, Stein E, et al. Low concentrations of rhFVIIa or FEIBA significantly and rapidly reverse the anticoagulant effect of supratherapeutic edoxaban. Poster at the ASH Congress. San Diego (CA), December 10, 2011.

28. Godier A, Miclot A, Le Bonniec B, et al. Evaluation of prothrombin complex concentrate and recombinant activated factor VII to reverse rivaroxaban in a rabbit model. Anesthesiology 2012;116:94–102.

29. Escolar G, Arellano-Rodrigo E, Reverter JC, et al. Coagulation factor concentrates restore alterations in hemostasis induced by a high dose of apixaban: studies in vitro with circulating human blood. Blood 2012;120:Abstract: 2263.

30. Gruber A, Marzec UM, Buetehorn U, et al. Activated factor VII and activated prothrombin complex for reversal of the antihemostatic effects of rivaroxaban in primates. Br J Haematol 2009;145:Abstract: 80.

31. Levi M, Levy JH, Andersen HF, et al. Safety of recombinant activated factor VII in randomized clinical trials. N Engl J Med 2010;363(19):1791–800.
32. Eerenberg ES, Kamphuisen PW, Levi M, et al. Reversal of rivaroxaban and dabigatran by prothrombin complex concentrate: a randomized, placebo-controlled, cross-over study in healthy subjects. J Thromb Haemost 2011;9:657.
33. Levi M, Moore KT, Levy JH, et al. Comparison of three-factor and four-factor prothrombin complex concentrates regarding reversal of the anticoagulant effects of rivaroxaban in healthy volunteers. J Thromb Haemost 2014;12:1428–36.
34. Dibu JR, Weimer JM, Ahrens C, et al. The role of FEIBA in reversing novel oral anticoagulants in intracerebral hemorrhage. Neurocrit Care 2016;24(3):413–9.
35. Dzik WH. Reversal of oral factor Xa inhibitors by prothrombin complex concentrates: a re-appraisal. J Thromb Haemost 2015;13(S1):S187–94.
36. Siegal DM, Cuker A. Reversal of novel oral anticoagulants in patients with major bleeding. J Thromb Thrombolysis 2013;35(3):391–8.
37. Pollack CV Jr, Reilly PA, Eikelboom J, et al. Idarucizumab for dabigatran reversal. N Engl J Med 2015;373(6):511–20.
38. Siegal DM, Curnutte JT, Connolly SJ, et al. Andexanet alfa for the reversal of factor Xa inhibitor activity. N Engl J Med 2015;373(25):2413–24.
39. Laulicht B, Bakhru S, Jiang X, et al. Antidote for new oral anticoagulants: mechanism of action and binding specificity of PER977. Journal of Thrombosis and Hemostasis 11(Suppl 2);1322.
40. van Ryn J, Sieger P, Kink-Eiband M, et al. Adsorption of dabigatran etexilate in water or dabigatran in pooled human plasma by activated charcoal in vitro. Blood 2009;144(22):1065.
41. Chang DN, Dager WE, Chin AI. Removal of dabigatran by hemodialysis. Am J Kidney Dis 2013;61:487–9.
42. Fuster V, Ryden LE, Cannom DS, et al. ACC/AHA/ESC 2006 guidelines for the management of patients with atrial fibrillation. Circulation 2006;114:e257–354.
43. Douketis JD. Perioperative management of patients who are receiving warfarin therapy: an evidence-based and practical approach. Blood 2011;117(19):5044–9.
44. Man-Son-Hing M, Nichol G, Lau A, et al. Choosing antithrombotic therapy for elderly patients with atrial fibrillation who are at risk for falls. Arch Intern Med 1999;159:677–85.
45. You JH. Novel oral anticoagulants versus warfarin therapy at various levels of anticoagulation control in atrial fibrillation—a cost-effectiveness analysis. J Gen Intern Med 2014;29(3):438–46.
46. Witt DM, Delate T, Garcia DA, et al. Risk of thromboembolism, recurrent hemorrhage, and death after warfarin therapy interruption for gastrointestinal tract bleeding. Arch Intern Med 2012;172(19):1484–91.
47. Nielsen PB, Larsen TB, Skjøth F, et al. Restarting anticoagulant treatment after intracranial hemorrhage in patients with atrial fibrillation and the impact on recurrent stroke, mortality, and bleeding: a nationwide cohort study. Circulation 2015;132(6):517–25.
48. Karamatsu JB, Gerner ST, Schellinger PD, et al. Anticoagulant reversal, blood pressure levels, and anticoagulant resumption in patients with anticoagulation-related intracerebral hemorrhage. JAMA 2015;313(8):824–36.

Rib Fracture Fixation
Indications and Outcomes

Lara Senekjian, MD, MSCI*, Raminder Nirula, MD, MPH

KEYWORDS

- Rib fracture • Chest trauma • Flail chest • Surgical fixation

KEY POINTS

- Thoracic trauma is common and rib fractures are frequently identified after blunt injury.
- History, physical, and symptoms may suggest fracture, but computed tomography scan is the best imaging modality to diagnose rib fractures.
- Rib fractures increase the risk of complications including pneumonia, prolonged ventilator days, and increased hospital stay. Rib fracture management requires significant resources, especially in the elderly.
- Treatment of rib fractures currently involves pain control and respiratory therapy.
- There is some evidence that surgical fixation may improve outcomes, but well-designed clinical trials with sufficient sample size are warranted to confirm these results.

INTRODUCTION

Managing patients with multiple rib fractures or flail chest requires significant health care resources. These patients may require critical care, ventilator management, and intensive pain control to minimize the risk of complications. Frequently seen in patients who sustain thoracic trauma, patients with rib fractures may also be diagnosed with blunt cardiac injury, pulmonary contusion, or great vessel injury. Patients with thoracic trauma, in particular with rib fractures, may develop complications such as pneumonia, prolonged ventilator times, prolonged hospitalization, and chronic debilitating pain after discharge. Current evidence indicates that a greater number of rib fractures is associated with an increased risk for pneumonia and death, particularly in the elderly. Treatment of rib fractures is controversial, but the goal of management is to prevent or minimize associated complications.

The authors have no financial conflicts of interest pertaining to the content of this article.
Department of Surgery, University of Utah, 50 North Medical Drive, Salt Lake City, UT 84132, USA
* Corresponding author.
E-mail address: lara.senekjian@hsc.utah.edu

Crit Care Clin 33 (2017) 153–165
http://dx.doi.org/10.1016/j.ccc.2016.08.009
criticalcare.theclinics.com

PATIENT EVALUATION
Epidemiology of Thoracic Trauma and Rib Fractures

It is common for patients with thoracic trauma to present to the emergency department with severe injury. Often chest trauma includes rib fractures. In 2000, the National Center for Healthcare Statistics estimated that more than 300,000 people were treated for rib fractures in the emergency department.[1] Of these roughly 180,000 were admitted to the hospital with multiple fractures with total hospital charges close to $8 billion dollars.[2] More than one-third of these patients are over the age of 65. The elderly population has a disproportionately higher degree of morbidity, mortality and cost of care after sustaining multiple rib fractures compared with younger patients. Elderly patients with similar fracture pattern have a 33% incidence of major pulmonary complications compared with 12% in younger patients.[3]

Flail chest is radiographically defined as multiple consecutive rib fractures (>4) on 1 side of the chest with fractures in 2 or more locations. Clinically, flail chest is defined as a segment of the chest wall exhibiting paradoxic movement with inspiration. As expected, this fracture pattern has greater impact on patient outcomes than individual rib fracture.[4] A metaanalysis of 29 studies of blunt thoracic trauma identified that age 65 years and older, 3 or more rib fractures, the presence of preexisting disease, and the development of pneumonia after injury were significant risk factors for mortality.[5] The mean number of mechanical ventilation days required for patients with multiply displaced rib fractures or flail chest ranges from 7 to 30 days in several studies.[6–9] Nosocomial pneumonia occurs significantly more frequently in elderly patients than in their younger counterparts in a dose–response relationship, showing higher rates of nosocomial pneumonia in those with greater numbers of ribs fractures (**Fig. 1**).[3]

Not surprisingly, there is a disproportionate use of resources among elderly patients when evaluating the number of ribs fractured. The elderly have a much higher complication rate than the younger population.[3] Elderly flail chest patients (>64 years of age) incur a mean hospital charge that is $39,125 greater and a hospital duration of stay that is 3.2 days longer than younger flail chest patients (18–44 years of age). As many as 40% of patients with multiple rib fractures require critical care resources,

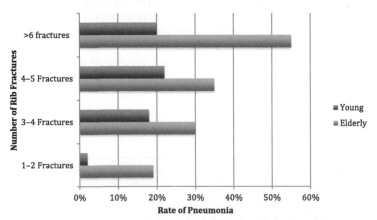

Fig. 1. Relationship between pneumonia and number of rib fractures. The pneumonia rate increases as the number of rib fractures increases, most notably for the elderly group. (*From* Bulger EM, Arneson MA, Mock CN, et al. Rib fractures in the elderly. J Trauma 2000;48(6):1040–6. [discussion: 1046–7].)

with the elderly forming a large portion of this group (68%).[10] Between 35% and 60% of elderly rib fracture patients are eventually discharged to other care facilities instead of their home, which further increases the cost of care for these individuals. Multiple rib fractures leads to reduced productivity and chronic disability. Many patients with flail chest still complain of thoracic cage pain, tightness, and dyspnea 12 months after injury (89%, 84%, and 63% respectively).[6] The mean number of days before return to work for individuals with multiple fractures was 70 days in 1 study.

Symptoms of Chest Trauma

Chest trauma is a common presentation in the emergency department.[1,5,11] Patient symptoms are a poor indicator of injury severity in chest trauma as the "classic" indicators of rib fractures are nonspecific. These include but are not limited to point tenderness, focally referred pain with compression, splinting, crepitus, and ecchymosis.[12] The most common ribs fractured are the 4th through 10th ribs. Ribs 1 to 3 are associated with nerve or vascular injury. Ribs 10 to 12 are often associated with injuries to the abdominal cavity, including the spleen, liver, and retroperitoneum.

Rib fractures are frequently seen with other thoracic injuries. Pneumothorax and hemothorax are common. One series found that more than half of patients with rib fracture had underlying pneumothorax or hemothorax.[13] Pulmonary contusion can be seen in 30% to 70% of patients with blunt thoracic trauma. As expected, worse outcomes are seen in patients who have both contusion and rib fracture.[14] Other thoracic injuries seen with rib fracture can include ruptured diaphragm, aortic rupture, tracheobronchial injury, cardiac contusion, pericardial injuries, and great vessel injuries. Many of these associated injuries are deadly, for example, of patients with aortic rupture it is estimated that only 20% survive more than 1 hour from injury.[13] Thus, rib fractures carry their associated risk of complications but also act as marker for mere serious and devastating injuries.

Causes of Rib Fracture

Although rib fracture is seen in penetrating trauma, blunt trauma is by far the more common cause of multiple rib fractures most often secondary to motor vehicle crash (60%–70%).[10,13] Seatbelt impingement leading to localized thoracic loading can displace rib fractures.[15] Any trauma patient that sustained moderate force to the chest via fall or motor vehicle crash should increase suspicion for rib fractures.

Diagnosis of Rib Fractures in Thoracic Trauma

Chest radiographs

Various imaging modalities have been used with varying accuracy in the diagnosis of rib fractures. As part of the Advanced Trauma Life Support guidelines, all patients who have a potential for a chest injury should get a chest radiograph as part of the secondary survey.[16] However, chest radiography is not a perfect test with more than 50% of fractures being missed on standard chest radiography.[1] Chest radiographs also miss 10% to 50% of pneumothoraces that are subsequently seen on computed tomography (CT) of the chest.[17] Fractures located in the arc of the rib are the most frequently missed fractures on chest radiograph.[18] Sensitivity of chest radiograph has been as low as 15% depending on the location of the fracture.[18] Therefore, some authors advocate for a rib series beyond the classic chest film.[12] This series would include oblique views with a marker over the area of interest with optimal exposure and multiple views. The time and positioning of involved with this technique make this impractical for the trauma patient where spine precautions must be maintained.

Ultrasound imaging

Ultrasonography (US) is as an alternative test to radiography. Advantages include lack of radiation, and in experienced hands is more sensitive than plain film to diagnose fracture.[12] However, US is not only time consuming it is more costly and painful to the patient. The quality of the US is variable, moreover rib cortex and pleura can appear similar on studies.[19] Thus, fractures may be overdiagnosed on US alone. US may have a place to diagnose rib pathology; however, it has not been universally accepted as the diagnostic test of choice for trauma. Ten times more fractures are diagnosed on US than radiography.[19] US can also demonstrate costal cartilage injury where chest radiograph cannot. However, US has disadvantages, because it requires the patient to move from supine to decubitus positions, causing pain. US also cannot see posterior fractures deep to the scapula. Therefore, US has little value for the diagnosis of rib fractures in trauma patients.[19]

Computed tomography scan

According to 1 study, chest CT scanning alters management in 20% of patients with abnormal initial chest radiograph.[17] If a patient has a severe mechanism and a normal chest radiograph, 39% will have chest injury findings on a subsequent chest CT scan.[18] Advantages of CT scanning include the ability to diagnose a costal cartilage injury as well as more accurate diagnosis of rib fractures themselves. CT scanning can also diagnose other underlying injury to the lung parenchyma or great vessels in patients with polytrauma.[12] In patients with penetrating injury or major trauma that are stable enough for imaging CT scan is the test of choice to fully evaluate the severity and number of rib fractures.[12]

PHARMACOLOGIC TREATMENT OPTIONS

The goal in the management of patients with rib fractures is to optimize chest wall mechanics to minimize their sequelae.[20] In the acute period, pain limits patient's cough, which results in sputum retention, atelectasis, and reduced functional residual capacity.[21] This sequence leads to hypoxemia, VQ mismatch, altered lung compliance, and respiratory failure. Pain after trauma has significant long-term impact on all patients with chest trauma. At a 30-day follow-up, 70% of patients with multiple rib fractures continued to use narcotics.[22] Hence, pain management is vital to improving function and chest wall mechanics.

Nonsteroidal Antiinflammatory Drugs

Pain control includes nonsteroidal antiinflammatory drugs (NSAIDs). Advantages of NSAIDs include ease of use and accessibility.[21] NSAIDs also have no impact on central nervous system function or respiratory drive. Hospitalization is unnecessary if patients have good pain control with oral NSAIDs. However, patients with peptic ulcer disease or platelet dysfunction should not use these medications, and there is a risk of renal damage with any use of NSAIDs.[21]

Opioids

The use of opioids is often part of the pain control regimen for rib fracture.[23] Opioids can be administered orally, via intermittent intravenous injections, or via patient-controlled delivery systems. Patients who have severe pain may need continuous infusions, although often these patients are in the intensive care unit (ICU) and have multiple injuries that require management with opioid analgesia. Like NSAIDs, opioids are often used for pain management given the accessibility and familiarity of these medications.[21,22] Disadvantages of opioids include central nervous system depression, respiratory depression, nausea, opioid-induced ,constipation and the development of tolerance.

Local Anesthesia

Intercostal nerve block has shown some benefit in patients with rib fractures.[21] Injection of local agents (such as bupivacaine) can last 8 to 12 hours. This is advantageous, because it has no central nervous system depression or risk of dependence. However, the injection requires palpation of the rib or ribs that are fractured causing increase in pain, as well as need for injection above and below the fracture site given overlapping intercostal nerves. Intercostal block is also time consuming and only temporary; thus, multiple injections are needed for long-term pain management. With each injection there is an increase in the risk of pneumothorax.[21]

Epidural anesthesia includes agents (bupivacaine) with or without opioids (fentanyl) administered via lumbar or thoracic route.[21,24] Advantages over intercostal block include bilateral pain relief, lower dosage requirements, and increased functional residual capacity. Studies have demonstrated improved dynamic lung compliance, increased vital capacity and decreased airway resistance with the use of epidural aenesthesia.[25] In a randomized study comparing patients with and without epidurals, 18% of patients with an epidural versus 38% without an epidural developed pneumonia demonstrating the impact that pain control can have on respiratory outcomes. Epidural anesthesia is technically demanding and time intensive to get proper analgesia. Disadvantages can include hypotension, urinary retention, delayed respiratory depression, and risk of spinal cord injury.[21] Epidurals are also contraindicated in patients with elevated intracranial pressure, making this method of delivery undesirable for some trauma patients.

NONPHARMACOLOGIC TREATMENT OPTIONS

Historically, treatment of rib fractures and flail chest required mandatory ventilatory support.[14] Patients with flail chest were thought to have altered respiratory mechanics in which chest wall stabilization and mechanical ventilation were the required treatment. "Internal pneumatic stabilization" was required for patients with no regard to patient baseline pulmonary function. In 1981, Shackford and colleagues[26] demonstrated worse survival in patients who were ventilated owing to complications of mechanical ventilation. They concluded that mechanical ventilation should be used for abnormal gas exchange and not chest wall instability. Since that time, mandatory mechanical ventilatory support has been abandoned and Eastern Association for the Surgery of Trauma (EAST) guidelines state that "obligatory mechanical ventilation should be avoided."[14]

Aggressive treatment by involving respiratory therapy is now part of the usual management of patients with rib fractures. Todd and colleagues[23] describe a volume expansion protocol as part of the clinical pathway. Included in this pathway are aggressive pulmonary toilet, positive airway pressure systems, incentive spirometery and coughing to encourage volume expansion. Currently, the use of positive pressure and incentive spirometery are incorporated into the multidisciplinary approach to rib fractures, although pain management is generally the most effective nonoperative treatment.

SURGICAL TREATMENT OPTIONS

Surgical treatment of rib fractures involves open reduction and internal fixation of the fracture or fractures. This management has evolved over the years. Initially described in the first century, surgeons described resection of rib fractures to improve pain.[4] The technique of closed stabilization of fractures was then described in the 1500s. Surgical treatment then gained popularity in Europe and Asia in the 1950s.[14]

The invention and popularity of mechanical ventilation made internal fixation fall out of favor at that time, but select surgeons assumed that some patients would benefit from internal fixation.[4] Attempts at internal fixation gained popularity in the United Sates after World War II. Only those who failed mechanical ventilation were chosen for fixation. Currently, however, some data suggest that a wider population may benefit from fixation.

Specific indications for fixation remain to be elucidated. Some indications that have been adopted include flail chest, symptomatic fracture with displacement, or fixation of the way out from thoracotomy for other reasons (**Box 1**).[20] However, trauma surgeons debate the true benefit for surgical rib fracture fixation.

Evidence for Rib Fracture Surgical Fixation

Currently, 3 randomized controlled trials with 123 study participants, conducted outside the United States indicate decreased rates of pneumonia and shorter time on the ventilator when patients with rib fractures are treated with surgical fixation.[6,27,28] A recent metaanalysis[29] of these 3 studies reported no statistically significant difference in the primary outcome of death (relative risk [RR], 0.56; 95% confidence interval [CI], 0.13–2.42; $P = 0.7$). For secondary outcomes, all 3 studies reported pneumonia but none provided a definition for pneumonia. There was a statistically significant difference favoring the surgical group (RR, 0.36; 95% CI, 0.15–0.85; $P = 0.05$). Among patients randomized to surgery, reductions in pneumonia (RR, 0.36; 95% CI, 0.15–0.85; 3 studies, 123 participants, although pneumonia definitions not provided), chest deformity (RR, 0.13; 95% CI, 0.03–0.67; 2 studies, 86 participants), and tracheostomy (RR, 0.38; 95% CI, 0.14–1.02; $P = 0.05$, 2 studies, 83 participants) were noted. Duration of ventilation and of ICU/hospital stays were widely variable for all 3 studies, and could not be combined.

The randomized trials to date have been too small and with generally poor quality (particularly related to allocation concealment) to make definitive conclusions. Larger high-quality multicenter randomized controlled trials are needed to address this research question, which has significant clinical implications for appropriate care of thoracic trauma patients.

A recent single-institution prospective study[30] compared 1 year (2013) of nonoperative management with a second year (2014) of surgical rib fracture fixation for specific

---

Box 1
Potential indications and inclusion criteria for rib fracture repair

Potential indications for fixation

- Flail chest
- Reduce pain and disability
- Chest wall deformity
- Symptoms associated with nonunion
- On the way out (alternative reason for thoracotomy)

Data from Nirula R, Diaz JJ Jr, Trunkey DD, et al. Rib fracture repair: indications, technical issues, and future directions. World J Surg 2009;33(1):14–22.

indications (flail chest, ≥3 fractures with bicortical displacement, ≥30% hemithorax volume loss, and either severe pain or respiratory failure despite optimal medical management). The surgical group had a significantly lower likelihood of both respiratory failure (odds ratio, 0.24; 95% CI, 0.06–0.93; P = 0.03) and tracheostomy (odds ratio, 0.18; 95% CI, 0.04–0.78; P = 0.03). Duration of ventilation was significantly lower in the operative group (P<.01). Narcotic requirements were comparable between groups. There were no mortalities. In contrast, another recent study from 2 regional Canadian trauma centers[31] compared operative versus nonoperative rib fracture patients and reported significantly better outcomes (pneumonia, ventilator days, ICU and hospital durations of stay) in the nonoperative patient cohort. Given the available data to date, each patient must be evaluated individually regarding potential risks and benefits of rib fracture/flail chest surgical fixation.

Preoperative evaluation requires specific surgical planning. Patients typically need a CT scan to localize the fractures if a lesser invasive approach is to be employed rather than a full thoracotomy. CT with 3-dimensional reconstruction (**Figs. 2–5**) is very helpful in planning the optimal surgical approach to rib fracture fixation.[20] It assists with determination of the optimal surgical incisions, and attempts to keep surgical incisions as small as possible with fixation of as many rib fractures as possible through the same surgical site. Because hardware is to be placed, ensuring minimal bacterial contamination is vital and some authors advocate removal of chest tubes if appropriate clinically, although this is not mandatory.[32]

Surgical treatment is aimed at restoring chest wall stability and reducing deformity (see **Figs. 2–5**) while allowing normal breathing mechanics. Specifically, the goal of stabilizing the fracture must be balanced with the ability to maintain breathing mechanics and to not create a restrictive chest wall with excessive fixation.[14] Optimal timing of surgical treatment is also unclear. Some authors have suggested that fixation should take place soon after injury when physiologically feasible, but timing, much like patient selection, has not been clearly elucidated.

Surgical management is technically demanding owing to rib anatomy and fracture pattern variability. Inferior to the rib are intercostal nerve and artery, which must be preserved during fixation. Bony ribs are of variable thickness with a thin cortex and an abnormal contour. Ribs thus have poor stress tolerance and do not hold fixation

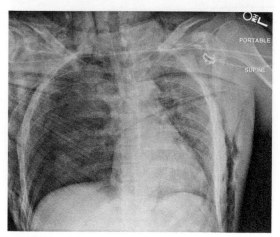

Fig. 2. Patient with multiple right-sided rib fractures, pneumothorax, and subcutaneous emphysema.

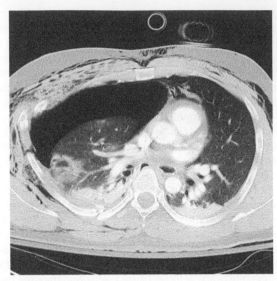

Fig. 3. Computed tomography scan of the same patient showing right chest deformity.

devices like other stronger bone.[20] Rib fractures are also irregular as far as the pattern of the fracture itself. Oblique comminuted fractures at multiple levels are not uncommon. There have been several devices that have been described to stabilize the chest with internal fixation.

Although the goal of fixation is always to stabilize the rib, many techniques have been described. The best method for surgical rib fracture fixation is unclear, but likely related to surgeon skill and preference. Anterior plates are made of a malleable metal

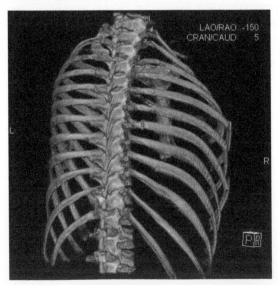

Fig. 4. Three-dimensional reconstruction of the same patient showing flail chest and angular deformity.

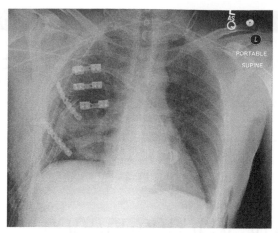

Fig. 5. Same patient with improved chest wall stabilization using 2 different plating systems.

that historically were attached to the rib using wire cerclage (**Fig. 6**).[20] These wires were prone to breaking and plate dislodgement was not uncommon. Wrapping the wire around the rib led to nerve impingement and chronic pain. Bicortical screws with anterior plates are now used because they can stabilize the plate without the risk of nerve impingement or breaking. Locking screw designs where threads lock into the plate are useful in softer bone and may result in less plate migration.[20]

Intramedullary nailing uses a single plate that spans the fracture internally in the medullary cavity of the rib. This technique is very technically demanding and there is no rotational stability after fixation. Finally, this technique carries risk of wire migration and has become an unpopular method of fixation.[20]

Judet struts and U-plating provide greater stabilization, theoretically, than straight anterior plates. Judet struts grab the rib above and below while spanning the fracture without transcortical screws. U-plates grasp the rib on the superior surface and span the fracture and screws secure the plate on the anterior and posterior portion of the rib.[20] The technology continues to develop with plating systems that contain right-angled screwdrivers to access the subscapular areas and percutaneous devices for reduction to facilitate minimally invasive approaches. At present, there is no evidence to support a specific type of rib fracture fixation method as optimal. Additional clinical studies are required to determine this.

COMPLICATIONS RELATED TO THORACIC TRAUMA AND RIB FRACTURE FIXATION

Postoperative complications related to rib fracture fixation are a rare but real concern. Trauma patients often require blood transfusions or otherwise immunocompromising interventions where complications will be poorly tolerated. Potential complications related to rib fracture fixation include surgical site infection, empyema, hematoma, or persistent effusion.[20] Complications that may be related to thoracic trauma in general include pneumonia, prolonged ventilation, prolonged hospitalization, or death.[7,27,28,33–37] It is difficult to discern whether or not the observed complications are related to the surgical rib fracture fixation or the thoracic injury itself.

Several studies have attempted to elucidate the risk of complications and rib fracture fixation when comparing operative with nonoperative management of patients

5. Battle CE, Hutchings H, Evans PA. Risk factors that predict mortality in patients with blunt chest wall trauma: a systematic review and meta-analysis. Injury 2012;43(1):8–17.

6. Tanaka H, Yukioka T, Yamaguti Y, et al. Surgical stabilization of internal pneumatic stabilization? A prospective randomized study of management of severe flail chest patients. J Trauma 2002;52(4):727–32 [discussion: 732].

7. Balci AE, Eren S, Cakir O, et al. Open fixation in flail chest: review of 64 patients. Asian Cardiovasc Thorac Ann 2004;12(1):11–5.

8. Voggenreiter G, Neudeck F, Aufmkolk M, et al. Operative chest wall stabilization in flail chest–outcomes of patients with or without pulmonary contusion. J Am Coll Surg 1998;187(2):130–8.

9. Ahmed Z, Mohyuddin Z. Management of flail chest injury: internal fixation versus endotracheal intubation and ventilation. J Thorac Cardiovasc Surg 1995;110(6): 1676–80.

10. Sirmali M, Turut H, Topcu S, et al. A comprehensive analysis of traumatic rib fractures: morbidity, mortality and management. Eur J Cardiothorac Surg 2003;24(1): 133–8.

11. Battle C, Hutchings H, Lovett S, et al. Predicting outcomes after blunt chest wall trauma: development and external validation of a new prognostic model. Crit Care 2014;18(3):R98.

12. Bhavnagri SJ, Mohammed TL. When and how to image a suspected broken rib. Cleve Clin J Med 2009;76(5):309–14.

13. Shorr RM, Crittenden M, Indeck M, et al. Blunt thoracic trauma. Analysis of 515 patients. Ann Surg 1987;206(2):200–5.

14. Simon B, Ebert J, Bokhari F, et al. Management of pulmonary contusion and flail chest: an Eastern Association for the surgery of trauma practice management guideline. J Trauma Acute Care Surg 2012;73(5 Suppl 4):S351–61.

15. Kent R, Woods W, Bostrom O. Fatality risk and the presence of rib fractures. Ann Adv Automot Med 2008;52:73–82.

16. American College of Surgeons. ATLS student course manual: advanced trauma life support. 9th edition. Chicago (IL): American College of Surgeons; 2012.

17. Peters S, Nicolas V, Heyer CM. Multidetector computed tomography-spectrum of blunt chest wall and lung injuries in polytraumatized patients. Clin Radiol 2010; 65(4):333–8.

18. Cho SH, Sung YM, Kim MS. Missed rib fractures on evaluation of initial chest CT for trauma patients: pattern analysis and diagnostic value of coronal multiplanar reconstruction images with multidetector row CT. Br J Radiol 2012;85(1018): e845–50.

19. Griffith JF, Rainer TH, Ching AS, et al. Sonography compared with radiography in revealing acute rib fracture. AJR Am J Roentgenol 1999;173(6):1603–9.

20. Nirula R, Mayberry JC. Rib fracture fixation: controversies and technical challenges. Am Surg 2010;76(8):793–802.

21. Karmakar MK, Ho AM. Acute pain management of patients with multiple fractured ribs. J Trauma 2003;54(3):615–25.

22. Kerr-Valentic MA, Arthur M, Mullins RJ, et al. Rib fracture pain and disability: can we do better? J Trauma 2003;54(6):1058–63 [discussion: 1063–4].

23. Todd SR, McNally MM, Holcomb JB, et al. A multidisciplinary clinical pathway decreases rib fracture-associated infectious morbidity and mortality in high-risk trauma patients. Am J Surg 2006;192(6):806–11.

24. Dehghan N, de Mestral C, McKee MD, et al. Flail chest injuries: a review of outcomes and treatment practices from the National Trauma Data Bank. J Trauma Acute Care Surg 2014;76(2):462–8.
25. Dittmann M, Keller R, Wolff G. A rationale for epidural analgesia in the treatment of multiple rib fractures. Intensive Care Med 1978;4(4):193–7.
26. Shackford SR, Virgilio RW, Peters RM. Selective use of ventilator therapy in flail chest injury. J Thorac Cardiovasc Surg 1981;81(2):194–201.
27. Granetzny A, Abd El-Aal M, Emam E, et al. Surgical versus conservative treatment of flail chest. Evaluation of the pulmonary status. Interact Cardiovasc Thorac Surg 2005;4(6):583–7.
28. Marasco SF, Davies AR, Cooper J, et al. Prospective randomized controlled trial of operative rib fixation in traumatic flail chest. J Am Coll Surg 2013;216(5): 924–32.
29. Cataneo AJ, Cataneo DC, de Oliveira FH, et al. Surgical versus nonsurgical interventions for flail chest. Cochrane Database Syst Rev 2015;7:CD009919.
30. Pieracci FM, Lin Y, Rodil M, et al. A prospective, controlled clinical evaluation of surgical stabilization of severe rib fractures. J Trauma Acute Care Surg 2016; 80(2):187–94.
31. Farquhar J, Almahrabi Y, Slobogean G, et al. No benefit to surgical fixation of flail chest injuries compared with modern comprehensive management: results of a retrospective cohort study. Can J Surg 2016;59(4):515.
32. Mayberry JC, Terhes JT, Ellis TJ, et al. Absorbable plates for rib fracture repair: preliminary experience. J Trauma 2003;55(5):835–9.
33. Leinicke JA, Elmore L, Freeman BD, et al. Operative management of rib fractures in the setting of flail chest: a systematic review and meta-analysis. Ann Surg 2013;258(6):914–21.
34. Bhatnagar A, Mayberry J, Nirula R. Rib fracture fixation for flail chest: what is the benefit? J Am Coll Surg 2012;215(2):201–5.
35. Nirula R, Allen B, Layman R, et al. Rib fracture stabilization in patients sustaining blunt chest injury. Am Surg 2006;72(4):307–9.
36. Majercik S, Cannon Q, Granger SR, et al. Long-term patient outcomes after surgical stabilization of rib fractures. Am J Surg 2014;208(1):88–92.
37. Slobogean GP, MacPherson CA, Sun T, et al. Surgical fixation vs nonoperative management of flail chest: a meta-analysis. J Am Coll Surg 2013;216(2): 302–11.e1.
38. Mayberry JC, Ham LB, Schipper PH, et al. Surveyed opinion of American trauma, orthopedic, and thoracic surgeons on rib and sternal fracture repair. J Trauma 2009;66(3):875–9.
39. Chen J, Jeremitsky E, Philp F, et al. A chest trauma scoring system to predict outcomes. Surgery 2014;156(4):988–93.
40. Pressley CM, Fry WR, Philp AS, et al. Predicting outcome of patients with chest wall injury. Am J Surg 2012;204(6):910–3 [discussion: 913–4].
41. Pape HC, Remmers D, Rice J, et al. Appraisal of early evaluation of blunt chest trauma: development of a standardized scoring system for initial clinical decision making. J Trauma 2000;49(3):496–504.

Postinjury Inflammation and Organ Dysfunction

Angela Sauaia, MD, PhD[a],*, Frederick A. Moore, MD[b], Ernest E. Moore, MD[c]

KEYWORDS

- Organ dysfunction • Postinjury inflammation • SIRS • CARS • SARS • PICS

KEY POINTS

- The development of organ dysfunction (OD) is related to the intensity and balance between trauma-induced simultaneous, opposite inflammatory responses.
- Early proinflammation via innate immune system activation may cause early OD, whereas early antiinflammation, via inhibition of the adaptive immune system and apoptosis, may induce immunoparalysis, impaired healing, infections, and late OD.
- Patients discharged with low-level OD may develop the persistent inflammation-immunosuppression catabolism syndrome (PICS), which may cause an indolent death.
- The incidence of multiple organ failure (MOF) has decreased over time, but MOF remains morbid, lethal, and resource intensive. Single OD, especially acute lung injury, remains frequent.
- At this time, treatment of OD is limited, and prevention via adequate resuscitation, ventilation, and nutritional support remains the mainstay strategy.

HISTORICAL PERSPECTIVE: EVOLVING CONCEPTS ON THE PATHOGENESIS OF MULTIPLE ORGAN FAILURE

As advances in prehospital and acute hospital care conquered the so-called golden hour, multiple organ failure (MOF) emerged as the leading cause of late trauma death.[1–3] Eiseman and colleagues[4] coined the term MOF in 1977, with a clinical description of 42 patients with progressive organ dysfunction (OD). By the 1990s, Moore and colleagues[5]

Disclosures: Drs A. Sauaia and E.E. Moore received funding from the National Institute of General Medical Sciences grant P50 GM049222 and the National Heart, Lung, and Blood Institute grant UM1 HL120877. Dr Frederick A. Moore received funding from the National Institute of General Medical Sciences grant P50 GM111152. The content of this article is solely the responsibility of the authors and does not necessarily represent the official views of the NIGMS, NHLBI, or National Institutes of Health. The authors have no commercial or financial conflicts of interest.

[a] University of Colorado Denver, 655 Broadway #365, Denver, CO 80203, USA; [b] University of Florida, PO BOX 100108, Gainesville, FL 32610, USA; [c] Denver Health Medical Center, University of Colorado Denver, 655 Broadway #365, Denver, CO 80203, USA
* Corresponding author.
E-mail address: Angela.Sauaia@ucdenver.edu

Crit Care Clin 33 (2017) 167–191
http://dx.doi.org/10.1016/j.ccc.2016.08.006
0749-0704/17/© 2016 Elsevier Inc. All rights reserved.

proposed that MOF was a bimodal phenomenon. In the 1-event model, a massive traumatic insult induces intense systemic inflammation response syndrome (SIRS) and precipitates OD. In the 2-event model, patients initially resuscitated into moderate SIRS become vulnerable to a second activating event (infections, embolism, transfusions, secondary operations, etc.) during the so-called compensatory antiinflammatory response syndrome (CARS) and could develop late MOF.

Modern hypotheses propose that injury triggers simultaneous, opposite responses: the proinflammation response (SIRS) and the antiinflammation response, previously misnamed compensatory (CARS) (**Fig. 1**).[6] OD is related to the intensity and the balance between these opposing trauma-induced inflammatory responses. Severe SIRS, a proinflammation via activation of the innate immune system, causes early OD, whereas early antiinflammation, via inhibition of the adaptive immune system and apoptosis, limits proinflammation and creates a preconditioned state to protect against second hits and hasten healing. When countering unbalanced proinflammation, persistent antiinflammation leads to the severe systemic antiinflammatory response syndrome (SARS; a more appropriate term than CARS), setting the stage for immunoparalysis, impaired healing, infections, and late OD.[6,7] This process was confirmed in a 2011 study by the Inflammation and Host Response to Injury Large-Scale Collaborative Research Program (Glue Grant) showing that alterations in the genomic expression of the classic inflammatory and antiinflammatory responses occurred simultaneously.[8]

As MOF began to recede as a result of aggressive prevention, a new OD phenotype emerged among patients discharged after lengthy intensive care unit (ICU) stays to long-term facilities, where they developed a persistent inflammation-immunosuppression catabolism syndrome (PICS).[7] Although the phenotypes and epidemiology of postinjury OD have changed considerably over the past 20 years, it remains morbid, lethal, and resource intensive, as described later.[9]

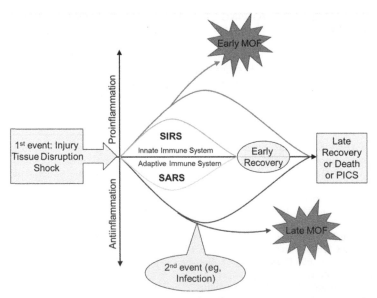

Fig. 1. Theoretic framework for postinjury MOF: The synchronous immunoinflammatory model. PICS, persistent inflammation-immunosuppression catabolism syndrome; SARS, systemic antiinflammatory response syndrome.

DEFINING MULTIPLE ORGAN FAILURE

The Denver score (**Table 1**)[10] and the Multiple Organ Dysfunction Score (MODS)[11–13] are among the most common validated definitions in trauma studies. For others, readers are referred to Baue's[14] excellent review. The Denver score grades the dysfunction of 4 systems (pulmonary, renal, hepatic, and cardiovascular), whereas the MODS grades 6 organ systems (pulmonary, renal, hepatic, cardiovascular, hematologic, and neurologic). Both scores have good predictive performance, but the MODS tends to be more sensitive (high incidence of MOF, low case-fatality rate), whereas the Denver score tends to be more specific (low incidence, high case-fatality rate).

Table 1
Denver postinjury MOF score

Organ System	Grade 0	Grade 1	Grade 2	Grade 3
Pulmonary				
Pao_2/Fio_2 ratio	>250	250–200	200–100	≤100
Renal				
Creatinine (mg/dL)	≤1.8	1.9–2.5	2.51–5.0	>5.0
Creatinine (μmol/L)	<159	160–221	222–442	>442
Hepatic				
Bilirubin (mg/dL)	≤2.0	2.0–4.0	4.1–8.0	>8.0
Bilirubin (μmol/L)	<34	34–68	69–137	>137
Cardiac	No inotropes	Only 1 inotrope at a small dose[a]	Any inotrope at moderate dose or >1 agent, all at small doses[a]	Any inotrope at large dose or >2 agents at moderate doses[a]

	Small	Moderate	Large
Milrinone	<0.3	0.4–0.7	>0.7
Vasopressin	<0.03	0.03–0.07	>0.07
Dopamine	<6	6–10	>10
Dobutamine	<6	6–10	>10
Epinephrine	<0.06	0.06–0.15	>0.15
Norepinephrine	<0.11	0.11–0.5	>0.5
Phenylephrine	<0.6	0.6–3	>3

Abbreviation: Fio_2, fraction of inspired oxygen.
[a] Inotrope doses (in μg/(kg min)).

EPIDEMIOLOGY AND CLINICAL RELEVANCE

US and Australian studies have shown a steady decline in MOF incidence over the past decade.[9,15–17] In contrast, a large German study reported an increase in MOF incidence.[18] However, most studies agree that MOF-associated mortality and morbidity remain high.[9,15,16,18–23] We recently studied MOF temporal trends in the Glue Grant data set, a prospective study including adults with severe blunt torso injuries and hemorrhagic shock, enrolled from 2003 to 2010 in several US trauma centers sharing standard operating procedures.[9,24] MOF, defined by the Denver score, was diagnosed in 223 patients (13.6%), of whom 36% died. **Table 2** details the distribution of admission risk factors, fluids, transfusions, complications, and outcomes over time. After adjustment for risk factors, MOF incidence decreased over time, whereas MOF-related mortality persisted at high levels (**Fig. 2**). Patients with MOF continued to need lengthy ventilator and critical care support. Applying the MODS definition produced similar trends.

The risk factors for developing MOF included demographic characteristics (advanced age, male sex, obesity), injury severity, and physiologic derangement on admission (acidosis, number of transfused units of red blood cells [RBCs] within 12 hours). MOF-related death was positively associated with female sex, injury severity, and RBC units transfused within the first 12 hours postinjury. The time interval between MOF onset and death was usually short, with death ensuing in 2 days in 58% of the cases. Early MOF (<3 days) carried a higher mortality than late MOF (**Fig. 3**).

Lung failure incidence decreased significantly over time, but remained the most common OD over the study period, affecting more than half of these patients (see **Table 1**). Cardiovascular dysfunction also became significantly less frequent, whereas renal and liver failures persisted at low, similar levels. The mortality was highest for cardiovascular dysfunction (39%), followed by failure of the kidneys (38%), liver (19%), and lungs (12%). There was a decrease in the progression from lung dysfunction to MOF over time.[25] MOF without lung dysfunction was rare: only 8% of the patients with MOF did not have lung involvement.

THE BURDEN OF MULTIPLE ORGAN FAILURE

In the abovementioned study, we showed that MOF survivors were responsible for 20% of the total ICU and mechanical ventilation days despite being only 9% of the total population.[9] Based on national estimates of daily critical care costs,[26] the total cost of the critical care delivered to patients with MOF in this dataset was estimated at $19,990,420, or 22% of the total ICU cost for this population. The estimated median cost per patient with MOF was $77,202, double the presumed cost of caring for patients without MOF ($38,442).

PATHOPHYSIOLOGY

Fig. 4 shows a framework for the response to trauma. SIRS is the manifestation of the immunoinflammatory activation in response to ischemia/reperfusion (I/R) injury and factors released from disrupted tissue, mediated by inherent genetic and environmentally determined host characteristics.

The 1994 danger theory of the inflammatory response following trauma or infection proposed that the immunologic system's role was to protect the body from danger.[27–32] In this theory, immunologic responses are triggered by specific types of cell death. If a healthy, undamaged cell dies an apoptotic death, it is scavenged without triggering an immune response. In contrast, cell lysis or apoptosis via trauma or infection releases intracellular contents and signals danger, triggering both innate and adaptive responses.[28,30,33]

The injured cell releases endogenous damage-associated molecular patterns (DAMPs), analogous to the microbial pathogen-associated molecular patterns (PAMPs), released in sepsis, both of which activate the innate immunity.[32,34,35] PAMPs

Table 2
Population characteristics, admission risk factors, resuscitation fluids and blood transfusions, outcomes, and complications of 1643 adult patients with blunt trauma admitted to 4 US trauma centers (Glue Grant data set)

Variable	2003–2004 N = 335			2005–2006 N = 506			2007–2008 N = 546			2009–2010 N = 256			P value[a]
	Median or %	LQ	UQ	Median or %	LQ	UQ	Median or %	LQ	UQ	Median or %	LQ	UQ	
Demographic													
Age (y)	40	26	54	41	26	54	43	28	57	45.5	25.5	58	.0246
Body mass index (kg/m^2)	25.7	23.1	29.9	26.7	23.7	31.4	27.1	23.8	31.3	27.3	24.1	32.0	.0017
Male sex (%)	64.5	—	—	66.6	—	—	67.2	—	—	67.6	—	—	.3940
Comorbidity index $\geq$2 (%)	8.4	—	—	12.9	—	—	8.4	—	—	10.2	—	—	.8276
Antiplatelet therapy (%)[b]	6.6	—	—	7.1	—	—	10.1	—	—	8.2	—	—	.1414
Injury													
Moderate TBI (%)[c]	30.2	—	—	18.0	—	—	21.6	—	—	18.0	—	—	.0037
Injury severity score	29	22	41	32	22	41	34	24	41	34	22	43	.0622
Prehospital GCS	13	4	15	14	10	15	14	9	15	14	9	15	<.0001
Prehospital SBP (lowest)	89.0	72.5	104.5	86.0	71.0	102.0	88.0	73.0	108.0	85.0	74.0	100.0	.8425
Prehospital HR (beats/min; highest)	116	95	131	118	100	130	115	97	130	118	102	132	.4810
Admission GCS	6	3	15	10	3	15	11	3	15	3	3	15	.1534
Admission SBP (mm Hg)	110	93	135	111	90	132	110	90	131	109.5	89	128	.0429
Admission SBP $\leq$90 mm Hg	22.1	—	—	25.9	—	—	26.7	—	—	29.9	—	—	.0350
Admission HR (beats/min)	108	86	127	110	90	126	109	91	127	110	92	127.5	.2080
Fluids/Blood													
RBC units/12 h	5	3	11	6	3	12	5	2	9	5	2	9	.0739
FFP units/12 h	3	0	8	3	0	8	2	0	6	3	0	7	.0798
0–6 h RBC/FFP ratio	0.6	0	1.5	0.5	0	1.6	0	0	1.5	0.6	0	1.4	.1224

(continued on next page)

Table 2
(continued)

Variable	2003–2004 N = 335			2005–2006 N = 506			2007–2008 N = 546			2009–2010 N = 256			P value[a]
	Median or %	LQ	UQ	Median or %	LQ	UQ	Median or %	LQ	UQ	Median or %	LQ	UQ	
Platelet units/12 h	0	0	1	0	0	1	0	0	1	0	0	1	.4160
Prehospital crystalloids(ml)	1.6	0.6	3.0	1.8	0.7	3.3	1.4	0.5	2.9	1.8	0.7	3.1	.3504
Crystalloids (mL)/12 h	10.3	7.2	15.7	10.0	7.6	13.6	8.7	5.9	12.3	9.0	6.3	12.0	<.0001
Laboratorial Tests													
ED base excess (mEq/L)	−8.9	−11.4	−6	−8.4	−11.2	−6	−7.6	−0.8	−5	−8	−11.1	−5.35	.0012
ED lactate (mg/dL)	4.3	3	5.9	3.9	2.7	5.6	3.6	2.4	5.2	4	2.4	6	.0016
Day 1 platelet 1000/μL	100	79	129	95	76	123	107	87	133	101	84	128.5	.0028
Pao$_2$/Fio$_2$ ratio/12 h	119	66	213	161	86.5	256	158	89	269	163	79	285	.0003
ED hemoglobin (g/dL)	10.9	9.33	13	11.3	9.5	13.1	11.9	10	13.3	11.5	9.6	12.9	.0217
ED INR	1.2	1.1	1.5	1.3	1.1	1.5	1.21	1.1	1.5	1.3	1.1	1.5	.3152
Complications													
Nonseptic complication (%)	44.5	—	—	47.2	—	—	44.1	—	—	40.4	—	—	.2365
Surgical site infection (%)	13.1	—	—	16.4	—	—	14.8	—	—	8.2	—	—	.1180
VAP (%)	26.6	—	—	26.5	—	—	24.4	—	—	23.1	—	—	.2335
Outcomes													
MOF (%)	17.0	—	—	15.0	—	—	11.9	—	—	9.8	—	—	.0033
Lung failure (%)	57.6	—	—	56.5	—	—	55.3	—	—	50.8	—	—	.1073
Cardiac failure (%)	20.9	—	—	17.6	—	—	16.1	—	—	12.5	—	—	.0064
Liver failure (%)	15.2	—	—	16.2	—	—	13.4	—	—	14.1	—	—	.3762

	Median	LQ	UQ	Median	LQ	UQ	Median	LQ	UQ	Median	LQ	UQ	P value
Renal failure (%)	10.1	—	—	10.7	—	—	11.9	—	—	12.5	—	—	.2804
ICU days	8	4	19	9	4	17	10	5	18	9	5	17	.1070
ICU-free days	11	0	21	15	4	23	15	3	22	17	8	22	.0002
Ventilator days	6	2	14	5	2	13	7	2	13	6	2	12	.8414
Ventilator-free days	16	0	24	19	7	25	20	8	25	21	12	25	<.0001
Mortality (%)	23.9	—	—	15.4	—	—	12.3	—	—	10.5	—	—	<.0001
MOF-related Outcomes													
Case-fatality (%)	33.3	—	—	38.2	—	—	36.9	—	—	36.0	—	—	.7800
ICU days	22	9	34	17	8.5		15	9	27	19	10	24	.1889
ICU-free days	0	0	4	0	0	8	0	0	10	0	0	7	.2289
Ventilator days	20	9	26	15	6.5	27	12	7	21	13	6	19	.0642
Ventilator-free days	0	0	8	0	0	11.5	0	0	14	4	0	14	.1969
MOF-related Complications													
Nonseptic complication (%)	77.2	—	—	75.0	—	—	83.1	—	—	80.0	—	—	.4481
Surgical site infection (%)	22.8	—	—	27.6	—	—	16.9	—	—	20.0	—	—	.4042
VAP (%)	47.3	—	—	43.4	—	—	50.8	—	—	44.0	—	—	.8946

Data are expressed as median and lower quartile (LQ) and upper quartile (UQ) or percentages.

Abbreviations: ED, emergency department; FFP, fresh frozen plasma; GCS, Glasgow Coma Scale; HR, heart rate; INR, international normalized ratio, RBC, packed red blood cells; SBP, systolic blood pressure; TBI, traumatic brain injury; VAP, ventilator-associated pneumonia.

[a] Cochran-Armitage trend test was used for categorical variables and the nonparametric Spearman correlation coefficient and test for continuous variables; negative correlation coefficients indicate values decreased over time, whereas positive coefficients indicate values increased over time; significance set at $P<.01$ to account for the large number of comparisons.

[b] Antiplatelet medication before injury.

[c] Moderate TBI: Head Abbreviated Injury Scale greater than 3 with Glasgow Coma Scale motor component greater than 3.

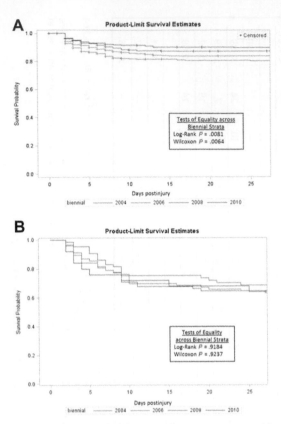

Fig. 2. Kaplan-Meyer curves for MOF incidence and outcomes across biennial periods from 2003 to 2010 in 1643 adult patients with blunt trauma admitted to 4 US trauma centers (Glue Grant data set). (*A*) MOF incidence. (*B*) Mortality in patients with MOF. Stratum 2004 = 2003 to 2004; stratum 2006 = 2005 to 2006; stratum 2008 = 2007 to 2008; stratum 2010 = 2009 to 2010.

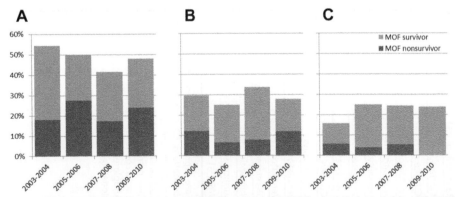

Fig. 3. MOF onset and respective case-fatality rates. (*A*) MOF onset 3 days or less. (*B*) MOF onset 4 to 7 days. (*C*) MOF onset greater than 7 days.

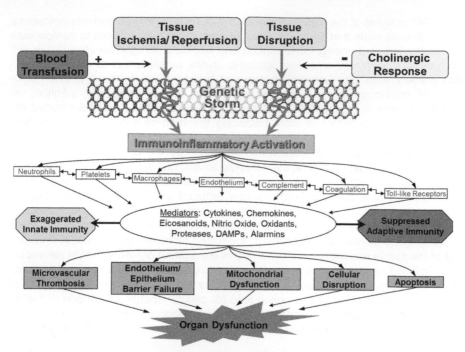

Fig. 4. Response to trauma: hemostatic, inflammatory, endocrine, and neurologic systems interaction. DAMPs, damage-associated molecular patterns.

are exogenous microbial molecules that alert the organism to pathogens and are recognized by cells of the innate and acquired immunity system, primarily through toll-like receptors (TLRs), and activate several signaling pathways (eg, nuclear factor kappa-B [NF-κB]).[27] DAMPs include HMGB1 (high mobility group box protein-1), heat-shock proteins, uric acid, and DNA. HMGB1, a nuclear protein that binds to nucleosomes and promotes DNA bending, has been associated with SIRS and end-organ damage in animals. In humans, it has been shown to be at high levels as early as 1 hour postinjury.[27,36,37] Zhang and colleagues[34] showed that injury releases mitochondrial DAMPs into the circulation, which create a sepsis-like state and may be the key link between trauma, inflammation, and SIRS.

Most proteins identified in the plasma of patients with blunt trauma are intracellular molecules that could function as DAMPS/alarmins and trigger pattern recognition receptors.[38] Our laboratory was the first to describe the proteome of human mesenteric lymph collected from critically ill or injured patients using a label-free semiquantitative mass spectrometry (MS).[39] A total of 477 proteins were identified, including markers of hemolysis, extracellular matrix components, and general tissue damage in addition to the classic serum proteins. Postinjury hemolysis releases hemoglobin to the extracellular environment, where it becomes a redox-reactive DAMP molecule that can bind to PAMPs, trigger TLR-mediated signal transduction, and generate reactive oxygen species (ROS), potentially affecting innate immunity.[40] In the mesenteric lymph, we showed several markers of tissue damage and mitochondrial proteins suggestive of lysed mitochondria.[39] Circulating mitochondrial DNA and formyl peptides may mediate OD through polymorphonuclear neutrophil [PMN] activation.[34]

Our MS analysis of the plasma metabolome of severely injured patients indicated a hypercatabolic state that could provide carbon and nitrogen sources to compensate for trauma-induced energy consumption and negative nitrogen balance.[41] Our MS analysis also confirmed an altered lipidomic profile, a hallmark of metabolic adaptation to injury, with fatty acid mobilization and lipid breakdown, resulting in accumulation of anionic compounds (eg, ketone bodies) and acidosis.[41] In addition, we noted increases in proinflammatory arachidonate metabolites, which supported the immunomodulatory effect of diets balancing the ratio of omega-3/omega-6 fatty acids.[42]

We observed significant proteolysis, as shown by the accumulation of several amino acids (alanine, aspartate, cysteine, glutamate, histidine, lysine, and phenylalanine) and cyclic dipeptide cyclo (glu-glu), which stimulates T lymphocytes.[41] Glutamate and cysteine buildup could fuel new reduced glutathione synthesis, thereby serving as physiologic protection from the increase in trauma-dependent oxidative stress. There was significant nucleoside breakdown, as shown by increased levels of purines and pyrimidine catabolites.[41] Increased nicotinamide, a breakdown product of the purine metabolite NAD, may signal exhaustion of NAD+/NADH reservoirs, potentially compromising many energy and redox-related processes that depend on these cofactors. Notably, there was no glutamine accumulation, possibly because of enhanced consumption of this amino acid for cellular energy production or fueling transamination reactions.[41] Glutamine supplementation in critically ill patients has been a long-sought therapeutic approach, but there is no evidence to date showing its benefit.[43]

Succinate, in particular, has elicited much interest in I/R injury-related states.[44–46] Levels of this intermediate metabolite, normally produced during cellular respiration, become increased after ischemia because of 2 potential mechanisms: (1) an interesting activity reversal of the enzyme succinate dehydrogenase, which, during normal oxygen conditions, breaks down succinate; and (2) macrophage activation leading to glutamine metabolism and succinate production.[46] During reperfusion, succinate is oxidized with the now abundant oxygen, and drives a reversal of the electron transport through complex 1, which produces ROS. Succinate has inflammatory signaling capacity, leads to interleukin (IL)-1-beta production and activates immune cells.[46,47] Chouchani and colleagues[44] showed that preventing increased succinate levels protected against I/R injury in mouse models of brain and heart ischemia. Binding of succinate to a specific receptor (SUCNR1) in dendritic cells (antigen-presenting cells with an important role in initiating immune responses) seems to enhance the production of proinflammatory factors, suggesting that succinate may have a role in alerting the innate system to danger.[46,48]

Specifically in the lungs, succinate has been shown to mediate stabilization of the hypoxia-inducible factor 1-alpha, a transcription factor that, when stabilized by hypoxia (and also by mechanically stretched lung epithelia), mediates several protective actions during low oxygen availability. This process provides a direct role for succinate in lung protection during acute lung injury.[49–51]

In one of the few clinical studies of patients with acute respiratory distress syndrome (ARDS), large increases in the levels of precursors of uric acid (hypoxanthine, xanthine, guanosine) were observed, suggesting that the pathway was activated (although no uric acid was detected).[52] Uric acid has previously been shown to be a major endogenous danger signal in the lung, activating the NALP3 inflammasome and leading to IL-1β production.[53] Bos and colleagues[54,55] suggested that metabolomic analyses targeting lung injury focus on exhaled air, namely breathomics. This group used an electronic nose (sNOSE) to detect patterns in volatile organic compounds (VOCs) through gas chromatography and MS, which discriminated ICU patients with and without acute lung injury (ALI) with 92% accuracy. These investigators identified 3 VOCs in patients with ARDS within the first 24 hours after ICU admission: acetaldehyde (potentially from neutrophil infiltration in the lungs), octane, and 3-methylheptane (the last 2 possibly related to lipid peroxidation caused by oxidative stress).[55]

The Glue Grant study suggested that severe blunt trauma produced a genomic storm in the expression of more than 80% of the leukocyte transcriptome across the first 28 days compared with healthy subjects.[8] The overexpressed genes were related to both the innate and adaptive immunity, whereas genes related to T-cell function and antigen presentation had decreased expression. The genomic response to blunt injury was remarkably similar to the response observed in burns and endotoxemia. Postinjury complications were associated with greater and prolonged overexpression, although there were no major differences in which genes were invoked. Despite providing compelling evidence, the abovementioned investigation had limitations, including a small sample, inclusion of only blunt torso trauma, and focus on circulating leukocytes.[8] It is conceivable that different tissues have specific, localized inflammation expression patterns.

Patients with PICS have manageable OD with a long, eventful postinjury clinical course with recurrent inflammatory insults and infections, progressive loss of lean body mass (despite good nutritional support), poor wound healing, and decubitus ulcers.[7] Their laboratory tests show persistent neutrophilia and lymphopenia. Discharged to long-term care facilities, patient with PICS die an indolent death or experience sepsis recidivism and ICU readmission. Elderly patients with baseline comorbidities and sarcopenia are especially prone to this refractory clinical phenotype. Often, the long-term outcome involves impairment of cognitive and functional status from which recovery is uncertain.[7,56] Clinically, PICS is defined as long ICU stay (>14 days), persistent inflammation (C-reactive protein concentration >150 μg/dL and retinol binding protein concentrations <10 μg/dL), immunosuppression (total lymphocyte count <800/mm^3), and a catabolic state (serum albumin level <3.0 mg/dL, creatinine height index <80%, and weight loss >10% or body mass index <18 kg/m^2 during the current hospitalization). Studies are underway to better define the phenotype, its true significance, and novel interventions to prevent it or its progression. As the population ages, PICS is likely to be the next challenge in surgical critical care.

Role of the Gut

Initially, the dominant hypothesis linking the gut to MOF was related to bacterial translocation. However, inconsistent results led to experiments showing that the mesenteric lymph acted as a bridge between the gut and the systemic circulation, allowing gut-derived inflammatory mediators to reach the systemic circulation.[57–59] Via the thoracic duct, these mediators reach the lungs before other organs, which is consistent with human studies showing that respiratory dysfunction almost always precedes other ODs.[60]

Role of Polymorphonuclear Neutrophils and Macrophages

Although most postinjury patients develop neutrophilia at 3 hours postinjury, patients with MOF show a rapid neutropenia between 6 and 12 hours postinjury suggesting end-organ sequestration.[61] PMN margination in end organs causes direct local cytotoxic cellular effects via degranulation and release of nitric oxide (NO), ROS, and proinflammatory mediators (IL-6, IL-8, tumor necrosis factor alpha [TNF-α]).[62]

Following trauma there is an immediate increase in adhesion molecules, including L-selectin and CD18, which allow PMNs to slow and roll along the endothelium and marginate out of circulation.[63] Antibodies directed against the CD11b/CD18 components of the adhesion receptor complex between leukocytes and endothelium significantly attenuate lung injury and prevent the neutropenia associated with tissue sequestration during experimental sepsis.[63] Circulating monocytes and tissue macrophages also become primed after severe injury and the microvascular endothelium has an important role in priming of the innate inflammatory response.[62]

Role of Platelets

Thrombocytopenia, especially when persistent, is a predictor of postinjury OD.[64,65] Gawaz and colleagues[66] observed that irreversible degranulation of granule glycoproteins correlated positively with OD severity. Platelet-neutrophil interaction has been shown to be important in models of ALI[67] and blocking it reverses ALI in animal models.[68] In a rat model of trauma/hemorrhagic shock, the authors observed that pretreatment with a platelet P2Y12 receptor antagonist protected from postinjury ALI.[69] Furthermore, isoflurane, an ether that interferes with platelet-granulocyte aggregation, attenuated ALI partially through platelet ADP pathway inhibition.[70]

Preinjury antiplatelet therapy has been associated with a decreased risk of ALI, MOF, and mortality in transfused patients with blunt trauma and in patients with ARDS.[71,72] The multicenter trial Lung Injury Prevention with Aspirin (LIPS-A, NCT01504867) should provide evidence on the therapeutic use of this antiplatelet agent.

Cytokines

Cytokines can be proinflammatory (TNF-α, Macrophage Inflammatory Proteins, granulocyte-macrophage colony-stimulating factor [GM-CSF], interferon gamma [IFN-γ], IL-1, IL-2, IL-6, IL-8, IL-17, and so forth) and antiinflammatory (IL-4, IL-10, IL-13).[63] Jastrow and colleagues[73] showed that, compared with patients without MOF, patients with MOF had higher levels of IL-1 receptor antagonist, IL-8, eotaxin, granulocyte colony-stimulating factor, GM-CSF, inducible protein 10, monocyte chemotactic protein-1, and macrophage inflammatory protein-1. Adams and colleagues[74] showed that IL-8 can activate PMNs via 2 different receptors, and differential early expression of these receptors explained higher MOF risk.

Although inflammatory mediators' levels vary greatly according to injury and individual characteristics, most studies agree that the changes start very early postinjury.[75] A 2009 study from Germany found that IL-6, IL-8, and IL-10 levels predicted MOF within 90 minutes of injury.[75]

Toll-like Receptors

TLRs are transmembrane proteins present in most body cell types, that form the major pattern recognition receptors that transduce signals in response to DAMPs after I/R.[76] Innate immune system responses are then initiated, including NF-κB activation and proinflammatory cytokine production. Inhibition of TLR2 or TLR4 seems to be protective for I/R injury in liver, kidneys, brain, and heart, but not in the gut. Because the gut mucosa is continuously exposed to local bacterial endotoxins, local TLRs may be uniquely regulated to prevent inflammation.

Complement

The complement system is a major component of the innate immunity response, enhances the adaptive response, and links the immune system with the coagulation system.[29,77,78] Complement system activation occurs immediately after trauma, with production of proinflammatory activation products C3a, C3b, and C5a and generation of the terminal C5b-C9 complex (the complement membrane-attack complex), which leads to lysis of the target cells.[29,35] Complement activation also results in the production of oxygen free radicals, arachidonic acid metabolites, and cytokines. However, excessive intravascular C5a may lead to neutrophil function paralysis, rendering them incapable of responding to C5a or other chemoattractants.[79] Complement activation, especially serum C3 and C3a levels as well as C5a, seems to reflect severity and treatment of injury and OD.[80–83]

Complement regulatory proteins (CD55, CD46, CD55, CD59), the C5a receptor (CD88) inhibitors of complement, such as C4b-binding protein (C4BP) and factor I, modulate the complement cascade and protect against complement-mediated tissue destruction. Several studies in patients with polytrauma indicate that these regulatory factors are significantly altered postinjury, suggesting a trauma-induced complementopathy.[83–85]

Oxidative Stress

Excessive reactive oxygen intermediates (ROIs) cause direct oxidative injury to cellular proteins and nucleic acids, and disrupt cell membranes by inducing lipid peroxidation.[76,86] I/R leads to significant disturbances in ROI production.[35,76] ROIs secreted from PMNs after I/R injury induce cytokines, chemokines (IL-8), heat shock proteins, and adhesion molecules (P-selectin, Intercellular Adhesion Molecule 1) leading to cell and tissue damage.[35]

Under normal conditions, NO production greatly exceeds O_2^- production in the endothelial cell.[87] However, with reperfusion, the balance between NO and O_2^- shifts in favor of O_2^-, leaving little NO available to reduce arteriolar tone, prevent platelet aggregation, and minimize PMN adhesion to endothelium.[88] In addition, NO seems to upregulate the production of proinflammatory cytokines.[87] Thus, altering the cell's redox state may contribute to the ongoing inflammatory cytokine production and progression to MOF. ROIs also play a role as second messengers in the intracellular signaling pathways of inflammatory cells, in particular activation of NF-κB and activator protein 1 (AP-1), which can be activated by both oxidants and antioxidants depending on the cell type and on intracellular conditions.[86]

Endogenous antioxidant defenses, including enzymatic (superoxide dismutase, catalase, glutathione peroxidase) and nonenzymatic (vitamins E and C, provitamin A, glutathione, bilirubin, urate) groups, were the focus of interventions to modulate the inflammatory response. However, the REDOX (Reducing Deaths due to Oxidative Stress)[89–91] and MetaPlus[92] trials showed harm in systemic administration of antioxidants.[43] For both glutamine and antioxidants, the greatest potential for harm was renal dysfunction in patients with MOF.[91]

Later Risk Factors

Several conditions can serve as secondary stimuli that precipitate OD. Abdominal compartment syndrome (ACS), now in frank decline, leads to high ventilator pressures, decreased cardiac output, and impaired renal function.[93] Although ACS physiologic effects usually reverse on decompression, the immunomodulatory effects may persist and trigger MOF.[94]

Although judicious blood transfusions have contributed to lower MOF incidence, early transfusion remains one of the most powerful independent risk factors for postinjury MOF.[9,21] Blood products are immunoactive, contain proinflammatory cytokines and lipids, and have an early immunosuppressive effect predisposing to SARS, infection, and late MOF.[95] Transfusing stored RBC older than 3 weeks early postinjury is associated with higher MOF rates compared with units with shorter storage.[96] Leukodepletion does not remove the potential for blood to act as a second hit, because red blood cells contain proinflammatory mediators. Biologically active lipids, capable of PMN priming, accumulate in stored blood and so-called passenger leukocytes have been implicated as pivotal components. Proposed mechanisms include induction of T-cell anergy in the recipient, decreased natural killer cell function, altered ratio of T-helper to T-suppressor cells, and soluble proinflammatory cytokines produced by leukocytes during storage.[95]

Other blood-derived products (platelets, plasma, and coagulation factors) are also immunoactive.[97] Proteomic analyses of platelet supernatants of healthy donors suggested a storage and sex-dependent impairment of blood coagulation mediators, proinflammatory complement components and cytokines, energy and redox metabolic enzymes, as well as platelet activation.[98,99]

Infections remain important predictors of late MOF. In the late 1970s, intra-abdominal abscess was a frequent inciting event,[100] while currently, nosocomial pneumonia is the principal infection associated with MOF.[101] Although SARS limits potentially autodestructive inflammation, it is associated with immunosuppression predisposing the host to infections.[102]

The secondary operations can be considered controlled traumatic events.[63] Although early definitive fracture fixation decreases postinjury morbidity and improves recovery,[103] it has consequences when performed within the priming window. A 2003 randomized controlled trial (RCT) showed that early external fixation followed by delayed conversion to intramedullary instrumentation was associated with a decreased inflammatory response to the operative fixation.[104] The same group compared damage control orthopedics (DC; femoral fracture stabilized with an external fixator) and primary intramedullary nailing (IMN) and showed that, despite more severe injuries, DC patients had less postoperative SIRS compared with IMN.[105]

Our group showed that DC was a safer initial approach, significantly decreasing the initial operative exposure and blood loss compared with early total care with IMN for patients with multiple injuries with femoral shaft fractures.[106] We observed similar beneficial effects regarding pulmonary complications, infections, mechanical ventilation, and ICU stay in spine fractures.[107]

INTERVENTIONS

Preventing the onset of MOF through therapies directed at modulating the balance of SIRS and SARS offers more practical benefit than efforts to treat MOF once established, when the treatment is largely supportive.[9]

Protective Resuscitation Techniques

Certain resuscitative strategies protect against distant OD after periods of gut I/R.[57] Resuscitation with isotonic crystalloids in the late 1960s decreased mortality and renal failure, but contributed to the emergence of ARDS. There is still controversy about the use of isotonic crystalloids compared with colloids. The 2004 multicenter, randomized Saline versus Albumin Fluid Evaluation (SAFE) Study[108] and a 2012 large RCT[109] found similar outcomes, which were confirmed in a 2013 Cochrane Systematic Review.[110]

A 2007 systematic review comparing hypertonic with isotonic crystalloid solutions for trauma/burns resuscitation did not provide enough data to determine a difference in outcomes.[111] Hypertonic resuscitation was compared with lactated Ringer solution in adult patients with blunt trauma in a 2011 RCT,[112] which was stopped at an interim analysis for potential safety concern (increased mortality in the subgroup of nontransfused patients receiving hypertonic saline) and futility. It showed no significant difference in ARDS-free survival (hazard ratio, 1.01; 95% confidence interval, 0.6–1.6). A subsequent analysis of patients in severe shock suggested that hypertonic saline was associated with hyperfibrinolysis.[113]

Hypertonicity has an effect on multiple immune response functions, which may translate into improved outcomes when administered locally (as opposed to systemically) or using alternative modes of administration.[114] To test this hypothesis, we are conducting a phase I trial of nebulized hypertonic saline in moderately injured patients (NCT01667666).

In addition, the ALM (adenosine, lidocaine, magnesium) resuscitation has shown protective effects in animal models of sepsis and injury as well as in a few clinical trials in cardiac surgery patients.[115,116] Specifically, the combination of these 3 agents seems to confer cardiovascular protection, improvement of coagulation (presumably by inducing a shift in thrombin substrate specificity from the profibrinolytic protein C pathway to the antifibrinolytic TAFI [thrombin activatable fibrinolysis inhibitor] pathway at the endothelial thrombomodulin-thrombin complex level), reduction of proinflammatory factors (eg, TNF-α), and increase of antiinflammatory cytokine levels (eg, IL-10). However, the mechanisms through which ALM exerts the abovementioned beneficial effects remain elusive.

Judicious Use of Blood Transfusions

A 12-year analysis of our Denver trauma data set suggests that reduction in blood use contributed to the decreased incidence of MOF.[21] Current transfusion guidelines support the safety of restrictive transfusion practices in patients with trauma.[117,118] Other techniques to reduce the deleterious effects of packed RBCs (PRBCs) are washed PRBCs and prestorage leukoreduction.[95] Washed PRBCs have benefits but implementing them is an unrealistic practice in most settings. Prestorage leukoreduction trials have shown modest improvements in outcomes, except for cardiac surgery patients, among whom mortality was halved.[119,120]

Blood substitutes have offered promising results in trauma. Two hemoglobin substitutes have been studied extensively in injured patients: the diaspirin cross-linked hemoglobin (Hemassist, Baxter Corporation) and the polymerized, pyridoxylated human hemoglobin (PolyHeme Northfield Laboratories).[95,121,122]

Our experience in the trauma setting with PolyHeme suggests it provides an immunologic advantage relative to blood in injured patients by diminishing PMN priming and decreasing IL-6 and IL-8 levels.[123] Although PolyHeme has been associated with outcomes comparable with standard of care and with more adverse events, the benefit/risk ratio of PolyHeme was favorable when blood was needed but not available.[124] As of 2015, the US Food and Drug Administration (FDA) has not approved any blood substitutes, but Hemopure was approved in South Africa for use in acute anemia in 2001 and in Russia for use in the treatment of acute anemia in adults in 2010.[121]

Protective Lung Ventilation

Positive pressure ventilation can result in lung injury that is functionally and histologically identical to that seen in ARDS. Areas of low compliance (pulmonary contusion, edema, or infection) force tidal volumes to areas of high compliance, resulting in increased alveolar pressures, overdistension, and injury to uninvolved lung tissue. Mechanical injuries to the lung (barotrauma, atelectrauma, volutrauma) initiate a local inflammatory reaction and biotrauma with release of inflammatory mediators from damaged cells and recruitment of PMNs. Mechanical stresses on the living cell are

available at www.isrctn.com and www.c4ts.qmul.ac.uk/organ-failure–protection/top-art, Accessed December 18, 2015).

REFERENCES

1. Baker CC, Oppenheimer L, Stephens B, et al. Epidemiology of trauma deaths. Am J Surg 1980;140(1):144–50.
2. Sauaia A, Moore FA, Moore EE, et al. Epidemiology of trauma deaths: a reassessment. J Trauma 1995;38(2):185–93.
3. Pang JM, Civil I, Ng A, et al. Is the trimodal pattern of death after trauma a dated concept in the 21st century trauma deaths in Auckland 2004. Injury 2008;39(1): 102–6.
4. Eiseman B, Beart R, Norton L. Multiple organ failure. Surg Gynecol Obstet 1977; 144(3):323–6.
5. Moore F, Moore E. Evolving concepts in the pathogenesis of postinjury multiple organ failure. Surg Clin North Am 1995;75(2):257–77.
6. Moore FA, Moore EE. The evolving rationale for early enteral nutrition based on paradigms of multiple organ failure: a personal journey. Nutr Clin Pract 2009; 24(3):297–304.
7. Gentile LF, Cuenca AG, Efron PA, et al. Persistent inflammation and immunosuppression: a common syndrome and new horizon for surgical intensive care. J Trauma Acute Care Surg 2012;72(6):1491–501.
8. Xiao W, Mindrinos MN, Seok J, et al. A genomic storm in critically injured humans. J Exp Med 2011;208(13):2581–90.
9. Sauaia A, Moore EE, Johnson JL, et al. Temporal trends of postinjury multiple-organ failure: still resource intensive, morbid, and lethal. J Trauma acute Care Surg 2014;76(3):582–93.
10. Moore FA, Sauaia A, Moore EE, et al. Postinjury multiple organ failure. J Trauma Inj Infect Crit Care 1996;40(4):501–12.
11. Marshall JC, Cook DJ, Christou NV, et al. Multiple organ dysfunction score: a reliable descriptor of a complex clinical outcome. Crit Care Med 1995;23(10):1638–52.
12. Marshall JC. A scoring system for the multiple organ dysfunction syndrome (MODS). In: Reinhart K, Eyrich K, Sprung C, editors. Sepsis: current perspectives in pathophysiology and therapy. Berlin: Springer-Verlag; 1994. p. 38–49.
13. Sauaia A, Moore EE, Johnson JL, et al. Validation of postinjury multiple organ failures scores. Shock 2009;31(5):438–47.
14. Baue AE. MOF, MODS, and SIRS: what is in a name or an acronym? Shock 2006;26(5):438–49.
15. Dewar DCMB, Tarrant SMMBB, King KLRNMN, et al. Changes in the epidemiology and prediction of multiple-organ failure after injury. J Trauma Acute Care Surg 2013;74(3):774–9.
16. Benns M, Carr B, Kallan MJ, et al. Benchmarking the incidence of organ failure after injury at trauma centers and nontrauma centers in the United States. J Trauma Acute Care Surg 2013;75(3):426–31.
17. Minei JP, Cuschieri J, Sperry J, et al. The changing pattern and implications of multiple organ failure after blunt injury with hemorrhagic shock. Crit Care Med 2012;40(4):1129–35.
18. Fröhlich M, Lefering R, Probst C, et al. Epidemiology and risk factors of multiple-organ failure after multiple trauma: an analysis of 31,154 patients from the TraumaRegister DGU. J Trauma Acute Care Surg 2014;76(4):921–8.

19. Laudi S, Donaubauer B, Busch T, et al. Low incidence of multiple organ failure after major trauma. Injury 2007;38(9):1052–8.
20. Nast-Kolb D, Aufmkolk M, Rucholtz S, et al. Multiple organ failure still a major cause of morbidity but not mortality in blunt multiple trauma. J Trauma 2001;51(5):835–41.
21. Ciesla DJ, Moore EE, Johnson JL, et al. 12-year prospective study of postinjury multiple organ failure: has anything changed? Arch Surg 2005;140(5):432–8.
22. Durham RM, Moran JJ, Mazuski JE, et al. Multiple organ failure in trauma patients. J Trauma 2003;55(4):608–16.
23. Wafaisade A, Lefering R, Bouillon B, et al. Epidemiology and risk factors of sepsis after multiple trauma: an analysis of 29,829 patients from the Trauma Registry of the German Society for Trauma Surgery. Crit Care Med 2011;39(4):621–8.
24. Cuschieri J, Johnson JL, Sperry J, et al. Benchmarking outcomes in the critically injured trauma patient and the effect of implementing standard operating procedures. Ann Surg 2012;255(5):993–9.
25. Ciesla DJ, Moore EE, Johnson JL, et al. Decreased progression of postinjury lung dysfunction to the acute respiratory distress syndrome and multiple organ failure. Surgery 2006;140(4):640–7.
26. Dasta JF, McLaughlin TP, Mody SH, et al. Daily cost of an intensive care unit day: the contribution of mechanical ventilation. Crit Care Med 2005;33(6):1266–71.
27. Bianchi ME. DAMPs, PAMPs and alarmins: all we need to know about danger. J Leukoc Biol 2007;81(1):1–5.
28. Matzinger P. Tolerance, danger, and the extended family. Annu Rev Immunol 1994;12:991–1045.
29. Self KJ. Non-self, and danger: a complementary view. In: Lambris J, editor. Current topics in complement, vol. 586. Boston (MA): Springer US; 2006. p. 71–94.
30. Hwang PF, Porterfield N, Pannell D, et al. Trauma is danger. J Transl Med 2011;9:92.
31. Hirsiger S, Simmen H-P, Werner CML, et al. Danger signals activating the immune response after trauma. Mediators Inflamm 2012;2012:315941.
32. Lord JM, Midwinter MJ, Chen Y-F, et al. The systemic immune response to trauma: an overview of pathophysiology and treatment. Lancet 2014; 384(9952):1455–65.
33. Matzinger P. An innate sense of danger. Semin Immunol 1998;10(5):399–415.
34. Zhang Q, Raoof M, Chen Y, et al. Circulating mitochondrial DAMPs cause inflammatory responses to injury. Nature 2010;464(7285):104–7.
35. Tsukamoto T, Chanthaphavong RS, Pape H-C. Current theories on the pathophysiology of multiple organ failure after trauma. Injury 2010;41(1):21–6.
36. Levy RM, Mollen KP, Prince JM, et al. Systemic inflammation and remote organ injury following trauma require HMGB1. Am J Physiol Regul Integr Comp Physiol 2007;293(4):R1538–44.
37. Peltz ED, Moore EE, Eckels PC, et al. HMGB1 is markedly elevated within 6 hours of mechanical trauma in humans. Shock 2009;32(1):17–22.
38. Liu T, Qian W-J, Gritsenko MA, et al. High dynamic range characterization of the trauma patient plasma proteome. Mol Cell Proteomics 2006;5(10):1899–913.
39. Dzieciatkowska M, Wohlauer MV, Moore EE, et al. Proteomic analysis of human mesenteric lymph. Shock 2011;35(4):331–8.
40. Lee SK, Ding JL. A perspective on the role of extracellular hemoglobin on the innate immune system. DNA Cell Biol 2013;32(2):36–40.
41. Peltz EDDO, D'Alessandro AP, Moore EEMD, et al. Pathologic metabolism: an exploratory study of the plasma metabolome of critical injury. J Trauma Acute Care Surg 2015;78(4):742–51.

42. Moore FA, Moore EE, Kudsk KA, et al. Clinical benefits of an immune-enhancing diet for early postinjury enteral feeding. J Trauma 1994;37(4):607–15.

43. van Zanten AR, Hofman Z, Heyland DK. Consequences of the REDOXS and METAPLUS trials: the end of an era of glutamine and antioxidant supplementation for critically Ill patients? JPEN J Parenter Enteral Nutr 2015;39(8):890–2.

44. Chouchani ET, Pell VR, Gaude E, et al. Ischaemic accumulation of succinate controls reperfusion injury through mitochondrial ROS. Nature 2014;515(7527):431–5.

45. D'Alessandro A, Slaughter AL, Peltz ED, et al. Trauma/hemorrhagic shock instigates aberrant metabolic flux through glycolytic pathways, as revealed by preliminary (13)C-glucose labeling metabolomics. J Transl Med 2015;13:253.

46. O'Neill LAJ. Biochemistry: succinate strikes. Nature 2014;515(7527):350–1.

47. Tannahill GM, Curtis AM, Adamik J, et al. Succinate is an inflammatory signal that induces IL-1beta through HIF-1alpha. Nature 2013;496(7444):238–42.

48. Rubic T, Lametschwandtner G, Jost S, et al. Triggering the succinate receptor GPR91 on dendritic cells enhances immunity. Nat Immunol 2008;9(11):1261–9.

49. Eltzschig HK, Bratton DL, Colgan SP. Targeting hypoxia signalling for the treatment of ischaemic and inflammatory diseases. Nat Rev Drug Discov 2014; 13(11):852–69.

50. Vohwinkel CU, Hoegl S, Eltzschig HK. Hypoxia signaling during acute lung injury. J Appl Physiol (1985) 2015;119(10):1157–63.

51. Eckle T, Brodsky K, Bonney M, et al. HIF1A reduces acute lung injury by optimizing carbohydrate metabolism in the alveolar epithelium. PLoS Biol 2013; 11(9):e1001665.

52. Stringer KA, McKay RT, Karnovsky A, et al. Metabolomics and its application to acute lung diseases. Front Immunol 2016;7:44.

53. Gasse P, Riteau N, Charron S, et al. Uric acid is a danger signal activating NALP3 inflammasome in lung injury inflammation and fibrosis. Am J Respir Crit Care Med 2009;179(10):903–13.

54. Bos LDJ, Sterk PJ, Schultz MJ. Measuring metabolomics in acute lung injury: choosing the correct compartment? Am J Respir Crit Care Med 2012;185(7):789.

55. Bos LDJ, Weda H, Wang Y, et al. Exhaled breath metabolomics as a noninvasive diagnostic tool for acute respiratory distress syndrome. Eur Respir J 2014;44(1): 188–97.

56. Ulvik A, Kvåle R, Wentzel-Larsen T, et al. Multiple organ failure after trauma affects even long-term survival and functional status. Crit Care 2007;11(5):R95.

57. Magnotti LJ, Deitch EA. Burns, bacterial translocation, gut barrier function, and failure. J Burn Care Rehabil 2005;26(5):383–91.

58. Magnotti LJ, Upperman JS, Xu DZ, et al. Gut-derived mesenteric lymph but not portal blood increases endothelial cell permeability and promotes lung injury after hemorrhagic Shock. Ann Surg 1998;228(4):518–27.

59. Moore FA, Moore EE, Poggetti R, et al. Gut bacterial translocation via the portal vein: a clinical perspective with major torso trauma. J Trauma 1991;31(5): 629–36 [discussion 636–28].

60. Ciesla DJ, Moore EE, Johnson JL, et al. The role of the lung in postinjury multiple organ failure. Surgery 2005;138(4):749–57.

61. Botha AJ, Moore FA, Moore EE, et al. Postinjury neutrophil priming and activation states: therapeutic challenges. Shock 1995;3(3):157–66.

62. Moore EE, Moore FA, Harken AH, et al. The two-event construct of postinjury multiple organ failure. Shock 2005;24(Suppl 1):71–4.

63. Giannoudis PV. Current concepts of the inflammatory response after major trauma: an update. Injury 2003;34(6):397–404.

64. Sauaia A, Moore FA, Moore EE, et al. Multiple organ failure can be predicted as early as 12 hours after injury. J Trauma 1998;45(2):291–301.
65. Nydam TL, Kashuk JL, Moore EE, et al. Refractory postinjury thrombocytopenia is associated with multiple organ failure and adverse outcomes. J Trauma 2011; 70(2):401–6 [discussion 406–07].
66. Gawaz M, Fateh-Moghadam S, Pilz G, et al. Severity of multiple organ failure (MOF) but not of sepsis correlates with irreversible platelet degranulation. Infection 1995;23(1):16–23.
67. Matthay MA, Ware LB, Zimmerman GA. The acute respiratory distress syndrome. J Clin Invest 2012;122(8):2731–40.
68. Zarbock A, Singbartl K, Ley K. Complete reversal of acid-induced acute lung injury by blocking of platelet-neutrophil aggregation. J Clin Invest 2006;116(12):3211–9.
69. Harr JN, Moore EE, Wohlauer MV, et al. Activated platelets in heparinized shed blood: the "second hit" of acute lung injury in trauma/hemorrhagic shock models. Shock 2011;36(6):595–603.
70. Harr JN, Moore EE, Stringham J, et al. Isoflurane prevents acute lung injury through ADP-mediated platelet inhibition. Surgery 2012;152(2):270–6.
71. Harr JN, Moore EE, Johnson J, et al. Antiplatelet therapy is associated with decreased transfusion-associated risk of lung dysfunction, multiple organ failure, and mortality in trauma patients. Crit Care Med 2013;41(2):399–404.
72. Boyle A, Di Gangi S, Hamid U, et al. Aspirin therapy in patients with acute respiratory distress syndrome (ARDS) is associated with reduced intensive care unit mortality: a prospective analysis. Crit Care 2015;19(1):109.
73. Jastrow KM, Gonzalez EA, McGuire MF, et al. Early cytokine production risk stratifies trauma patients for multiple organ failure. J Am Coll Surg 2009; 209(3):320–31.
74. Adams JM, Hauser CJ, Livingston DH, et al. Early trauma polymorphonuclear neutrophil responses to chemokines are associated with development of sepsis, pneumonia, and organ failure. J Trauma 2001;51(3):452–6.
75. Bogner V, Keil L, Kanz KG, et al. Very early posttraumatic serum alterations are significantly associated to initial massive RBC substitution, injury severity, multiple organ failure and adverse clinical outcome in multiple injured patients. Eur J Med Res 2009;14(7):284.
76. Arumugam TV, Okun E, Tang S-C, et al. Toll-like receptors in ischemia-reperfusion injury. Shock 2009;32(1):4–16.
77. Carroll MC. The complement system in regulation of adaptive immunity. Nat Immunol 2004;5(10):981–6.
78. Kenawy HI, Boral I, Bevington A. Complement-coagulation cross-talk: a potential mediator of the physiological activation of complement by low pH. Front Immunol 2015;6:215.
79. Gerard C. Complement C5a in the sepsis syndrome — too much of a good thing? N Engl J Med 2003;348(2):167–9.
80. Roumen RM, Redl H, Schlag G, et al. Inflammatory mediators in relation to the development of multiple organ failure in patients after severe blunt trauma. Crit Care Med 1995;23(3):474–80.
81. Hecke F, Schmidt U, Kola A, et al. Circulating complement proteins in multiple trauma patients–correlation with injury severity, development of sepsis, and outcome. Crit Care Med 1997;25(12):2015–24.
82. Donnelly TJ, Meade P, Jagels M, et al. Cytokine, complement, and endotoxin profiles associated with the development of the adult respiratory distress syndrome after severe injury. Crit Care Med 1994;22(5):768–76.

83. Huber-Lang M, Kovtun A, Ignatius A. The role of complement in trauma and fracture healing. Semin Immunol 2013;25(1):73–8.

84. Amara U, Kalbitz M, Perl M, et al. Early expression changes of complement regulatory proteins and C5a receptor (CD88) on leukocytes after multiple injury in humans. Shock 2010;33(6):568–75.

85. Burk A-M, Martin M, Flierl MA, et al. Early complementopathy after multiple injuries in humans. Shock 2012;37(4):348–54.

86. Bulger EM. Antioxidants in critical illness. Arch Surg 2001;136(10):1201–7.

87. Mittal M, Siddiqui MR, Tran K, et al. Reactive oxygen species in inflammation and tissue injury. Antioxid Redox Signal 2014;20(7):1126–67.

88. Galkina SI, Dormeneva EV, Bachschmid M, et al. Endothelium-leukocyte interactions under the influence of the superoxide-nitrogen monoxide system. Med Sci Monit 2004;10(9):BR307–16.

89. Heyland DK, Dhaliwal R, Day AG, et al. REducing Deaths due to OXidative Stress (The REDOXS© Study): rationale and study design for a randomized trial of glutamine and antioxidant supplementation in critically-ill patients. Proc Nutr Soc 2006;65(03):250–63.

90. Heyland D, Muscedere J, Wischmeyer PE, et al. A randomized trial of glutamine and antioxidants in critically ill patients. N Engl J Med 2013;368(16):1489–97.

91. Heyland DK, Elke G, Cook D, et al. Glutamine and antioxidants in the critically ill patient: a post hoc analysis of a large-scale randomized trial. JPEN J Parenter Enteral Nutr 2015;39(4):401–9.

92. van Zanten AH, Sztark F, Kaisers UX, et al. High-protein enteral nutrition enriched with immune-modulating nutrients vs standard high-protein enteral nutrition and nosocomial infections in the ICU: a randomized clinical trial. JAMA 2014;312(5):514–24.

93. Madigan MC, Kemp CD, Johnson JC, et al. Secondary abdominal compartment syndrome after severe extremity injury: are early, aggressive fluid resuscitation strategies to blame? J Trauma 2008;64(2):280–5.

94. Balogh Z, McKinley BA, Cox CSJ, et al. Abdominal compartment syndrome: the cause or effect of postinjury multiple organ failure. Shock 2003;20(6):483–92.

95. Silliman CC, Moore EE, Johnson JL, et al. Transfusion of the injured patient: proceed with caution. Shock 2004;21(4):291–9.

96. Zallen G, Moore EE, Ciesla DJ, et al. Stored red blood cells selectively activate human neutrophils to release IL-8 and secretory PLA2. Shock 2000;13(1):29–33.

97. Johnson JL, Moore EE, Kashuk JL, et al. Effect of blood products transfusion on the development of postinjury multiple organ failure. Arch Surg 2010;145(10):973–7.

98. Dzieciatkowska M, D'Alessandro A, Burke TA, et al. Proteomics of apheresis platelet supernatants during routine storage: gender-related differences. J Proteomics 2015;112:190–209.

99. Dzieciatkowska M, D'Alessandro A, Hill RC, et al. Plasma QconCATs reveal a gender-specific proteomic signature in apheresis platelet plasma supernatants. J Proteomics 2015;120:1–6.

100. Fry DE, Pearlstein L, Fulton RL, et al. Multiple system organ failure. The role of uncontrolled infection. Arch Surg 1980;115(2):136–40.

101. Sauaia A, Moore FA, Moore EE, et al. Pneumonia: cause or symptom of postinjury multiple organ failure? Am J Surg 1993;166(6):606–10.

102. Elster E. Trauma and the immune response: strategies for success. J Trauma 2007;62(6):S54–5.

103. Bone LB, Johnson KD, Weigelt J, et al. Early versus delayed stabilization of femoral fractures. A prospective randomized study. J Bone Joint Surg Am 1989;71(3):336–40.

104. Pape HC, Grimme K, Van Griensven M, et al. Impact of intramedullary instrumentation versus damage control for femoral fractures on immunoinflammatory parameters: prospective randomized analysis by the EPOFF Study Group. J Trauma 2003;55(1):7–13.

105. Harwood PJ, Giannoudis PV, van Griensven M, et al. Alterations in the systemic inflammatory response after early total care and damage control procedures for femoral shaft fracture in severely injured patients. J Trauma 2005;58(3):446–52 [discussion 452–444].

106. Tuttle MS, Smith WR, Williams AE, et al. Safety and efficacy of damage control external fixation versus early definitive stabilization for femoral shaft fractures in the multiple-injured patient. J Trauma 2009;67(3):602–5.

107. Stahel PF, VanderHeiden T, Flierl MA, et al. The impact of a standardized "spine damage-control" protocol for unstable thoracic and lumbar spine fractures in severely injured patients: a prospective cohort study. J Trauma Acute Care Surg 2013;74(2):590–6.

108. Finfer S, Bellomo R, Boyce N, et al, The SAFE Study Investigators. A comparison of albumin and saline for fluid resuscitation in the intensive care unit. N Engl J Med 2004;350(22):2247–56.

109. Myburgh JA, Finfer S, Bellomo R, et al. Hydroxyethyl starch or saline for fluid resuscitation in intensive care. N Engl J Med 2012;367(20):1901–11.

110. Perel P, Roberts I, Ker K. Colloids versus crystalloids for fluid resuscitation in critically ill patients. Cochrane Database Syst Rev 2013;(2):CD000567.

111. Bunn F, Roberts I, Tasker R, et al. Hypertonic versus near isotonic crystalloid for fluid resuscitation in critically ill patients. Cochrane Database Syst Rev 2004;(3):CD002045.

112. Bulger EM, May S, Kerby JD, et al. Out-of-hospital hypertonic resuscitation after traumatic hypovolemic shock: a randomized, placebo controlled trial. Ann Surg 2011;253(3):431–41.

113. Delano MJ, Rizoli SB, Rhind SG, et al. Prehospital resuscitation of traumatic hemorrhagic shock with hypertonic solutions worsens hypocoagulation and hyperfibrinolysis. Shock 2015;44(1):25–31.

114. Ciesla DJ, Moore EE, Biffl WL, et al. Hypertonic saline activation of p38 MAPK primes the PMN respiratory burst. Shock 2001;16(4):285–9.

115. Dobson GPP, Letson HLM. Adenosine, lidocaine, and Mg2+ (ALM): from cardiac surgery to combat casualty care–teaching old drugs new tricks. J Trauma Acute Care Surg 2016;80(1):135–45.

116. Granfeldt A, Letson HL, Dobson GP, et al. Adenosine, lidocaine and Mg2+ improves cardiac and pulmonary function, induces reversible hypotension and exerts anti-inflammatory effects in an endotoxemic porcine model. Crit Care 2014; 18(6):682.

117. Napolitano LM, Kurek S, Luchette FA, et al. Clinical practice guideline: red blood cell transfusion in adult trauma and critical care. Crit Care Med 2009;37(12): 3124–57.

118. West MA, Shapiro MB, Nathens AB, et al. Inflammation and the host response to injury, a large-scale collaborative project: patient-oriented research core-standard operating procedures for clinical care. IV. Guidelines for transfusion in the trauma patient. J Trauma 2006;61(2):436–9.

119. Bilgin YM, van de Watering LM, Brand A. Clinical effects of leucoreduction of blood transfusions. Neth J Med 2011;69(10):441–50.

120. Blajchman MA. The clinical benefits of the leukoreduction of blood products. J Trauma 2006;60(6 Suppl):S83–90.

121. Chen J-Y, Scerbo M, Kramer G. A review of blood substitutes: examining the history, clinical trial results, and ethics of hemoglobin-based oxygen carriers. Clinics (Sao Paulo) 2009;64(8):803–13.

122. Lewis CJ, Ross JD. Hemoglobin-based oxygen carriers: an update on their continued potential for military application. J Trauma Acute Care Surg 2014; 77(3 Suppl 2):S216–21.

123. Johnson JL, Moore EE, Gonzalez RJ, et al. Alteration of the postinjury hyperinflammatory response by means of resuscitation with a red cell substitute. J Trauma 2003;54(1):133–9.

124. Moore EE, Johnson JL, Moore FA, et al. The USA multicenter prehospital hemoglobin-based oxygen carrier resuscitation trial: scientific rationale, study design, and results. Crit Care Clin 2009;25(2):325–56.

125. Dolinay T. Gene expression profiling of target genes in ventilator-induced lung injury. Physiol Genomics 2006;26(1):68–75.

126. Ventilation with lower tidal volumes as compared with traditional tidal volumes for acute lung injury and the acute respiratory distress syndrome. The Acute Respiratory Distress Syndrome Network. N Engl J Med 2000;342(18):1301–8.

127. Petrucci N, De Feo C. Lung protective ventilation strategy for the acute respiratory distress syndrome. Cochrane Database Syst Rev 2013;(2):CD003844.

128. Guillamondegui O, Cotton B, Diaz J, et al. Acute adrenal insufficiency may affect outcome in the trauma patient. Crit Care Med 2005;33(Suppl):A43.

129. Offner PJ, Moore EE, Ciesla D. The adrenal response after severe trauma. Am J Surg 2002;184(6):649–53.

130. Marik PE, Pastores SM, Annane D, et al. Recommendations for the diagnosis and management of corticosteroid insufficiency in critically ill adult patients: consensus statements from an international task force by the American College of Critical Care Medicine. Crit Care Med 2008;36(6):1937–49.

131. Wiener RS, Wiener DC, Larson RJ. Benefits and risks of tight glucose control in critically ill adults: a meta-analysis. JAMA 2008;300(8):933–44.

132. Sperry JL, Frankel HL, Vanek SL, et al. Early hyperglycemia predicts multiple organ failure and mortality but not infection. J Trauma 2007;63(3):487–93.

133. Langley J, Adams G. Insulin-based regimens decrease mortality rates in critically ill patients: a systematic review. Diabetes Metab Res Rev 2007;23(3): 184–92.

134. Chin TL, Sauaia A, Moore EE, et al. Elderly patients may benefit from tight glucose control. Surgery 2012;152(3):315–21.

135. Kudsk KA. Beneficial effect of enteral feeding. Gastrointest Endosc Clin North Am 2007;17(4):647–62.

136. Kang W, Kudsk KA. Is there evidence that the gut contributes to mucosal immunity in humans? JPEN J Parenter Enteral Nutr 2007;31(3):246–58.

137. Korff S, Loughran P, Cai C, et al. Eritoran attenuates tissue damage and inflammation in hemorrhagic shock/trauma. J Surg Res 2013;184(2):e17–25.

138. Thompson CM, Park CH, Maier RV, et al. Traumatic injury, early gene expression, and gram-negative bacteremia. Crit Care Med 2014;42(6):1397–405.

139. Flohe S, Lendemans S, Selbach C, et al. Effect of granulocyte-macrophage colony-stimulating factor on the immune response of circulating monocytes after severe trauma. Crit Care Med 2003;31(10):2462–9.

140. Lendemans S, Kreuzfelder E, Waydhas C, et al. Differential immunostimulating effect of granulocyte-macrophage colony-stimulating factor (GM-CSF), granulocyte colony-stimulating factor (G-CSF) and interferon γ (IFNγ) after severe trauma. Inflamm Res 2007;56(1):38–44.
141. Monsel A, Zhu YG, Gennai S, et al. Cell-based therapy for acute organ injury: preclinical evidence and ongoing clinical trials using mesenchymal stem cells. Anesthesiology 2014;121(5):1099–121.
142. Wilson JG, Liu KD, Zhuo H, et al. Mesenchymal stem (stromal) cells for treatment of ARDS: a phase 1 clinical trial. Lancet Respir Med 2015;3(1):24–32.
143. Zheng G, Huang L, Tong H, et al. Treatment of acute respiratory distress syndrome with allogeneic adipose-derived mesenchymal stem cells: a randomized, placebo-controlled pilot study. Respir Res 2014;15:39.
144. Sordi R, Nandra KK, Chiazza F, et al. Artesunate protects against the organ injury and dysfunction induced by severe hemorrhage and resuscitation. Ann Surg 2016. [Epub ahead of print].

Trauma Quality Improvement

Mark R. Hemmila, MD*, Jill L. Jakubus, PA-C, MHSA

KEYWORDS

- ACS-TQIP • MTQIP • Trauma • Benchmarking • Quality improvement
- Collaborative • Outcomes • Comparative effectiveness

KEY POINTS

- Performance improvement is local.
- Access to data is essential.
- Collaboration allows diversity of ideas and rapid dissemination of information.

INTRODUCTION

Patients enter the hospital acutely following traumatic injury with the intention of restoring their previous health. From the patient's perspective, the most desirable healing pathway is one that takes the shortest time, results in the least discomfort, and produces the fewest complications. Traditional quality improvement measures have focused on rates of mortality and morbidity; objective statistical numbers. An alternative approach involves pivoting this focus toward processes of care received by the patient and the avoidance of life-altering problems. For example, if a patient is able to avoid developing a deep venous thrombosis (DVT) this lessens the patient's risk of sudden death from a pulmonary embolus. Moreover, ongoing treatment with therapeutic anticoagulation is not required and the suffering associated with post-thrombotic syndrome is averted. DVT avoidance optimizes the patient's health and decreases consumption of short-term resources, which translates into reduced long-term costs to the patient and health care system.

Value in health care is defined as outcomes relative to costs multiplied by appropriateness.[1,2]

$$Value = \left(\frac{Outcomes}{Costs}\right) \times Appropirateness$$

Disclosure: Support for the Michigan Trauma Quality Improvement Program is provided by Blue Cross Blue Shield of Michigan and Blue Care Network, a nonprofit mutual insurance company.
Department of Surgery, University of Michigan Medical School, North Campus Research Complex, Building 16, Room 139E, 2800 Plymouth Road, Ann Arbor, MI 48109-2800, USA
* Corresponding author.
E-mail address: mhemmila@umich.edu

Value is an essential measure of health care efficiency in relation to quality because cost reduction without concern for achieved outcomes leads to self-defeating cost savings at the expense of effective clinical care. No matter how positive the outcome or how low the cost, if the procedure was not needed (appropriateness) then it is of zero value. Concern regarding the relationship between variation in quality and its impact on increasing health care expenditures has led to recent heath care policy initiatives focused on achieving high-quality care with the efficient use of scarce health care resources.[3] In layman's terms, this equates to providing the right care, at the right time, to the right patient.

Over the past decade, quality programs to support clinical benchmarking of surgical outcomes have grown dramatically. These initiatives include programs administered by the American College of Surgeons (ACS): the ACS National Surgical Quality Improvement Program, ACS Trauma Quality Improvement Program (ACS-TQIP), Metabolic and Bariatric Surgery Accreditation and Quality Improvement Program, National Accreditation Program for Breast Centers, Commission on Cancer Accreditation Program, and ACS Surgeon Specific Registry.[4] Commercial proprietary programs to record and assess surgical outcomes are also available. The University Health Consortium and The Leapfrog Group are the two best-known commercial programs.

ACS-TQIP (https://www.facs.org/quality-programs/trauma/tqip) is a national trauma quality improvement program, with more than 450 participating trauma centers across the United States.[5] ACS-TQIP uses risk-adjusted benchmarking to provide hospitals with accurate national comparisons via benchmark reports, with the goal to improve the quality of care for patients with trauma in all trauma centers. They also provide education and training, including the evidence-based ACS-TQIP Best Practice Guidelines. These guidelines offer recommendations for managing specific patient populations. Guidelines are currently available guidelines for geriatric trauma, massive transfusion, traumatic brain injury, and orthopedic trauma (https://www.facs.org/quality-programs/trauma/tqip/best-practice). Analyses of ACS-TQIP data allows for identification of common practices at participating trauma centers[6] and provides evidence to support best practices in the treatment of patients with trauma.[7]

Regionally based quality improvement programs serve as adjuncts to large national programs with the potential advantages of grassroots participation, agile collaborative synergy, and accessible program management. Examples of these include formal statewide trauma systems, third-party payer sponsored organizations, and physician-led voluntary surveillance systems. The Northern New England Cardiovascular Disease Study Group in New England and The Surgical Care and Outcomes Assessment Program (SCOAP) in Washington are examples of regional voluntary consortiums.[8,9] Blue Cross Blue Shield of Michigan and Blue Care Network (BCBSM/BCN) has sponsored many innovative examples of collaborative quality initiatives (CQI) on a statewide basis as part of its Value Partnerships Program (Table 1).[10] To focus on improving the quality of care delivered to patients with trauma, BCBSM/BCN supports the Michigan Trauma Quality Improvement Program (MTQIP).[11]

The MTQIP is a collaborative initiative that connects trauma centers within a geographic region to focus on quality improvement efforts in a nonpunitive manner. The program provides participants with a means to meet on a frequent basis to share information and experiences. Trauma centers can access their own data online and make comparisons with the collaborative as a whole. Robust patient-level drill-down capability is also built into the Web-based analytical platform. Mutual

Table 1
Blue Cross Blue Shield of Michigan/Blue Care Network sponsored, registry-based, collaborative quality initiatives

CQI Name	Specialty	Basis
Anesthesiology Performance Improvement and Reporting Exchange	Anesthesia	Hospital
BCBSM Cardiovascular Consortium-Percutaneous Coronary Intervention	Interventional cardiology	Hospital
BMC2-Vascular Interventions Collaborative	Vascular interventions	Hospital
Genetic Testing Resource and Quality Consortium	Genetic testing	Professional
Integrated Michigan Patient-centered Alliance on Care Transitions	Physician organizations	Professional
Michigan Anticoagulation Quality Improvement Initiative	Vascular medicine	Hospital
Michigan Arthroplasty Registry Collaborative for Quality Improvement	Orthopedic surgery	Hospital
Michigan Bariatric Surgery Collaborative	Bariatric surgery	Hospital
Michigan Breast Oncology Quality Initiative	Breast cancer	Hospital
Michigan Emergency Department Improvement Collaborative	Emergency medicine	Hospital
Michigan Hospital Medicine Safety Consortium	Internal medicine	Hospital
Michigan Oncology Quality Consortium	Oncology	Nonregistry
Michigan Pharmacists Transforming Care and Quality	Physician organizations	Professional
Michigan Radiation Oncology Quality Consortium	Radiation oncology	Hospital
Michigan Society of Thoracic and Cardiovascular Surgeons Quality Collaborative	Cardiac surgery	Hospital
Michigan Spine Surgery Improvement Collaborative	Spine surgery	Hospital
Michigan Surgical Quality Improvement Collaborative	General and gynecologic surgery	Hospital
Michigan Trauma Quality Improvement Program	Trauma surgery	Hospital
Michigan Transitions of Care Collaborative	Physician organizations	Professional
Michigan Urologic Surgery Improvement Collaborative	Urologic surgery	Professional
Michigan Value Collaborative	Hospital administration	Nonregistry

Abbreviation: CQI, continuous quality improvement.

opportunities for quality improvement are identified and selected with associated prospective targets. Interval progress for these measures is then monitored within the collaborative over time. Trust is gained through coordinating center transparency, ongoing data validation efforts, and information sharing.

PROGRAM STRUCTURE

MTQIP consists of 29 ACS Committee on Trauma (ACS-COT) level I and II verified hospitals delivering trauma care in the state of Michigan. BCBSM/BCN sponsors MTQIP by providing support for the coordinating center and to each participant hospital. The program began in 2008 as a voluntary pilot and was formalized in July of 2010 with the provision of sustained support and expansion of enrollment. MTQIP provides comprehensive risk-adjusted benchmark reports to participants in paper form and online. Face-to-face collaborative meetings are held 3 times per year. Trauma centers participate in global performance improvement projects (venous thromboembolism prophylaxis, hemorrhage control and blood product use, brain injury management). In addition, each center selects an individual performance improvement project. Based on their current data, the center sets target values for quality improvement. All MTQIP trauma centers also enroll in ACS-TQIP and receive the full benefits of national quality improvement program participation and benchmarking.

MTQIP relies on the following core personnel for operation of the coordinating center. The program director is a trauma surgeon and devotes dedicated effort to MTQIP. The program director is also a board-certified general surgeon who practices in acute care surgery. His background is in comparative effectiveness research, engineering, and statistical methods. There are 2 program managers. One is a nurse by training with advanced professional degrees, long-term experience as a trauma program manager, and hospital administration experience. The other is a physician assistant with a degree in health services administration and prior quality improvement program experience. The 2 program managers direct participant administration, data management, information technology, vendor interactions/contracts, and meeting coordination. The biostatistician is employed at 50% effort and provides specific analyses for meetings, support for data queries, and ongoing efforts to investigate new quality reporting metrics. The program is supported by a full-time administrative assistant.

COMPONENTS
Data Collection

Data are collected using the existing trauma registry at participating hospitals. The MTQIP data dictionary is published online and updated annually.[12] Trauma registrars and data abstractors from participating trauma centers complete training in MTQIP and National Trauma Data Standard data definitions. Each MTQIP center undergoes an annual data validation audit. Written feedback reports detailing the audit performance and areas for improvement are provided. Data elements beyond those collected in the standard registry and outlined in the National Trauma Data Standard are collected in the trauma registry software using add-on modules.

Data Management

New trauma registry data are transmitted to the coordinating center every 4 months. The data from each individual participant trauma center are cleaned and undergo audit checks. MTQIP uses a feedback loop that allows trauma centers to correct data submission errors before using the data. The cleaned registry data are then collated and added to the master data set maintained at the coordinating center. The master data set is transmitted to a third-party vendor for uploading into a Web-based analytical platform. MTQIP is actively working with trauma registry software vendors to simplify and automate the data submission process.

Data Analysis and Reporting

Routine data analysis is performed using the Web-based analytical platform. Trauma centers can create their own reports, query the data, and drill down to the patient level. Hard-copy reports are distributed 3 times per year at the collaborative meetings on a standard grouping of trauma outcomes and processes (**Fig. 1**). Specialty analyses and new report development are performed by the coordinating center biostatistician. For example, a recently implemented specialty analysis is the reporting of risk-adjusted antibiotic days (**Fig. 2**). In addition to the detailed 40-page feedback report, a

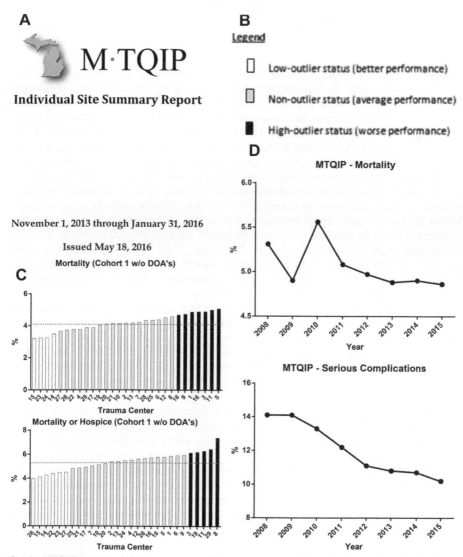

Fig. 1. MTQIP reports. (*A*) Report cover, (*B*) report legend, (*C*) risk-adjusted and reliability-adjusted mortality, (*D*) trend graphs for risk-adjusted rates of mortality and serious complications. DOA, dead on arrival; w/o, without.

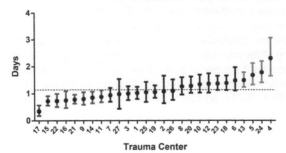

Fig. 2. Risk-adjusted antibiotic days.

dashboard detailing select outcome results and compliance with performance measures is provided (**Fig. 3**). Lists of specific patients along with results are created to provide feedback on blood product resuscitation performance, outcomes and interventions for patients in shock, and interventions for patients with traumatic brain injury.

MTQIP performs risk and reliability adjustment using a 2-stage approach. Multivariate logistic regression modeling is used to account for differences in baseline characteristics and injury severity, thereby allowing risk adjustment at the patient level. Potential predictors of the outcome of interest are entered into the model. A logit equation is derived based on the significant covariates using forward selection. Separate models for each outcome are constructed and the order of variable entry is determined by the c-index, which measures the ability of a parameter to discriminate outcome. Reliability adjustment uses a Bayesian random effects model to account for sample size differences between hospitals. Logit equations resulting from second-stage models are used to calculate expected outcome risk. Adjusted rates for each trauma center are then calculated by multiplying the rate ratio of observed to expected events by the overall collaborative rate.

In some instances, specific incidents have missing values for potentially important covariates (eg, Glasgow Coma Scale [GCS] motor score, systolic blood pressure, and pulse rate). To minimize bias, these values are imputed using multiple or single imputation techniques because missing data are frequently not missing at random. In other models, missing data are represented by use of an indicator variable. The final models and analyses include all of the incidents that meet MTQIP entry criteria for the cohort being examined.

Continuous data showing a right-skewed distribution, such as hospital length of stay, are natural log transformed. Multivariate analysis of hospital length of stay, intensive care unit (ICU) length of stay, and mechanical ventilator days is performed using multiple linear regression adjusting for significant covariates. After the regression analysis is conducted, the generated coefficient from the regression model is exponentiated to determine the percentage increase or decrease in length of stay relative to the risk-adjusted mean. Only patients who survived are considered in the hospital and ICU length of stay analysis to simplify this approach. To be included in the ICU length of stay or mechanical ventilator days analysis, patients must have at least 1 day of use for the resource being investigated.

Potential covariates entered into risk-adjustment models include age, gender, race, mechanism of injury, emergency department physiology, prehospital cardiopulmonary resuscitation, Injury Severity Score, injury severity by body region, transfer status,

M·TQIP

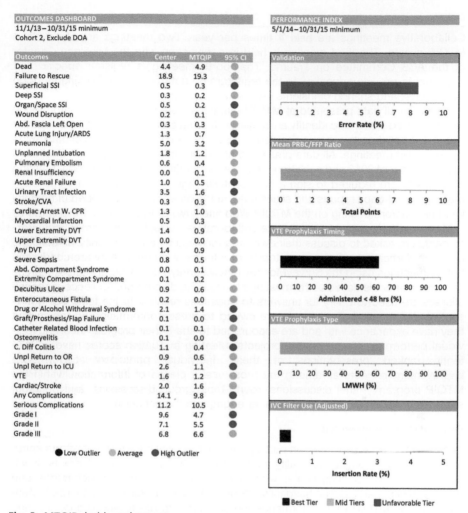

Outcomes	Center	MTQIP	95% CI
Dead	4.4	4.9	
Failure to Rescue	18.9	19.3	
Superficial SSI	0.5	0.3	
Deep SSI	0.3	0.2	
Organ/Space SSI	0.5	0.2	
Wound Disruption	0.2	0.1	
Abd. Fascia Left Open	0.3	0.3	
Acute Lung Injury/ARDS	1.3	0.7	
Pneumonia	5.0	3.2	
Unplanned Intubation	1.8	1.2	
Pulmonary Embolism	0.6	0.4	
Renal Insufficiency	0.0	0.1	
Acute Renal Failure	1.0	0.5	
Urinary Tract Infection	3.5	1.6	
Stroke/CVA	0.3	0.3	
Cardiac Arrest W. CPR	1.3	1.0	
Myocardial Infarction	0.5	0.3	
Lower Extremity DVT	1.4	0.9	
Upper Extremity DVT	0.0	0.0	
Any DVT	1.4	0.9	
Severe Sepsis	0.8	0.5	
Abd. Compartment Syndrome	0.0	0.1	
Extremity Compartment Syndrome	0.1	0.2	
Decubitus Ulcer	0.9	0.6	
Enterocutaneous Fistula	0.2	0.0	
Drug or Alcohol Withdrawal Syndrome	2.1	1.4	
Graft/Prosthesis/Flap Failure	0.1	0.0	
Catheter Related Blood Infection	0.1	0.1	
Osteomyelitis	0.1	0.0	
C. Diff Colitis	1.1	0.4	
Unpl Return to OR	0.9	0.6	
Unpl Return to ICU	2.6	1.1	
VTE	1.6	1.2	
Cardiac/Stroke	2.0	1.6	
Any Complications	14.1	9.8	
Serious Complications	11.2	10.5	
Grade I	9.6	4.7	
Grade II	7.1	5.5	
Grade III	6.8	6.6	

OUTCOMES DASHBOARD
11/1/13–10/31/15 minimum
Cohort 2, Exclude DOA

● Low Outlier   ● Average   ● High Outlier

PERFORMANCE INDEX
5/1/14–10/31/15 minimum

Validation — Error Rate (%)
Mean PRBC/FFP Ratio — Total Points
VTE Prophylaxis Timing — Administered < 48 hrs (%)
VTE Prophylaxis Type — LMWH (%)
IVC Filter Use (Adjusted) — Insertion Rate (%)

■ Best Tier   ■ Mid Tiers   ■ Unfavorable Tier

Fig. 3. MTQIP dashboard report.

comorbid conditions, intubation status, and payment mechanism. Risk-adjustment modeling and reporting development represents a combined effort between MTQIP analytical staff and a commercially contracted vendor (ArborMetrix). Newer reports/ analyses are provided directly by MTQIP to participant centers. More standardized metrics that are no longer new or in the development phase have their analytics/ reporting automated and are available online for direct access by centers. In addition to reporting on outcomes and utilization, MTQIP also tracks compliance with processes of care. Specialized reporting is provided in processes, interventions, and ACS-COT verification review committee prereview questionnaire metrics.

Poor quality data are dealt with at the time of data submission. Problems of out-of-range or missing data are identified during the data collation and cleaning process. These problems are then disclosed to the participant centers for correction before proceeding with final release of the data to analytics. A data validation program is in place to ensure compliance with the standardized data definitions.

Collaborative Meetings

Collaborative meetings are held 4 times per year. Two meetings are stand-alone MTQIP events. The third meeting is held in conjunction with the Michigan Chapter of the ACS Committee on Trauma. The fourth meeting is registrar specific and designed to provide education to the registrars on data collection, seeking input on data issues, and sharing of insights on data abstraction practices.

Originally, all data presented at MTQIP meetings were blinded and no information was conveyed that would identify an individual trauma center. In 2013, during the third year of the collaborative, it was decided to move forward with unblinding of data at the collaborative meetings. All data presented at MTQIP meetings have been unblinded since October of 2013 and each trauma center is identified by a 2-letter code. Meeting participants are required to sign a confidentiality agreement before entry into each meeting. Hard-copy reports and slides used at the meetings are scrubbed of hospital identifiers before posting on the MTQIP Web site (www.mtqip.org).

Many methods are used to promote collaborative interaction at the meetings. Participants are asked to discuss their own data followed by an opportunity for dialogue between participants. Surveys on topics of interest and controversy are conducted before meetings using the SurveyMonkey (www.surveymonkey.com) platform. These results are later displayed at the meetings to facilitate discussion. Audience response clickers are used to query for answers to questions relevant to the topic being presented at a meeting. Participants are invited to present information on topics that they have experience with and are encouraged to share their progress involving individual performance improvement projects. Meeting evaluation scores have consistently ranked presentations of these individual participant performance improvement projects as among the most useful pieces of information within the MTQIP program. Panel discussions, round-table group discussions, and breakout sessions are used as additional member engagement mechanisms.

Performance Improvement

Each trauma center is scored on participation and quality improvement efforts annually. The MTQIP continuous quality improvement (CQI) performance index is developed by the coordinating center with guidance from an advisory committee and discussed with participating hospital surgeon champions before being finalized. Measures on the MTQIP CQI performance index scorecard are reviewed annually, and updated if applicable, with increasing weight given to performance measures. When MTQIP initially began the BCBSM/BCN hospital CQI performance index scoring was based solely on participation (eg, timely data submission, participant attendance, completion of data validation visits). As MTQIP became more established, BCBSM/BCN requested a transition in the CQI scoring allocation of points from 100% for participation to a phased change over time to 30% for participation and 70% based on performance. For 2016, MTQIP has 50% of its scoring in participation and 50% in performance, and this will change to 30% participation and 70% performance in 2018.

The current MTQIP hospital performance index is detailed in **Table 2**. Performance-based point allocation includes the measures of data accuracy, center quality improvement, blood transfusion ratio compliance, timely venous thromboembolism prophylaxis administration, and prophylactic inferior vena cava filter use. Points for the quality of data submitted are based on the annual data validation error rate for the trauma center. To measure center-level quality improvement, participants must conduct and report on 1 individual trauma center performance improvement project using MTQIP data. Scoring of blood product transfusion ratio compliance is based on calculating the ratio of units of packed red blood cells to units of plasma for each patient receiving 5 or more units of packed red blood cells in the first 4 hours of an acute trauma resuscitation. Timely initiation of venous thromboembolism prophylaxis is tracked and is based on the first dose of drug administered. In addition, reduction in the use of prophylactic inferior vena cava filters in patients with trauma to a level of 1.5% or less is a group target for the entire collaborative.[13]

At the end of each calendar year, points are allocated within participation and performance categories on the MTQIP CQI performance index and total points achieved calculated for each participant hospital. Only the final total aggregate score from 0 to 100 is reported to BCBSM/BCN for use in their Value Partnerships Program. The BCBSM/BCN Value Partnerships Program rewards hospitals for improvement and achievement in quality and efficiency through a pay-for-performance program. Hospitals have the opportunity to earn up to 40% of the hospital pay-for-performance allocation based on their participation and performance in up to 10 CQI initiatives. This approach shifts payment from the traditional fee-for-service to a fee-for-value model. The structure and measures of the pay-for-performance program are developed in collaboration with hospitals through a Blue Cross Blue Shield of Michigan Hospital Pay-for-Performance Program workgroup.

Data Validation

MTQIP operates a robust data validation program that assesses the quality of data entered for MTQIP patients at each participant trauma center on an annual basis. The data validation program is completed by the MTQIP coordinating center to gauge inter-rater reliability. Each participant receives an annual audit visit and data validation feedback report. The MTQIP data definitions manual is published online, updated annually, and aligned with the National Trauma Data Standard definitions when possible.[12] Targeted selection criteria are used to query the submitted data for potentially high-yield charts to be abstracted during the validation visit. A total of 7 to 10 charts are reviewed and scored during a site validation visit. The feedback letter to participant MTQIP centers from a validation visit includes information of overall error rate, specific types of errors, and areas for data collection improvement.

Trauma Center Expectations

To participate in MTQIP, a facility must meet the following requirements: (1) have an active adult trauma program in place that is currently verified as an ACS-COT level I or II trauma center, (2) be signed up for a BCBSM/BCN Participating Hospital Agreement. To successfully participate in the MTQIP, each site is expected to do the following:

- Develop and maintain an organizational commitment to active participation in the MTQIP program with regard to facility administration and MTQIP program staff levels
- Commit to scheduled submission of data in a timely manner
- Identify a clinical champion who is a trauma surgeon
  - The surgeon champion will lead the hospital in MTQIP performance improvement efforts
  - The surgeon champion, or equivalent designee, will attend all triannual collaborative meetings

Table 2
Michigan Trauma Quality Improvement Program hospital performance index scoring for January 1 to December 31, 2016

Measure	Weight	Measure Description	Points	Participation (50%)
1	10	*Data Submission (Partial/Incomplete Submissions)*		
		On time and complete 3 of 3 times	10	
		On time and complete 2 of 3 times	5	
		On time and complete 1 of 3 times	0	
2	20	*Meeting Participation: Surgeon*		
		Participated in 3 of 3 meetings	20	
		Participated in 2 of 3 meetings	10	
		Participated in 1 of 3 meetings	5	
		Participated in 0 of 3 meetings	0	
3	15	*Meeting Participation: Clinical Reviewer or Program Manager*		
		Participated in 3 of 3 meetings	15	
		Participated in 2 of 3 meetings	10	
		Participated in 1 of 3 meetings	5	
		Participated in 0 of 3 meetings	0	
4	5	*Meeting Participation: Registrars (All Registrars Preferred)*		
		At least 1 registrar participated in the annual registrar-specific meeting	5	
		Did not participate	0	

		Data Accuracy	First Validation Visit Error Rate (%)	≥2 Validation Visits Error Rate (%)	Performance (50%)
5	10	5-Star Validation	0–4.5	0–4.5	10
		4-Star Validation	4.6–5.5	4.6–5.5	8
		3-Star Validation	5.6–8.0	5.6–7.0	5
		2-Star Validation	8.1–9.0	7.1–8.0	3
		1-Star Validation	>9.0	>8.0	0
6	10	Site-specific Quality Initiative (2/2016–2/2017)			
		Developed and implemented with evidence of improvement			10
		Developed and implemented with no evidence of improvement			5
		Not developed or implemented			0
7	10	Ratio of Red Blood Cells to Plasma in Patients Transfused ≥5 Units in First 4 h (1/1/15–6/30/16, 18 mo of Data)			
		Tier 1: ≤1.5			10
		Tier 2: 1.6–2.0			10
		Tier 3: 2.1–2.5			5
		Tier 4: >2.5			0
8	10	Venous Thromboembolism Prophylaxis Initiated ≤48 h After Arrival: Trauma Service Admissions, 1/1/15–6/30/16, 18 mo of Data (%)			
		>50			10
		≥40			5
		<40			0
9	10	Collaborative-wide Initiative: Inferior Vena Cava Filter Use, 1/1/15–6/30/16, 18 mo of Data (%)			
		≤1.5			10
		>1.5			0
Total (maximum points)	100				

- o If the trauma medical director is not the surgeon champion then the trauma medical director must be fully supportive of the program and the designated surgeon champion with regard to collaborative performance improvement efforts
- Identify an administrative lead/site coordinator
  - o The site coordinator will be the administrative lead for MTQIP at the facility (eg, trauma program manager)
  - o This person will also provide institutional support for full project participation
  - o The site coordinator or MTQIP clinical reviewer will attend all triannual collaborative meetings
- Assign a dedicated MTQIP clinical reviewer and trauma registrar to collect data:
  - o This should consist of a 1.0 full-time equivalent (FTE) person per 525 MTQIP cases
  - o The registrar should have access to an appropriate computer with high-speed Internet connectivity
- Focus on quality improvement:
  - o Enroll and maintain active program participation in ACS-TQIP
  - o Actively integrate MTQIP and ACS-TQIP into the existing trauma center performance improvement patient safety/quality improvement program
- Commit to using MTQIP and ACS-TQIP data elements and data definitions
  - o These are updated annually and are available on the MTQIP Web site
- Commit to using the Association for Advancement of Automotive Medicine 2005 with 2008 updates version of the Abbreviated Injury Scale (AIS) for injury coding in the trauma registry
- Collaborate with coordinating center:
  - o Participate in MTQIP coordinating center site visits and external data validation audits of patient data entered into the MTQIP database
  - o Commit to developing and implementing a site-specific quality improvement agenda, linked to the MTQIP quality improvement agenda, and also driven by opportunities specific to the facility based on its own experience
- Collaborate with other participating sites:
  - o Participate in process improvement, including sharing of and learning from best practices
  - o Be willing to share deidentified data
- Confidentiality and collegiality
  - o Strive to promote a friendly and collegial atmosphere
  - o Refrain from using MTQIP or ACS-TQIP data for competitive advantage or marketing

The MTQIP coordinating center staff conducts on-site customer service visits for participant trauma centers. These visits allow the trauma center and coordinating center personnel to have dialogue exchange, address questions, and get to know one another in a less hurried environment than the collaborative meetings. In addition, consultative services regarding interpretation of MTQIP and/or ACS-TQIP reports and data are offered if requested by a participant trauma center. The coordinating center also facilitates pairing of trauma centers that seek similar information or solutions to problems so that they can communicate with each other in a nonthreatening way.

Sponsorship and Support

BCBSM/BCN provides support for all of the operating costs of the MTQIP coordinating center. In addition, support is provided by BCBSM/BCN to each participant trauma center for registry license fees and an FTE MTQIP clinical reviewer for data abstraction/entry beyond the traditional trauma registry data elements. Face-to-face collaborative meetings are held 3 times per year in which benchmark reports are distributed, data are reviewed, results are discussed, and best practices are shared.

The regional collaboration model sponsored by BCBSM/BCN has the following unifying hallmarks across all CQI programs in Michigan.[14–16] The first is rigorous and efficient data collection with standardized data definitions and multitiered data auditing performed for completeness and accuracy. Second, a clinical champion is designated at each site with mandatory participation in collaborative meetings and commitment to performance improvement projects that examine the relationship between outcomes and processes of care required. Third, there is trust that grows within this safe environment. The outcomes data collected are not used to reward or punish participants; they are used to guide collaborative quality improvement efforts. Participants are encouraged to share data and experiences; however, BCBSM/BCN only has access to aggregated data to assess the effectiveness of the program at a region-wide level.

In 2016, the BCBSM Value Partnerships program offers hospitals the opportunity to earn 40% of the hospital pay for performance based on its participation and performance in up to 10 CQI initiatives. A hospital's score for each CQI is determined by its performance on specific measures related to that CQI. The measures and corresponding weights linked to each measure are referred to as the hospital's CQI performance index scorecard. Some measures are related to program participation and engagement, such as meeting attendance and timely data submission. Other measures are performance based and related to quality and clinical process improvement and outcomes, such as reductions in morbidity or surgical complications.

The goal is to move from a fragmented fee-for-service system with poorly aligned incentives to a value-based system that rewards collaboration and population-based improvement. The BCBSM/BCN value-based reimbursement model offers hospitals an opportunity to share in the year-over-year savings based on their efforts to keep population-level costs down while optimizing efficiency in the services they offer. BCBSM/BCN focuses on population-based performance because health care change moves faster when all providers responsible for a common patient population are given an incentive that is earned through better care coordination.

Advisory Committee

The MTQIP advisory committee is an essential group of colleagues within the CQI. Committee membership consists of 5 trauma surgeon champions from participant trauma centers and the coordinating center staff. The advisory committee meets in person 3 times per year, before each MTQIP meeting, and on an as-needed basis via conference calls. All essential MTQIP administrative matters, such as policy decisions, CQI scoring, benchmark report development, and program direction, are discussed and input sought from the advisory committee before rolling out to the entire CQI membership.

ADJUNCT COMPONENTS
American College of Surgeons Trauma Quality Improvement Program

Each participant trauma center is also enrolled in ACS-TQIP. Data are submitted separately to ACS-TQIP from the trauma center registry at each MTQIP trauma center using the National Trauma Data Bank mechanism. Trauma centers receive benchmark reports from ACS-TQIP twice per year, which detail their performance relative to national averages on a risk-adjusted basis. Benchmark reporting within ACS-TQIP differs from MTQIP in the following ways:

1. Injury scoring
   a. ACS-TQIP: crosswalking of International Classification of Diseases, Ninth Revision, or AIS 05/90 values to AIS 98.
   b. MTQIP: AIS 2005 with 2008 updates
2. Inclusion criteria
   a. ACS-TQIP: AIS 98 value greater than or equal to 3 in at least 1 body region
   b. MTQIP: Injury Severity Score greater than or equal to 5
3. Exclusion criteria
   a. ACS-TQIP:
      i. Exclude ED disposition home, other, left against medical advice, transfer
      ii. Exclude preexisting advance directive
      iii. Exclude patients with the following combinations of ED vitals:
         1. SBP = 0, and pulse = 0, and GCS Motor = 1
         2. SBP = NK/NR, and pulse = 0, and GCS Motor = 1
         3. SBP = 0, and pulse = 0, and GCS Motor = NK/NR
         4. SBP = 0, and pulse = NK/NR, and GCS Motor = 1
         5. SBP = NK/NR, and pulse = 0, and GCS Motor = NK/NR
   b. MTQIP: Exclude if length of stay is less than 24 hours and patient is alive

Vendors

MTQIP contracts with commercial software vendors for services essential to the program. Contracts are held with Digital Innovation Incorporated and Clinical Data Management for provision of MTQIP modules within their respective trauma registry software to collect custom data elements measuring outcomes and processes deemed essential to MTQIP participants. These two vendors also provide automated data transmission services to assist in uploading of trauma registry data from the participant hospitals to the coordinating center. The MTQIP module is revised and updated on an annual basis to reflect changes in the data elements to be captured and their associated definitions.

Online analytics is provided by ArborMetrix. The MTQIP collaborative data set is transferred to ArborMetrix using a secure file transfer protocol application. This advanced online platform is customized for MTQIP reporting and data query. Platform highlights include user-selected filters to guide cohort creation; ability to see non–risk-adjusted and risk-adjusted results; and comparisons with collaborative benchmarks for means, rank, and trends. Participants can also easily create reports detailing patient characteristics, outcomes, and performance on process measures. Drill-down reporting allows users to instantly examine data from the macroscopic outcome perspective to the microscopic patient-level perspective. Export capabilities allow downloading of graphs (picture format or PowerPoint slide) and data (Excel files) for trauma center usage.

An informational and organizational Web site (www.mtqip.org) is maintained for MTQIP by Medical School Information Services and provides information technology services to the University of Michigan Medical School. The Web site contains all of the documentation pertaining to the MTQIP program for becoming a member, policies, administrative agreements, data definitions, data validation procedures, schedules, and contact information. Educational materials are available in a searchable slide library, YouTube video channel, and as page document files. Links are provided to the ArborMetrix report site and to U-M Box, a secure file transfer program used to move information to and from the participant trauma centers and the MTQIP coordinating center.

RESULTS

Trauma centers participating in the MTQIP CQI produced a 40% decline in their rate of serious complications from 2008 to 2013 (14.9% to 9.1%; $P<.001$).[11] Mean risk-adjusted episode payments for pre-CQI hospitals were $38,752, and mean episode payments for post-CQI hospitals were $37,394, which resulted in an average saving of $1357 per episode ($P = .009$). There was a significant increase in payment relative to the risk-adjusted rate of serious complications within MTQIP trauma centers (**Fig. 4**). The authors believe that these changes are attributable to key components of this regional quality improvement program. First, risk-adjusted reports of mortality and morbidity outcomes were continuously provided to trauma centers over a 5-year

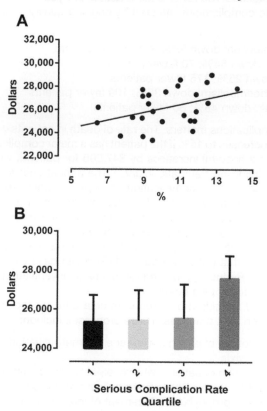

Serious Complication Rate vs. Payment

Fig. 4. Risk-adjusted serious complication rate versus 30-day episode payment. (A) Serious complication rate versus median payment for 26 MTQIP trauma centers ($P = .038$, slope of linear regression fitted line). (B) Median payment as a function of serious complication rate quartile ($P = .08$, Kruskal-Wallis test). (From Hemmila MR, Cain-Nielsen AH, Wahl WL, et al. Regional collaborative quality improvement for trauma reduces complications and costs. J Trauma Acute Care Surg 2015;78:84; with permission.)

period. Second, face-to-face meetings of the collaborative allowed discussion of common issues and targeting of global performance improvement initiatives. Third, annual trauma registry data validation audits ensured credibility and ongoing reductions in variability of the data.

To accomplish the task of reducing complications, it was important for trauma centers to focus on picking up small victories in multiple areas. Examples of complications and methods used to reduce their rates include:

- Pneumonia: hand washing, subglottic suctioning endotracheal tubes, timely and safe extubation
- Urinary tract infection: not placing a Foley catheter in every patient with trauma, early nurse-driven discontinuation of Foley catheter
- Return to ICU: education, use of step-down status beds
- Venous thromboembolism: timely initiation of prophylaxis, increasing the use of low-molecular-weight heparin as the preferred prophylaxis agent (**Fig. 5**)[17]
- *Clostridium difficile* colitis: handwashing, antibiotic stewardship

Deaths from trauma in MTQIP centers decreased from 4.9% (2010) to 4.1% (2015). This decrease translates to 158 fewer patient deaths per year in Michigan from traumatic injury. Specific complications affected by ongoing quality improvement efforts include:

- Urinary tract infection: down 58%, 429 fewer patients
- Severe sepsis: down 54%, 70 fewer patients
- Pneumonia: down 25%, 175 fewer patients
- Venous thromboembolism: down 35%, 109 fewer patients
- Decubitus ulcer: down 46%, 80 fewer patients.

Avoidance of complications matters. The rate of death in patients without a complication is 4%, but it increases to 15% if the patient has a major complication.[18] The median net payment to a hospital increases by $47,000 for patients who experience a major complication following traumatic injury.[18] The annual cost savings generated by MTQIP in preventing serious complications is approximately $16 million. Hospital length of stay was reduced by 9% or 0.5 days. This reduction translates into 9300 fewer days spent in the hospital per year for patients with trauma. ICU length of stay was reduced by 9% or 0.5 days. Hence, this has reduced the need for costly ICU care by 2367 d/y. The need for mechanical ventilation was reduced by 12% or 1.0 days, which means that patients required 1797 fewer days with breathing assistance from a machine. Reducing the need for mechanical ventilation usually reduces the risk of the patient developing pneumonia.

MTQIP has targeted specific processes in trauma care for focused collaborative improvement based on best practices. These processes include:

1. Increasing the proportion of patients who receive timely initiation of venous thromboembolism prophylaxis.
2. Increasing the proportion of patients who receive low-molecular-weight heparin as the preferred agent for venous thromboembolism prophylaxis.
3. Decreasing the use of prophylactic placement of inferior vena cava filters.
4. Increasing the proportion of patients with bleeding who receive an appropriate ratio of blood to plasma during resuscitation.

MTQIP has achieved several successes with these strategies:
- The proportion of patients who received timely initiation of venous thromboembolism prophylaxis increased by 29% or 2081 patients. Use of

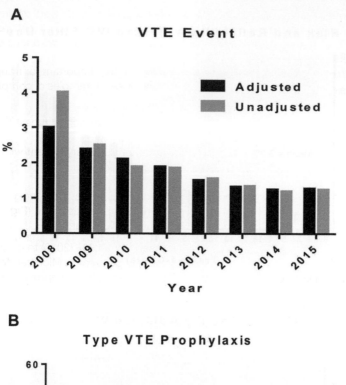

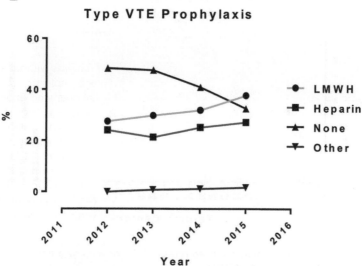

Fig. 5. (A) Venous thromboembolism event rate. (B) Frequency of use of venous thrombo-embolism pharmacoprophylaxis in patients hospitalized for 48 hours or longer. LMWH, low-molecular-weight heparin.

low-molecular-weight heparin as the preferred agent for venous thromboembolism prophylaxis increased by 11%. These two changes were associated with a 35% reduction in the number (109 fewer patients) of patients developing a life-threatening blood clot in their legs or lungs.

- Placement of a prophylactic inferior vena cava filter was reduced by 59% (**Fig. 6**); 210 fewer patients receive an inferior vena cava filter per year. Prophylactic

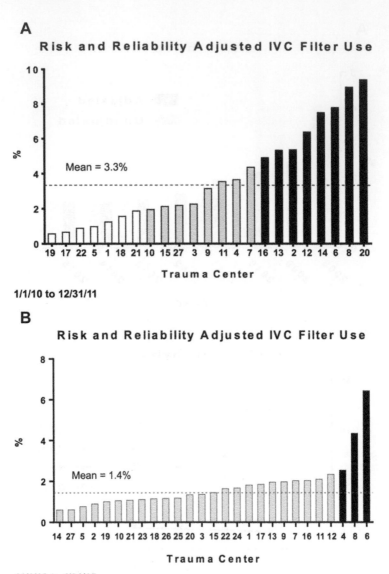

A

Risk and Reliability Adjusted IVC Filter Use

Mean = 3.3%

Trauma Center

19 17 22 5 1 18 21 10 15 27 3 9 11 4 7 16 13 2 12 14 6 8 20

1/1/10 to 12/31/11

B

Risk and Reliability Adjusted IVC Filter Use

Mean = 1.4%

Trauma Center

14 27 5 2 19 10 21 23 18 26 25 20 3 15 22 24 1 17 13 9 7 16 11 12 4 8 6

11/1/13 to 4/31/15

Fig. 6. Risk-adjusted and reliability-adjusted rates of inferior vena cava filter usage. (A) 1/1/2010 to 12/31/2011, (B) 11/1/13 to 4/31/15.

inferior vena cava filter placement in this patient population increases hospital costs by $10,000 per patient with no proven reduction in mortality risk.[13,19]

- The proportion of patients receiving an appropriate ratio of blood to plasma has increased by 13% or 26 patients, which means that, in patients with life-threatening hemorrhage, the resuscitation to help stop bleeding and keep the patient alive until surgical control of hemorrhage is achieved has been optimized. Shock and hemorrhage are the leading causes of early death in traumatically injured patients.

SUMMARY

MTQIP has improved the quality of care administered to patients with trauma by focusing on delivery of more appropriate care in a timely manner. The results achieved by the MTQIP collaborative have decreased patient deaths from traumatic injury, decreased costly and morbid complications, reduced consumption of costly hospital resources, and shown significant cost savings. Participation in a regional CQI program improves outcomes and reduces costs for patients with trauma. Support of regional collaborative quality improvement for trauma represents an effective investment to achieve health care value.

REFERENCES

1. Porter ME. What is value in healthcare? N Engl J Med 2010;363:2477–81.
2. Yong PL, Olsen LA, McGinnis JM, editors. Stakeholder perspectives on value. Value in health care: accounting for cost, quality, safety, outcomes, and innovation. Institute of Medicine (US) roundtable on value & science-driven health care. Washington, DC: National Academies Press (US); 2010.
3. Waljee JF, Birkmeyer NJ. Collaborative quality improvement in surgery. Hand Clin 2014;30:335–43.
4. American College of Surgeons. Quality programs [Internet]. Available at: http://www.facs.org/quality-programs. Accessed June 14, 2016.
5. Hemmila MR, Nathens AB, Shafi S, et al. The Trauma Quality Improvement Program: pilot study and initial demonstration of feasibility. J Trauma 2010;68(2):253–62.
6. Camazine MN, Hemmila MR, Leonard JC, et al. Massive transfusion policies at trauma centers participating in the American College of Surgeons Trauma Quality Improvement Program. J Trauma Acute Care Surg 2015;78(6 Suppl 1):S48–53.
7. Byrne JP, Mason SA, Gomez D, et al. Timing of pharmacologic venous thromboembolism prophylaxis in severe traumatic brain injury: a propensity-matched cohort study. J Am Coll Surg 2016. http://dx.doi.org/10.1016/j.jamcollsurg.2016.06.382.
8. Nnecdsg.org. Northern New England Cardiovascular Disease Study Group (NNECDSG) [Internet]. Available at: http://www.nnecdsg.org. Accessed June 14, 2016.
9. Scoap.org. SCOAP: Surgical Clinical Outcomes Assessment Program | A program of the Foundation for Health Care Quality [Internet]. Available at: http://www.scoap.org. Accessed June 14, 2016.
10. Valuepartnerships.com: Blue Cross Blue Shield of Michigan/Blue Care Network Value Partnerships [Internet]. Available at: http://www.valuepartnerships.com/. Accessed June 14, 2016.
11. Hemmila MR, Cain-Nielsen AH, Wahl WL, et al. Regional collaborative quality improvement for trauma reduces complications and costs. J Trauma Acute Care Surg 2015;78:78–87.
12. Mtqip.org: Michigan Trauma Quality Improvement Program [Internet]. Available at: http://mtqip.org/resources/data-resources/#data-dictionary. Accessed June 14, 2016.
13. Hemmila MR, Osborne NH, Henke PK, et al. Prophylactic inferior vena cava filter placement does not result in a survival benefit for trauma patients. Ann Surg 2015;262:577–85.
14. Birkmeyer NJ, Share D, Campbell DA Jr, et al. Partnering with payers to improve surgical quality: the Michigan plan. Surgery 2005;138:815–20.

15. Campbell DA Jr. Quality improvement is local. J Am Coll Surg 2009;209:141–3.
16. Share DA, Campbell DA, Birkmeyer N, et al. How a regional collaborative of hospitals and physicians in Michigan cut costs and improved the quality of care. Health Aff 2011;30:636–45.
17. Machado-Aranda D, Jakubus JL, Wahl WL, et al. Reduction in venous thromboembolism events: trauma performance improvement and loop closure through participation in a state-wide quality collaborative. J Am Coll Surg 2015;221:661–8.
18. Hemmila MR, Jakubus JL, Maggio PM, et al. Real money: complications and hospital costs in trauma patients. Surgery 2008;144:307–16.
19. Birkmeyer NJ, Share D, Baser O, et al, Michigan Bariatric Surgery Collaborative. Preoperative placement of inferior vena cava filters and outcomes after gastric bypass surgery. Ann Surg 2010;252:313–8.

Index

Note: Page numbers of article titles are in **boldface** type.

Crit Care Clin 33 (2017) 213–223
http://dx.doi.org/10.1016/S0749-0704(16)30104-X
0749-0704/17

criticalcare.theclinics.com

Moving?

Make sure your subscription moves with you!

To notify us of your new address, find your **Clinics Account Number** (located on your mailing label above your name), and contact customer service at:

Email: journalscustomerservice-usa@elsevier.com

800-654-2452 (subscribers in the U.S. & Canada)
314-447-8871 (subscribers outside of the U.S. & Canada)

Fax number: 314-447-8029

Elsevier Health Sciences Division
Subscription Customer Service
3251 Riverport Lane
Maryland Heights, MO 63043

*To ensure uninterrupted delivery of your subscription, please notify us at least 4 weeks in advance of move.

Printed and bound by CPI Group (UK) Ltd, Croydon, CR0 4YY

03/10/2024

01040394-0004